STRATEGIC HEALTHCARE MANAGEMENT

Stephen L. Walston

STRATEGIC HEALTHCARE MANAGEMENT

Planning and Execution

Second Edition

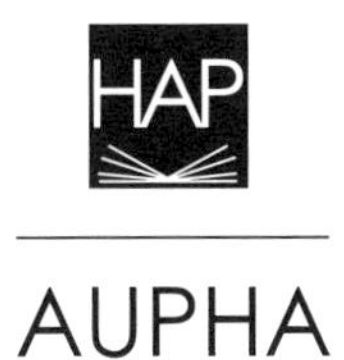

AUPHA

Health Administration Press, Chicago, Illinois

Association of University Programs in Health Administration, Washington, DC

Your board, staff, or clients may also benefit from this book's insight. For more information on quantity discounts, contact the Health Administration Press Marketing Manager at (312) 424-9450.

22 21 20 19 18 5 4 3 2 1

Library of Congress Cataloging-in-Publication Data

The paper used in this publication meets the minimum requirements of American National Standard for Information Sciences—Permanence of Paper for Printed Library Materials, ANSI Z39.48-1984. ∞™

Acquisitions editor: Janet Davis; Project manager: Theresa Rothschadl; Cover designer: James Slate; Layout: Cepheus Edmondson

Found an error or a typo? We want to know! Please e-mail it to hapbooks@ache.org, mentioning the book's title and putting "Book Error" in the subject line.

For photocopying and copyright information, please contact Copyright Clearance Center at www.copyright.com or at (978) 750-8400.

Health Administration Press
A division of the Foundation of the American
College of Healthcare Executives
One North Franklin Street, Suite 1700
Chicago, IL 60606-3529
(312) 424-2800

Association of University Programs
in Health Administration
1730 M Street, NW
Suite 407
Washington, DC 20036
(202) 763-7283

To my wife, Kathleen, and children,
who have supported and endured my careers and intellectual endeavors

BRIEF CONTENTS

DETAILED CONTENTS

Part V Plans for Achieving Mission and Vision

Part VI Implementing Strategies

PREFACE

The second edition of this book has been written for those interested in acquiring an updated, comprehensive, systematic understanding of strategy and strategic management of healthcare organizations. Although based on contemporary strategic theories, the text emphasizes the application of strategic principles to our rapidly changing healthcare environment. The target audience is graduate students in health services management and nursing programs. However, undergraduates, practicing healthcare executives, and healthcare providers also will find the content and structure useful for learning about strategic management and improving their strategy skills. The material is presented in a structured format that informs the reader of background strategy theories and options, teaches methods of crafting strategic plans, and provides methods for implementing strategies and monitoring strategic efforts.

This edition emphasizes learning through topical and timely case studies. It includes 13 long case studies that highlight strategic challenges healthcare leaders commonly face. These range from capitation and accountable care relationships to competitive positioning, dissolution of alliances, and vertical integration, among others. Each may be used to focus discussion and learning on relevant strategic topics. In addition, each chapter contains smaller cases and current healthcare examples. The reader will better understand strategic principles in the context of the contemporary healthcare industry.

Given the rapid and seemingly constant change in healthcare, skillful strategic planning and its implementation are essential to achieving organizational success. Developing and implementing strategy remains one of the most complicated and demanding jobs that leaders face because it integrates many competencies and skills, including communication, decision making, positioning, goal setting, and finance. Today, formulating and enacting strategies in a healthcare organization have become even more difficult because the changing, complicated, and diverse environment poses extreme challenges. This book provides a comprehensive overview to prepare future and current healthcare leaders for applying the strategic concepts that are critical to success today.

My background and experience lend this book a unique perspective. I have personally created and implemented strategies as a CEO at multiple hospitals; taught strategy to undergraduate and graduate students; and consulted nationally and internationally, formulating strategies for prominent healthcare organizations. The content, format, and sequence of the book and many of its featured examples and cases were informed by my experiences in these roles. I believe my perspective provides readers with unusual insight and a thorough understanding of strategic theory, as well as practical tools for the application of its principles.

Strategic Healthcare Management also differs from other strategy texts in that it promotes "mission advantage," which examines healthcare strategy from the premise that an organization's mission should direct its strategies. Much of the strategy literature has been focused on "competitive advantage," which is not always applicable to many sectors in healthcare. Although for-profit organizations exist in healthcare and are dominant in some healthcare fields (e.g., pharmaceuticals, insurance, medical devices), the strategy of many healthcare providers is not explicitly to gain advantage over competitors but to better fulfill their missions. Thus, this book focuses on gaining strategic "mission advantage," or *the ability to better achieve an organization's mission*—a concept applicable to both for-profit and not-for-profit healthcare organizations. Leaders seeking mission advantage will craft better strategies and make decisions that further their mission rather than seeking to best their competitors. I take a balanced, practical approach and highlight the need for both competitive and collaborative strategies that can maximize the achievement of one's mission.

The book is structured to provide readers necessary theoretical concepts and practical means of understanding, implementing, and monitoring strategies. It contains traditional strategic theories and common strategic methods along with tools for analyzing healthcare markets. Noteworthy features include chapters that highlight financial decision making, marketing, managing strategic change, and monitoring strategic actions. For evaluation of readers' learning, each chapter includes a thought-provoking introductory quotation, review questions, cases, and a suggested assignment. A list of competencies covered can be found at the conclusion of this preface. The end of the book features relevant case studies and an appendix. Upon completion of the text, readers will understand strategic principles and be able to apply them to make better decisions.

Stephen L. Walston, PhD
steve.walston@utah.edu

Competencies

Healthcare administrators' educational and professional environment, along with accrediting bodies, now strongly encourage—indeed, mandate—the use of competency-based learning models that seek to identify performance needs and demonstrate the value of learning. From an educational perspective, course curricula should provide students with the knowledge and skills required for future careers. Recognizing the wide variation of healthcare administration roles and professional settings, accrediting bodies such as the Commission on Accreditation of Healthcare Management Education allow individual programs to develop their own unique competencies.

Likewise, various professional organizations propose different sets of competencies for healthcare leaders. For example, the American College of Healthcare Executives (ACHE), the leading healthcare management professional organization, has adapted the competencies developed by the Healthcare Leadership Alliance (of which it is a part) to offer its members the ACHE Healthcare Executive 2017 Competencies Assessment Tool. This tool assists healthcare administrators in self-assessing their areas of strength and areas needing improvement (ACHE 2016). The assessment tool focuses on five areas of competence:

1. Communication and relationship management
2. Professionalism
3. Leadership
4. Knowledge of the healthcare environment
5. Business skills and knowledge

Given the wide variation of possible competencies, the author used the ACHE Healthcare Executive 2017 Competencies Assessment Tool to identify and develop competencies for inclusion in this book. The competencies found in each chapter are found in the following list. Instructors can quickly ascertain which competencies are covered in each chapter to develop their courses and syllabi appropriately, according to their competency-based curricula.

Competencies by Chapter

Chapter 1 Strategy and Strategic Management

Competencies
- Business skills and knowledge
  - General management
    - Ability to analyze and evaluate information to support a decision or recommendation
  - Strategic planning and marketing
    - Business planning, including case and exit-strategy development

Chapter 2 Understanding Market Structure and Strategy

Competencies

- Knowledge of the healthcare environment
  - Healthcare systems and organization
    - Managed care models, structures, and environment
  - Healthcare personnel
    - Healthcare sectors

Chapter 3 Business Models and Common Strategies

Competencies

- Knowledge of the healthcare environment
  - Community and environment
    - Organization and delivery of healthcare
- Business skills and knowledge
  - General management
    - Techniques for business plan development, implementation, and assessment
    - Justifying a new business model or business plan

Chapter 4 Growth and Integration Strategies

Competencies

- Knowledge of the healthcare environment
  - Healthcare systems and organization
    - Interdependency, integration, and competition among healthcare sectors

Chapter 5 Strategic Alliances

Competencies

- Business skills and knowledge
  - Organizational dynamics and governance
    - Building trust and cooperation among stakeholders
  - Strategic planning and marketing
    - Pursuing and establishing partnerships and strategic alliances

Chapter 6 Stakeholders, Values, Mission, and Vision

Competencies

- Communication and relationship management
  - Communication
    - Communicate organizational mission, vision, objectives, and priorities

  - Relationship management
    - Identifying stakeholder needs and expectations
- Leadership
  - Communicating vision
    - Establishing compelling organizational vision and goals
    - Encouraging a high level of commitment to the purpose and values of the organization
- Professionalism
  - Personal and professional accountability
    - Understanding consequences of unethical actions
    - Adhering to ethical business principles
- Business skills and knowledge
  - Strategic planning and marketing
    - Organizational mission, vision, objectives, and priorities

Chapter 7 The External Environment and Strategy

Competencies

- Knowledge of the healthcare environment
  - Healthcare systems and organization
    - Managed care models, structures, and environment
  - Healthcare personnel
    - Healthcare sectors
  - Community and Environment
    - Healthcare trends
    - Healthcare technological research and advancements
- Business skills and knowledge
  - General management
    - Collecting and analyzing data from internal and external sources relevant to each situation
    - Anticipating cause-and-effect relationships
    - Conducting needs analysis, identifying and prioritizing requirements
    - Defining problems or opportunities
    - Seeking information from a variety of sources
  - Risk management
    - Contingency planning

Chapter 8 The Internal Environment and Strategy

Competencies

- Business skills and knowledge

  - General management
    - Collecting and analyzing data from internal and external sources relevant to each situation
    - Conducting needs analysis; identifying and prioritizing requirements
    - Seeking information from a variety of sources
  - Organizational dynamics and governance
    - How an organization's culture influences its effectiveness

Chapter 9 Strategic Financial Analysis

Competencies

- Business skills and knowledge
  - General management
    - Measuring quantitative dimensions of systems and departmental effectiveness
  - Financial management
    - Financial management and analysis principles
    - Financial statements
    - Outcome measures and management
    - Principles of operating, project, and capital budgeting
    - Fundamental productivity measures

Chapter 10 Development and Execution of a Strategic Plan

Competencies

- Leadership
  - Managing change
    - Anticipating and planning strategies for overcoming obstacles
    - Anticipating the need for resources to carry out initiatives
- Business skills and knowledge
  - General management
    - Techniques for business plan development, implementation, and assessment
    - Defining problems or opportunities
  - Strategic planning and marketing
    - Business plan development and implementation process
    - Marketing principles and tools
    - Marketing plan development
    - Strategic planning processes development and implementation

Chapter 11 Business Plans and Strategic Management

Competencies

- Communication and relationship management
  - Communication skills
    - Preparing and delivering business communications, including meeting agendas, presentations, business reports, and project communication plans
- Business Skills and Knowledge
  - General management
    - Techniques for business plan development, implementation, and assessment
    - Justify a new business model or business plan
  - Strategic Planning and Marketing
    - Business plan development and implementation process

Chapter 12 Organizational Structure and Strategy

Competencies

- Communication and relationship management
  - Relationship management
    - Organizational structure and relationships
- Business skills and knowledge
  - Organizational dynamics and governance
    - Governance structure
    - Organizational dynamics, political realities, and culture
    - Constructing and maintaining governance systems

Chapter 13 Strategic Change Management

Competencies

- Leadership
  - Organizational climate and culture
    - Creating an organizational climate that encourages teamwork
  - Managing change
    - Promoting and managing change

Chapter 14 Strategic Leadership

Competencies

- Leadership
  - Leadership skills and behaviors

    - Potential impacts and consequences of decision making in situations both internal and external
    - Championing solutions and encouraging decision making
- Business skills and knowledge
  - General management
    - System thinking
  - Organizational dynamics and governance
    - How an organization's culture changes its effectiveness

Chapter 15 Implementing, Monitoring, and Evaluating Strategy

Competencies

- Leadership
  - Communicating vision
    - Holding self and others accountable for organizational goal attainment
- Business skills and knowledge
  - General management
    - Project management
    - Developing work plans
    - Performing audits of systems and operations
  - Financial management
    - Outcome measures and management
    - Developing and using performance monitoring metrics
  - Strategic planning and marketing
    - Managing projects and resources
    - Implementation planning
    - Strategic planning processes: development and implementation

Instructor Resources

This book's Instructor Resources include a test bank, PowerPoint slides for each chapter, answers to the chapter questions, and suggestions for presenting and discussing the cases.

For the most up-to-date information about this book and its Instructor Resources, go to ache.org/HAP and browse for the book's title or author name.

This book's Instructor Resources are available to instructors who adopt this book for use in their course. For access information, please e-mail hapbooks@ache.org.

ACKNOWLEDGMENTS

I appreciate the many people whose nurture and support provided me the ability to write the second edition of this book. Most important remains my family, especially my very patient spouse, who allowed me to quit in the middle of a successful career as a hospital chief executive and return to the University of Pennsylvania for my doctoral degree—then accompanied me across the United States and internationally. I also recognize those who have contributed to the cases. These include Erin Donnelly, director of strategic planning and business development at Primary Children's Hospital; Khanhuyen Vinh, manager of the hospitalist group MHCA; and Eric Connell, administrative fellow at Sanford Health (North Dakota). I have had the great honor of associating with these and many other good people and feel that my life and abilities have been greatly improved by these relationships. The completion of the second edition of this healthcare strategy text would have been impossible without their efforts and help.

PART

I

INTRODUCTION

Uncertainty clouds the direction of healthcare in the United States and across the world today. A thorough understanding of strategy in this uncertain world is critical for healthcare leaders to properly craft their organizations' strategies to position their firm within their market. All healthcare organizations—for-profit, governmental, and not-for-profit—struggle to gain what in this book is called *mission advantage*. Rather than the traditional competitive advantage advocated by most strategy books, this text integrates the concept of mission advantage and explores in depth the concepts, development, and implementation of strategy to achieve mission advantage. It provides both the theoretical concepts and the practical tools leaders need to make better strategic decisions. Part I features an overview of strategy and strategic management, and part II presents core concepts and theories. The section then transitions to a discussion on the development of strategic analyses. Part III examines the application of organizational purpose to strategy. Part IV discusses the need for environmental analyses, both external and internal, and proposes methods of evaluation. It also provides the financial tools needed to analyze organizations and direct decisions. Part V instructs readers on different plans that can be used to achieve an organization's mission and vision, including strategic plans, goals and objectives, project charters, marketing plans, and business plans. The book then advances to a discussion of the challenges inherent in implementing devised plans and describes methods of implementation. Part VI explores the importance of proper organizational structure, methods for managing strategic change, and strategic leadership. The last section, part VII, presents practical tools for implementing, monitoring, and evaluating strategic action.

CHAPTER 1

STRATEGY AND STRATEGIC MANAGEMENT

> For the past decade, Texas Health has been executing a strategic plan called the Ascent to the Summit. As the organization nears the end of that climb with a stronger strategic footing in place, the THR Promise continues to unify and strengthen us as we move into a journey toward becoming a high-reliability organization transforming the way healthcare is delivered. . . . In the past decade, Texas Health has shifted from an acute care hospital company to an integrated health system. In 2009, Texas Health Physicians Group was formed, creating a base of employed physicians who work with Texas Health on numerous objectives. Today, the group includes more than 830 physicians, physician assistants, nurse practitioners, and medical professionals dedicated to providing safe, quality care for its patients. The Texas Health Physicians Group's primary care and specialist network represents more than 50 medical specialties, with more than 250 locations spanning 11 North Texas counties. . . . Because of our culture, Texas Health was recognized in 2015 as the number one healthcare organization to work for in the United States by *Fortune*. We also were recognized as the number two workplace for women and the number three workplace for diversity in the nation, with one-third of our nurses from ethnically diverse backgrounds. We're proud to say we reflect the diversity of the communities we serve.
>
> —Barclay Berdan, "Climbing the Healthcare Summit," 2016

Learning Objectives

After reading this chapter, you will

- comprehend that *strategy* has many definitions, and its meaning depends on one's perspective;
- understand the role of strategy in moving a healthcare organization to achieve its goals, increase its business, and improve its performance;
- recognize the use of prospective and emergent strategies; and
- be aware that business strategies evolve over time as a result of changing circumstances and managerial modifications.

S*trategy*—integral to all businesses and life today—has different meanings to different people. Academics and consultants have suggested many diverse definitions. Little agreement on its meaning can be found in the business world, and it has been notoriously difficult to define (Luke, Walston, and Plummer 2004; Murray, Knox, and Bernstein 1994). For some, strategy is developing a formal plan. For others, strategy involves crafting a process or means for outwitting a competitor. Yet others see strategy as a way of doing business, positioning an organization, and determining competitive differences from a prospective or an emergent viewpoint (Mintzberg, Ahlstrand, and Lampel 1998; Porter 1985). Strategy tends to be a bit of all of these perspectives in that it involves processes and end goals but also constant adaptation to shifting conditions and circumstances in a world dominated by chance and uncertainty.

This text focuses on the importance of strategic thinking and strategic decision making. As the Texas Health Resource story in this chapter demonstrates, strategy is critical for organizations. At its foundation, strategy is about organizing information better to make better decisions. This text examines the fundamental components of strategy and methods for its implementation from both theoretical and practical perspectives. Theory is important to understanding strategy; as the great German general Carl von Clausewitz (1976, 141) stated, "Theory . . . becomes a guide to anyone who wants to learn about war from books; it will light his way, ease his progress, train his judgment, and help him avoid pitfalls." However, theories can provide only so much guidance, as we live in a world of incomplete information and often-limited knowledge of our competitors' strategic intentions and purposes. Likewise, strategies frequently emerge from the unintended, almost accidental results of decisions, as our earlier decisions commonly restrict the path of our choices and impose policies and actions that leaders initially would not have chosen (Murray, Knox, and Bernstein 1994).

Theoretically, an organization's established mission and vision should drive strategy formulation. The organization should first define what business it is in and what it wants to become and then establish goals, objectives, and tactics to achieve its mission and vision. This prospective approach is common to management-directed strategic planning. From this point of view, strategy establishes a path and direction toward an end state or outcome. In formal prospective planning processes, leaders often elaborately analyze the environment, set goals, and lay plans to achieve those aims. The strategic plan becomes management's action plan for running its business and operations. A management-driven organization's strategy addresses

- how management intends to grow the business,
- how the organization competes and collaborates with other organizations,

- how the functional components of the business relate and coordinate with each other,
- which services and programs the organization will emphasize and allocate greater resources to relative to other projects, and
- what the relationships and culture among employees will be.

This book primarily takes this perspective and elaborates on methods for better understanding and articulating organizational influences, purpose, and direction. Strategy and strategic thinking are important for all types of organizations. The text applies general business strategies to healthcare and examines their application to this growing, critical field.

History of Strategy

Derived from *strategos*, the Greek word signifying the planning of a military campaign, *strategy* literally means "the art of the general." The concept of strategy has been discussed for thousands of years, primarily with respect to aspects of war. Strategy was refined and articulated to further military purposes. Military campaigns encouraged the training of leaders to win battlefield conflicts. Millennia ago, generals recorded their experiences so that they could pass on their wisdom. Some of the first recorded strategy instruction originated in China during the period between 500 BCE and 700 CE and included significant treatises on warfare. The most familiar is Sun Tzu's *Art of War*, which has become one of the most important books on military strategy (Sawyer 2007). Sun Tzu taught the importance of positioning in military strategy—establishing objectives based on environmental conditions and the subjective beliefs of one's opponents.

Centuries later in the Mediterranean, modern military strategy developed under such leaders as Philip II (382–336 BCE), Alexander the Great (356–323 BCE) of Macedonia, and Hannibal (247–183 BCE) of Carthage. Philip II demonstrated how infantry, cavalry, engineers, and primitive artillery combine to form a trained, organized, and maneuverable fighting force. Later, Philip II's son Alexander and the great Carthage general Hannibal advanced military strategy by organizing open communication and supply lines, surprise tactics, better use of cavalry, and unity of command (Van Der Merwe 2002).

In 70 CE, Sextus Julius Frontinus, the Roman governor of Britain who subdued the hostile tribes in Wales, wrote a theoretical treatise on military science called *Stratagems*, which included a collection of examples of military strategies from Greek and Roman history. *Stratagems* did not exclusively denote acts of military ingenuity for the ancient Greeks and Romans but suggested a pattern of thinking to guide strategic behavior (Wheeler 1988).

The notion that strategy applied mostly to military warfare endured until the advent of the Industrial Revolution, when companies grew to a size that warranted more coordination and direction. In the early twentieth century, the need for explicit strategy was highlighted by executives at large companies, such as Alfred Sloan of General Motors and Chester Barnard of New Jersey Bell, who wrote about how to better organize and lead (Barnard 1968; Sloan 1963).

Today, strategy and strategic management are widely accepted. Courses about strategy are core in business schools, and strategic management is an integral part of leadership training. Teaching strategy can be a difficult task, involving both instruction on how to craft future-directed plans and, at the same time, development of intuitive insight and the ability to learn, adapt, and change (Burns 2002).

Strategy in Healthcare Today

The concept and importance of strategy expanded to healthcare in the 1970s. One factor motivating this expansion was the conversion of many hospitals and insurance companies, including health maintenance organizations, from not-for-profit to for-profit status. This change in ownership increased the level of competition among healthcare organizations.

Stimulated by governmental reimbursement changes and incentives, many national for-profit hospital companies, including Humana, Hospital Corporation of America, National Medical International, and American Medical International, aggressively sought to acquire hospitals across the country. These acquisitions dramatically changed the nature and behavior of local healthcare delivery and competition. For example, private, for-profit hospitals accounted for only 6.3 percent of US hospitals in 1975 (Gray 1986). As corporations formed extensive hospital chains, this percentage increased and competition grew; today, private, for-profit hospitals account for about 21 percent of US hospitals (American Hospital Association 2017). Likewise, physician practice continues to evolve. In 2000, about 24 percent of physicians worked for hospitals or integrated delivery systems (Medical Group Management Association 2005). However, by 2015, 38 percent of physicians were employed by hospitals or integrated delivery systems (Physicians Advocacy Institute 2016). As for-profit healthcare organizations became more prevalent and consolidation has occurred, the level of rivalry increased throughout the healthcare landscape, motivating organizations to adopt more competitive strategies.

Some maintain that there should be no difference in the application of strategic principles between the healthcare field and other sectors. While the general principles and techniques discussed in this book are relevant to healthcare, the field is distinct from many other sectors and a much higher percentage of its organizations are created for community or public benefit (often referred to as *not-for-profit organizations*). This difference in purpose or mission does not lessen the importance of applying strategy and its principles but should motivate more cooperative strategies to achieve missions.

As shown in exhibit 1.1, the purpose and mission of a healthcare organization should influence the emphasis it places on competitive versus collaborative strategies. Competition involves the effort of two of more parties seeking the rewards of a certain fixed contest. For example, a race or sports event may involve two or more teams that seek to win the contest. Likewise, companies submit bids for construction or other contracts, and only one contractor wins the job. As the story in exhibit 1.2 explains, competition involves outperforming one's competitor, which sometimes creates negative consequences for at least some members of the community. However, the dominant purpose of strategy in general business has been to gain competitive advantage at the detriment of competitors (Denning 2013). A common competitive strategy is to attract market share from competitors and, if possible, drive competitors out of the market. As a result, the community's access to products and services constricts and costs often increase.

Cooperative strategies, on the other hand, build on synergies and community good. As discussed in chapters 5 and 6, many healthcare organizations are now seeking to collaborate through cooperative strategies. Cooperation better uses community resources by reducing duplication and allows separate organizations to contribute their best competencies to achieving strategic goals.

EXHIBIT 1.1
Healthcare Organizations by Strategic Intent and Focus

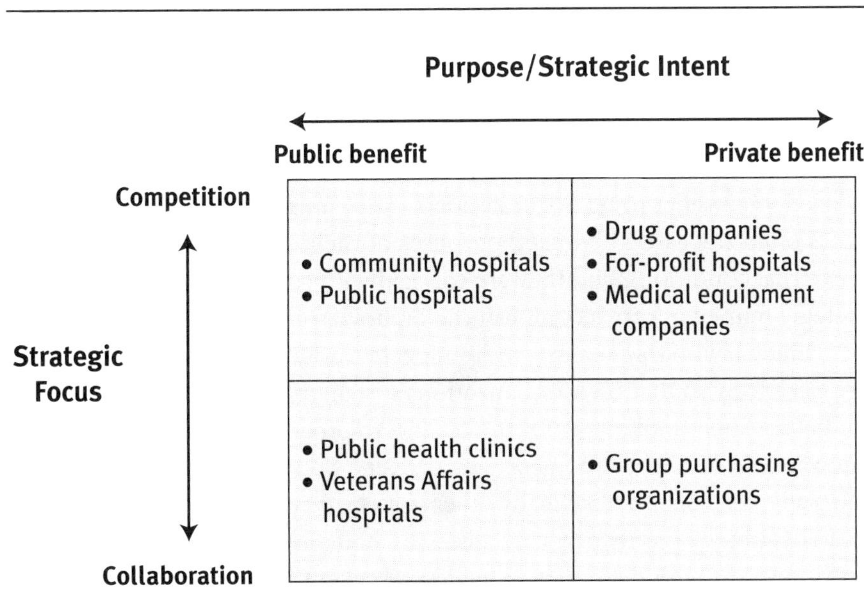

EXHIBIT 1.2
The Difference Between Competition and Collaboration

A salesperson had taken a client to the north country to camp and fish. They had taken off their shoes and were wading in a stream to cool their feet when a huge bear emerged from the trees and came charging toward them. The client, in his bare feet, ran fearfully out of the stream and up the rock-covered slope. He looked back and saw the salesperson quickly putting on his shoes. The client cried out to the salesperson that he must hurry because the bear was almost upon him. The salesperson said, "I'm okay. I don't have to outrun the bear—I only have to outrun you!"

Organizations' emphasis on competition and cooperation varies. Drug, medical equipment, and for-profit hospital companies typically demonstrate much more competitive strategies, while healthcare organizations working for the greater public benefit, such as public health clinics and the US Department of Veterans Affairs medical centers, use more collaborative strategies. Community hospitals, especially those in markets that include for-profit organizations, often adopt a more mixed strategy of competition and collaboration.

Why Study Healthcare Strategy and Strategic Management?

Healthcare organizations hire leaders to make decisions. Strategy and strategic management provide a solid framework for better decision making. Leaders ultimately have the responsibility and authority to make decisions and act. A key premise of successful leadership is that leaders must be good thinkers and deciders. For example, President Barack Obama was recognized by the magazine *Modern Healthcare* as its most influential person for three separate years during his presidency because of his actions on healthcare reform (Meyer 2016). Strategy and strategic management help leaders be mindful of the critical facts they need to consider to be better deciders. They must understand the purpose or, as is often the case, the mixed purposes of their organization and internal and external conditions, and they are charged with creating and implementing a strategic framework to accomplish the organization's purpose(s).

Leaders who think strategically allocate resources and minimize threats more effectively so that their organizations sustain mission advantage and perform better. Such thinking motivates leaders to proactively shape and craft the organization's business and inspires its delivery. Strategy is the road map and game plan for success. Unlike many other strategy texts, this book demonstrates that good strategy is only part of a successful equation. Good implementation must be added to good strategy to achieve excellent strategic outcomes. Both the creation and implementation of strategy are core functions of healthcare leaders.

Good strategy + Good strategy implementation =
Excellent strategic outcomes.

The importance of strategy in healthcare also is increasing because of the shift to value-based and patient-centered care in some states, which will require a complete restructuring of how healthcare is "organized, measured, and reimbursed" (Porter and Lee 2013). Change in healthcare is now driven by advancing technologies, demographic shifts, political debates, and global forces that directly affect the cost, access, and quality of healthcare. As these changes unfold, healthcare organizations require new, innovative strategies that may shift their direction and form new strategic thrusts. The following discussion highlights some of these changes and some strategies that have arisen as a result.

Healthcare Technology

Healthcare technology—especially diagnostic tools, information technology, and pharmaceuticals—has advanced rapidly in the past century. Radiological equipment, including computed tomography, magnetic resonance imaging, positron emission tomography, and ultrasound, has opened new diagnostic avenues. Radiologists' work has evolved from just reading X-rays to performing interventional procedures, operating outpatient facilities, and treating diseases that previously required major surgery. Hospitals and physician groups have reacted strategically by establishing centers for interventional radiology to compete with physician specialists, such as surgeons and cardiologists, who have traditionally provided these services. In addition, advances in molecular imaging will change needed services, as it will enable physicians to detect and treat disease at the cellular level.

Prescription drugs contribute an increasing burden to the cost of healthcare. The overall use of prescription drugs rose from 51 to 59 percent of the adult population between 1999 and 2012, with 15 percent of the overall population and 40 percent of adults 65 and older using five or more medications (Firger 2015). Because patents are time limited—the patents for seven of the ten most widely used prescription drugs expired in 2012–2016—(Anderson 2014), pharmaceutical companies' survival is tied directly to continuous research, discovery, and innovation. In 2015, global pharmaceutical research and development costs reached $150 billion (Statista 2017a). Yet big pharmaceutical companies spent more on marketing than research (Swanson 2015) and prescription drug prices have skyrocketed, with the cost of common brand-name drugs jumping 128 percent from 2008 to 2014 (Johnson 2015). In response to the changing environment—including declining drug-discovery success rates, expiration of blockbuster drug patents, cost and pricing pressures, and the subsequent rise of cheaper alternatives—drug companies have shifted their efforts toward greater consumer marketing, a focus on efficacy, targeted mergers, cost cutting, and research on biotech and therapeutic specialties, focusing on specific disease areas and populations (Deloitte 2016).

Advances in genomics and genetics may also transform much of medicine in the future. Developments in gene testing, gene therapy, and pharmacogenomics are now beginning to improve care for patients with AIDS and some cancers, and many predict they will have profound impact on healthcare in the coming decades (Wadhwa 2014).

Demographic Shifts

Demographic shifts occurring across the world are affecting the healthcare delivery system. Birth rates are falling in most countries, and populations are aging rapidly. In 1970, women had on average 4.5 children worldwide. By 2014, the birth rate had fallen to 2.5 children per woman. At the same time, global life spans have increased from 64.8 years in 1990 to about 70.0 years today (United Nations Population Fund 2017). While lower overall, birth rates in the United States remain higher among minority populations, and minority youth segments of the population are growing (Adamy 2016). This increasing diversity is driving innovative strategies and forcing healthcare organizations to be agile and adapt to the cultural and demographic needs of their constituents. Culture, race, ethnicity, and primary language have been shown to be associated with access-to-care issues and compliance with prevention and treatment of disease. As a result, many organizations emphasize culturally sensitive, linguistically appropriate care to ensure equity and quality across patient groups. Progressive health systems must take the lead in addressing these needs (Ubri and Artiga 2016).

The demographic trends in the United States will require different healthcare services. By the year 2050, almost one-third of the US population will be Hispanic, yet only 5 percent of physicians come from this group. Our citizens are getting older, as well as more racially, ethnically, and geographically diverse. People 65 years and older will grow from 14.5 percent of the American population in 2014 to almost 22 percent by 2040, and many will have multiple chronic diseases. These changes are creating significant challenges for healthcare planning in the United States, including deficits in geriatric care, fulfillment of ethnic needs, and treatment of chronic disease (Administration on Aging 2015). Globally, the number of people older than 65 is projected to grow by 1.6 billion and almost 16 percent of the population by the year 2050, while the number of young children will decline to approximately 7 percent of the total population (He, Goodkind, and Kowal 2016).

Political Forces

Political forces have a significant impact on healthcare. Legislation can substantially shift money, power, and regulation. Legislative bodies across the world continue to struggle to design laws that will curb the cost of healthcare while improving quality and access.

The politics affecting healthcare in the United States continues to be very significant. The Patient Protection and Affordable Care Act (ACA) signed into law by President Obama on March 23, 2010, triggered a seismic shift in the healthcare provider and payer communities with regard to organizational structure and operational work flows. The law provided greater drug coverage for seniors, diminished denial of insurance for preexisting conditions, mandated greater coverage of preventive services, shifted to a value-based orientation, and changed the mechanisms of provider payment. Value-based care sought to reimburse providers for the value patients received and not just quantity of services, which promoted approaches such as bundled payments and accountable care organizations. However, political representatives elected in 2016 have declared that this law will be overturned in 2017 and indicated an aversion to many of this law's components and results. What portions of the law will be retained and what will be changed remains highly uncertain (Bazzoli 2016).

Global Forces

Global forces affect all aspects of our lives today. Competition has broadened to include global players in healthcare. Patients increasingly are turning to new global alternatives to meet their healthcare needs, such as purchasing medications from other countries and seeking care abroad. Medical tourism is increasing steadily as US residents and others go to South America and Asia for surgeries and procedures that are more costly in their home country. Up to 750,000 US residents go abroad for medical care each year (Centers for Disease Control and Prevention 2016b).

Changes in the global healthcare market and politics are also affecting the number of foreign nationals who come to the United States for healthcare. For decades, the United States has attracted medical tourists because of the perception that it delivers the best healthcare in the world. In 2008, more than 400,000 non-US residents sought healthcare services in the United States, accounting for almost $5 billion in revenues and about 2 percent of total US healthcare services rendered that year. As global providers improve the quality of their care, this influx of patients may decline. The number of foreign patients coming to the United States has already fallen substantially since 2001, and the numbers of US residents traveling abroad for care could soon reach 23 million, spending almost $79 billion for services provided at international locations (Deloitte Center for Health Solutions 2008; Lee and Davis 2004; Patients Beyond Borders 2016).

Prospective and Emergent Strategies

Most large organizations engage in some type of planning process to analyze and design means to prospectively address the aforementioned issues and then produce some form of written document to guide their future decisions. This forward planning is called *prospective* or *prescriptive strategy*. This activity includes the general designing, planning, and positioning efforts of businesses to craft strategies for sustained competitive advantage.

A retrospective analysis of strategy, on the other hand, looks backward to see what actually happened. Constant experimentation and adaptation to new market conditions produce patterns identified retrospectively as *realized* or *emergent strategy*. Most organizations' strategy evolves incrementally over time, even in organizations that do prospective planning. This process also helps organizations understand their competitors' strategies. Chapters 2 and 7 discuss how understanding competitors' strategies contributes to an environmental analysis and to developing and forming more effective organizational strategies and tactics. Organizations often modify their plans, and the end results may vary significantly from those anticipated. Companies and individuals may abandon established strategies or introduce new initiatives. Furthermore, a retrospective analysis can help organizations better understand the effects of environmental factors and is important during times of upheaval and in industries subject to significant uncertainty and change.

Emergent strategy A pattern of actions that develop over time and become an organization's strategy de facto. This type of strategy is identified by examining decisions that were made and the patterns that occurred as a result. Also called *realized strategy*.

Both prospective and emergent views have merit; all strategy has both planned and unplanned components (Moncrieff 1999). Emergent strategy is more important in settings where greater environmental uncertainty and event randomness cause prospective strategies to be of little value in setting organizational direction. Emergent strategies may result from random choices, luck, the experience and reasoning of executives, or incremental decisions made by internal or external stakeholders. Scholars suggest that both deliberate action and nonlinear thought are needed for an organization to establish routines and processes while maintaining flexibility and ability to adapt (Burns 2002; Ghoshal and Bartlett 1995; Mintzberg, Ahlstrand, and Lampel 1998).

As shown in exhibit 1.3, **prospective strategy** can help to align an organization's actions with its mission and vision that will produce more relevant, appropriate outcomes (provided all goes according to plan). In addition, prospective strategy enables organizations to predict resource needs, identify and plan for major capital expenditures, recruit personnel, and attract other resources.

Prospective strategy A planning function that forecasts an organization's future situation and designs means to guide an organization's future decisions.

Planning for the future is a critical function of leaders. Healthcare organizations, such as pharmaceutical companies and hospitals, frequently invest millions in strategic projects involving buildings, equipment, and new hires that may take three to five years of development and effort before the new services, programs, or products become functional. Critical resources must be prospectively identified, accumulated, and organized so that they are available when needed. Likewise, prospective plans provide direction for proper resource allocation. Understanding what the future should look like allows leaders to

EXHIBIT 1.3
Value and Purpose of Prospective and Emergent Strategies

Prospective Strategy	Emergent Strategy
Align actions with mission/vision	Understand competitors' strategies
Predict resource needs	Evaluate own strategy
Allocate capital and personnel to projects	Enhance organizational learning
Position organization in competitive space	Adapt to uncertain environments

set aside appropriate capital and personnel prospectively for their strategic efforts. In addition, as Porter (1996) suggests, strategy directs an organization to choose a set of activities that will deliver a unique set of results. This prospective role actively guides an organization to differentiate itself to gain and maintain mission advantage.

On the other hand, as Winston Churchill (1931, 6) once stated, "There is always more error than design in human affairs." An emergent view of strategy acknowledges that prospective plans are often not translated into action, and designs frequently contain errors that prevent implementation. Many organizations do not begin with a defined strategy; as in Humana's case (see exhibit 1.4), their strategy and market position emerge through trial and error. Looking back, organizations can see how their strategy formed and understand the actions that created it. However, few would have predicted in the 1970s that Humana would become one of the largest health insurance companies in the United States.

An emergent perspective allows an organization to view its competitors' patterns of action and better understand their strategies. As discussed in chapter 2, knowing competitors' strategies helps an organization predict how it may react to strategic moves and better informs its prospective strategy. An organization may gather much more strategic information by observing its competitors' behavior and actions than it would by reading their written plans. Examining one's own strategy retrospectively is critical to learning from organizational successes and failures and providing feedback for future plans.

Strategy in many industries is emergent by nature; many avenues must be tried before a successful strategic direction is found. For example, in the past, pharmaceutical companies continuously searched for the next new blockbuster drug, and their discoveries drove their strategy. Chemical-driven experimentation dominated drug research. They tested hundreds of chemicals before finding one that might be effective for treating a disease. Today, their strategy is more prospective. Much of today's biomedical drug discovery is a process of first understanding how genes and proteins interact for a specific disease and then choosing a drug molecule to test. By using genomic markers to predict drug

EXHIBIT 1.4
Humana's Emergent Strategy

Humana is one of the larger insurance companies in the United States, but it was not always in this business. In fact, its strategies and focus evolved over time. In 1961, David Jones, Wendell Cherry, and others formed a partnership that grew to own seven nursing homes, going public in 1968. At the advent of Medicare, they decided to expand their for-profit company, Extendicare, into the hospital business. By 1972, they had divested their nursing homes and decided to concentrate on the growing hospital market.

Extendicare soon became one of the leading hospital companies. Reflecting its new direction, Extendicare was renamed Humana Inc. in 1974. Through the next two decades, Humana grew to encompass more than 80 hospitals in the United States and abroad. Humana was known for its centralized measurements and controls, and it sponsored innovative treatments, such as the first artificial heart. It also vertically integrated by creating the Humana Health Care Plan in 1984. The insurance arm was to help feed patients to Humana's hospitals, but by the 1990s, it seemed to create conflicts among the different divisions.

Humana again changed its strategies and focus. In 1993, the organization spun off its hospitals into a separate company called Galen Health Care Inc., which was shortly thereafter sold to Humana's for-profit competitor, Columbia/HCA. The company was left with only its health insurance business portfolio, which it leveraged to achieve a $32.3 billion market capitalization in 2016. That year, Aetna offered to purchase Humana for $37 billion.

Sources: Aetna (2015), E*TRADE (2017).

response, pharmacogenomics researchers can lower the cost of drug development and shorten drug development times (Cook, Hunter, and Vernon 2009; Thomson Reuters 2011).

Thus, organizations prospectively plan deliberate strategies and also realize emergent strategies retrospectively. Implementation of deliberate and emergent strategy may be influenced by many factors, including those shown in exhibit 1.5. Factors that influence the type of strategy an organization adopts include level of certainty, speed of change, degree of proactivity, clarity of mission, and time perspective. As exhibit 1.5 indicates, the greater the environmental uncertainty and change, the less clear the purpose or mission of the organization, and the shorter the time perspective, the more likely an organization will function from an emergent strategy.

Levels of Strategy

Strategy occurs at different levels in an organization. In today's world corporations, strategy is often divided into corporate, business, and functional levels. Most organizations—when they attain a large enough mass—create corporate

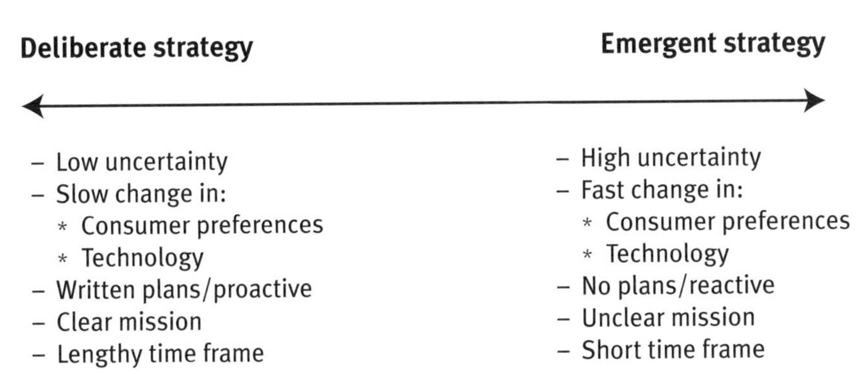

EXHIBIT 1.5 Factors Affecting Use of Strategy Type

structures with strategic business unit (SBU) subcomponents. As shown in exhibit 1.6, the corporate level—which consists of top executives, corporate staff, and generally a board of directors—is the apex of decision making in an organization. This corporate structure oversees the strategy for the complete organization. However, as discussed in chapter 12, the primary function of corporate strategy is to define the mission and overall strategic goals of the organization, allocate capital funds to the different SBUs, and decide which businesses to enter or exit.

For example, Merck & Co., Inc., is one of the largest pharmaceutical companies in the world, with approximately 68,000 employees, and it has robust corporate and SBU strategic planning and management. As shown in the organizational chart in exhibit 1.7, Merck's corporate structure in 2012 consisted of five large divisions: manufacturing, animal health, research laboratories, global human health, and consumer care. At the divisional level, the executives consider major acquisitions and divestiture. For example, in 2009,

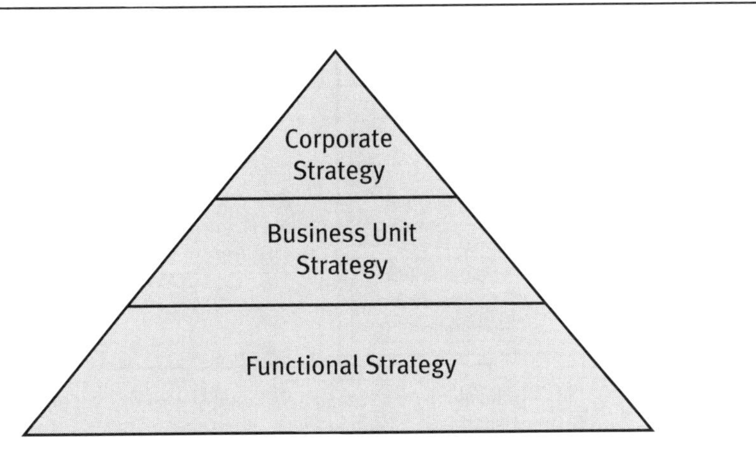

EXHIBIT 1.6 Levels of Organizational Strategy

Merck acquired Schering-Plough, another large pharmaceutical company, for $41 billion to create a more diverse portfolio of products and accelerate Merck's international growth (Reuters 2009). This acquisition was conceptualized, organized, and driven by **corporate-level strategy**. Likewise, Merck's mission and vision drive and derive from its corporate strategy (Merck 2017a):

Corporate-level strategy
The overall strategic scope and direction of a corporation. The primary function of corporate-level strategy is to allocate capital funds to SBUs and decide which businesses to enter or exit.

> **Vision:** To make a difference in the lives of people globally through our innovative medicines, vaccines, and animal health products. We are committed to being the premier, research-intensive biopharmaceutical company and are dedicated to providing leading innovations and solutions for today and the future.
>
> **Mission:** To discover, develop, and provide innovative products and services that save and improve lives around the world.

However, the Merck SBUs' business-level strategies focus on specific product lines, as demonstrated by the Merck Animal Health business unit (exhibit 1.8). At the SBU level, strategy focuses on more specific development projects, such as animal vaccines, pharmaceuticals, and diagnostics. Managers at this level usually receive the latitude to develop the best strategies for their areas of responsibility as long as those strategies fit into their corporate directives. Managers translate general statements of direction and intent from the

EXHIBIT 1.7
Merck & Co., Inc., Corporate Structure

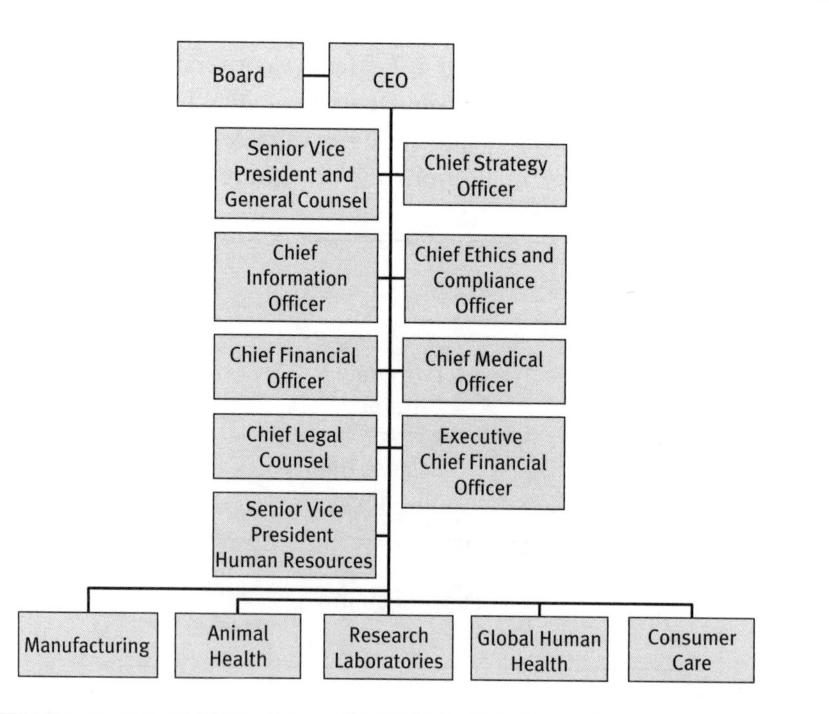

Source: Merck (2017c).

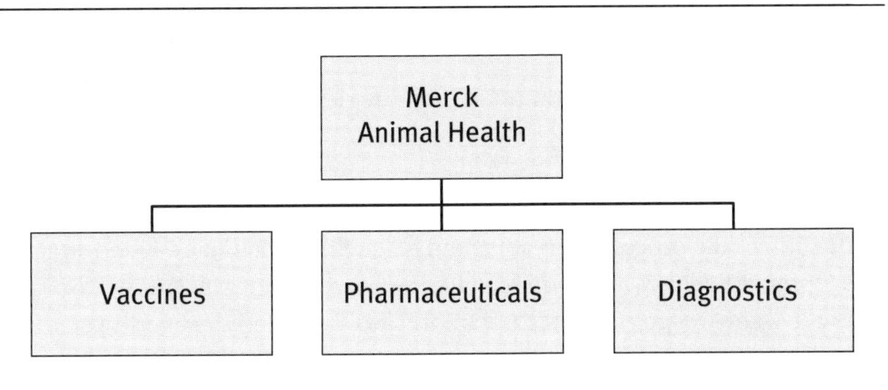

EXHIBIT 1.8
Merck & Co., Inc., Animal Health Division (SBU level) 2012

Source: Merck (2017b).

corporate level into concrete strategies for their individual businesses. Thus, while corporate strategy spans multiple businesses, **business-level strategy** focuses on a defined, specific business under the umbrella of corporate direction.

The functional level is the operating division, department, or project level. Here is where the rubber meets the road and the implementation of plans succeeds or fails. **Functional-level strategy** must support the business and corporate strategies. At this level, product or service line may be the drivers behind strategies. For example, Merck's Animal Health business unit (see exhibit 1.8) has a product-driven functional strategy that integrates research, marketing, production, and distribution to sell its products successfully. Hospitals may establish service line–driven functional strategies to promote their areas of specialty, such as oncology, cardiology, and obstetrics.

Each level's strategies must align with those of the other two. Misaligned plans may contradict the others' efforts and fail. Corporate strategies should cascade down the organization and be reflected in the lower levels' strategies and actions.

Business-level strategy
The strategic scope and direction of strategic business units (SBUs). SBUs focus on specific product/service lines while under the umbrella of corporate direction.

Functional-level strategy
Strategic scope and direction at the operating division, department, or project level. This type of strategy is driven by product or service line.

Text Overview

As shown in exhibit 1.9, this text explores in depth the concepts and tools needed to think strategically and develop and implement a strategic plan. Chapters 2 through 5 focus on strategy concepts; the remainder of the book seeks to answer the following questions:

- What is the purpose of the organization? (chapter 6)
- How well is the organization achieving its purpose? (chapters 7, 8, 9)
- What plans should the organization make to achieve its purpose more closely? (chapters 10 and 11)

- How should the organization act to better implement its strategies? (chapters 12, 13, 14)
- How can the organization tell if its strategies are having the desired effects? (chapter 15)

Building on the critical concepts presented in chapters 2 through 5, the text examines the process of creating and maintaining strategies. Good strategy development begins with an understanding of why an organization exists and where it wants to go. Chapter 6 explores how stakeholders and executives formulate an organization's strategic intent, including its values, mission, and vision. Next, an organization must look at its environment to understand the challenges it will need to overcome to achieve its strategic intent. Chapters 7 and 8 describe methods of analyzing the external and internal environments, and chapter 9 provides critical tools for strategic financial analyses.

EXHIBIT 1.9 The Text's Structure

Core Concepts of Strategy (Chapters 2–5)	
• Market structure • Business models • Generic and specialized strategies	• Growth strategies • Strategic alliances
What Is the Purpose of the Organization? (Chapter 6)	
• Stakeholders • Values	• Mission • Vision
How Well Is the Organization Achieving Its Purpose? (Chapters 7–9)	
• External environmental analyses • Internal environmental analyses	• Financial analyses
What Plans Should the Organization Make to Achieve Its Purpose Better? (Chapters 10–11)	
• Creation of strategic plans • Creation of goals and objectives • Creation of project charters	• Creation of marketing plans • Creation of business plans
How Should the Organization Act to Better Implement Its Strategies? (Chapters 12–14)	
• Proper organizational structure • Strategic change management	• Strategic thinking and strategic management
How Can the Organization Tell If Its Strategies Are Having the Desired Effects? (Chapter 15)	
• Engaging the right people • Monitoring strategic efforts	• Gantt charts • Strategy's interface with budgets

The book then shifts to the question of how organizations create strategic plans to better achieve their strategic intent. Chapter 10 explains how to engage key stakeholders in the planning process and outlines the structure and creation of strategic planning documents, including project charters and marketing plans. Chapter 11 discusses the use and creation of business plans. Chapters 12, 13, and 14 examine the organizational structure, change management, and strategic thinking critical to implementing strategy successfully. Chapter 15 concludes the text with a discussion on means of implementing and evaluating the strategic effort.

"The better conceived a company's strategy and the more competently it is executed, the more likely that company will be a standout performer in the marketplace" (Thompson et al. 2016, 17).

Chapter Questions

1. What is a prospective strategy?
2. What is an emergent strategy?
3. Why is it important to understand the difference between prospective and emergent strategies?
4. Why is there an imperfect matchup between prospective and emergent strategies?
5. What might interfere with the realization of a prospective strategy?
6. How might you manage the balance between design and emergence strategizing processes in an organization?
7. What are the major factors that distinguish levels of strategies in an organization?

Chapter Cases

Case Studies

In the case studies section at the end of this book, read "The Virulent Virus." Create teams of three to four students. Each team should reach a consensus and recommend a decision. This case encourages teams to explore risk preferences, environmental pressures, and differences in decision making and is an excellent activity for the first day of class.

(continued)

Repeal of Obamacare?

The ACA, signed into law in 2010, substantially changed the direction and strategies of most US healthcare organizations. The US Department of Health & Human Services was given the responsibility of implementing many of the provisions that sought to "expand coverage, emphasize prevention, improve the quality of health care and patient outcomes across health care settings, ensure patient safety, promote efficiency and accountability, and work toward high-value health care." The law instituted healthcare exchanges to facilitate purchasing insurance and banned lifetime dollar limits and discrimination based on preexisting conditions (Assistant Secretary for Planning and Evaluation 2016).

The law was designed to motivate care coordination and integration across the continuum of care by transitioning to a population health and value-based care focus. Healthcare organizations responded, among other ways, through mergers and acquisitions. Physicians merged into mega–group practices. Pharmaceutical and insurance companies consolidated (Singer 2016). Hospitals acquired other hospitals, as well as physician practices and insurance businesses. Providers opened accountable care organizations, which were established to take capitation that could function next to traditional fee-for-service models. Healthcare insurers merged to counterbalance the growing market power of hospitals. In sum, changes happened in and across all sectors in the healthcare field. Much of the consolidation has been blamed on the ACA, and in early 2016 these changes seemed inevitable (Gluck 2016).

However, few predicted the election of Donald Trump in the fall of 2016 and his effect on the direction the healthcare sector has taken. Trump signaled that on his first day in office he would "work immediately on repealing Obamacare" (Koronowski 2017). A full or even partial repeal of the ACA would have significant impact on the strategies of healthcare organizations. Although we may not know what the repeal means for some time, and the final shape of the healthcare field under a Trump administration may gradually evolve, most Americans support coverage guaranteed regardless of preexisting conditions yet oppose a mandate. The ACA also cut $700 billion from Medicare provider reimbursements, which will probably not be restored by Trump's reforms (Kapur 2016). Whatever the results, the political winds of change have roared through a healthcare sector that now must review and revise its plans.

Questions

1. Why does politics have such an important impact on strategy in the healthcare sector?
2. Why were healthcare organizations merging under the ACA? Why might these strategies need to be revisited under a Trump administration?
3. How does this case demonstrate the difficulty in only having a prospective strategy?

Chapter Assignment

After reading chapter 1, read the 1996 article by Michael Porter titled "What Is Strategy?" from *Harvard Business Review*, volume 74, issue 6, pages 61–79. After reading these materials and discussing them in class, write a one-page (single-spaced) paper on what strategy is to you and provide three examples of different types of strategies exhibited by healthcare organizations.

PART

CORE CONCEPTS OF STRATEGY

This section explores common strategy theories and concepts and applies them to the healthcare field. In chapter 2, readers learn that strategies must be aligned with an organization's environment and market structures. An organization's relationships to its environment and market structure directly affect its market power and ability to make strategic decisions. The chapter discusses the concepts of monopolies, oligopolies, monopolistic competition, and perfect competition, along with product life cycles and their impact on strategies.

Chapter 3 reviews the concept of business models and potential strategies. Business models define the core components of any company. Organizations must match the parts of their business model to their environment to succeed. Potential strategies include generic strategies that focus on low cost, or differentiation, or both. The advantages and disadvantages of being a first mover or an early entrant into a market also are discussed.

Chapter 4 examines a concept that has become critical in the healthcare field: the strategic use of vertical and horizontal expansion. *Vertical expansion*—connecting upstream and downstream components of an organization—has become a key strategy for many healthcare providers since the implementation of the Affordable Care Act and often calls for ownership and integration of hospitals, insurance products, physicians, and other healthcare businesses. *Horizontal expansion*—growth through mergers and acquisitions—continues to be a common healthcare strategy. The chapter explores the methods and challenges of both vertical and horizontal integration.

Chapter 5 considers *strategic alliances*—strategic nonowner relationships. Various types of alliances, their degree of interdependence, and requisite management skills are discussed. The chapter directly applies these concepts to the healthcare market and illustrates them through examples.

CHAPTER

2

UNDERSTANDING MARKET STRUCTURE AND STRATEGY

> Since the Affordable Care Act was signed into law, the American healthcare sector has experienced a frenzy of mergers and acquisitions. Regulators are currently reviewing two proposed mergers **that, if approved, would reduce the number of top national health insurers from five to just three gigantic companies.** Among hospitals, this trend is even more pronounced and could lead to significant price hikes. . . . Markets where hospitals have a monopoly are exposed to massive price hikes. Hospital prices in monopoly markets are 15.3 percent higher than in markets with four or more hospitals. Hospitals in duopoly markets charge prices that are 6.4 percent higher, and treatment in markets that have a hospital triopoly is 4.8 percent more expensive. . . . There are increasing signs that federal regulators are beginning to worry about the recent wave of hospital mergers.
>
> —Asher Schechter, "The True Price of Reduced Competition in Health Care: Hospital Monopolies Drastically Drive Up Prices," 2016

Learning Objectives

After reading this chapter, you will

- have an overview of the societal environment and its effect on the healthcare market,
- recognize the effect of technology on the demand for and provision of healthcare,
- know the components of an external environmental analysis,
- understand the basic concepts of the market structure of an industry,
- comprehend the principles of market position as it relates to market structure and competitors, and
- be familiar with two methods of measuring market concentration.

All organizations operate in an open system that involves continuous interaction with an external environment that directly and indirectly influences their success. The external environment comprises many components, including communities of people of different ages and cultures; governments and regulatory bodies; and competitive and collaborative industries and companies comprising numerous products, services, and providers. These influences generally fall into one of two categories: (1) societal factors and (2) market factors. The context in which an organization operates heavily influences its strategies and its ability to achieve its mission and vision. Organizations developing a strategic direction must recognize and understand their external environment to be successful.

The Societal Environment

Societal environment
The public and socioeconomic factors surrounding and influencing an organization, such as general economic conditions, population demographics, cultural values, governmental regulations, and technology.

The **societal environment** encompasses general economic conditions, population demographics, cultural values, governmental regulations, and technology. Healthcare is highly influenced by these factors. General economic conditions have a significant impact on healthcare. As economic conditions improve, people have more disposable income and insurance coverage, which can be used to obtain healthcare services. In the United States, more than half of health insurance policies for persons under age 65 are provided by employers. When the unemployment rate rises, many families lose their insurance coverage along with their jobs. As a result, people cut back on medications, preventive care, and visits to their doctor (Kaiser Family Foundation 2015). For example, the 2008 recession slowed the growth of healthcare spending to the lowest rate in almost 50 years (Hartman et al. 2010).

Population demographics are also important in healthcare. Healthcare spending varies dramatically by age, race, and gender. People older than 65 spend 3.6 times more on healthcare than those between the ages of 19 to 44. (Centers for Medicare & Medicaid Services [CMS] 2016). Across the world, the number of individuals 65 or older is increasing dramatically. There were more than 46 million older adults in the United States in 2014, or 14.5 percent of the population, but this figure is expected to grow to 98 million and 21.7 percent by 2060 (Administration on Aging 2015). Worldwide, 20 percent will be elderly by the middle of the twenty-first century. However, in developed, wealthy countries in Asia and Europe, this number is already much higher. For instance, in 2015, 33 percent of the population in Japan and 28 percent of the population in Germany were older than 60 (United Nations 2015). See exhibit 2.1 for more information.

As people age, they contract chronic conditions that require intensive treatments from acute care providers. In the United States, about half of all

EXHIBIT 2.1 Young Children and Older People as a Percentage of Global Population: 1950–2050

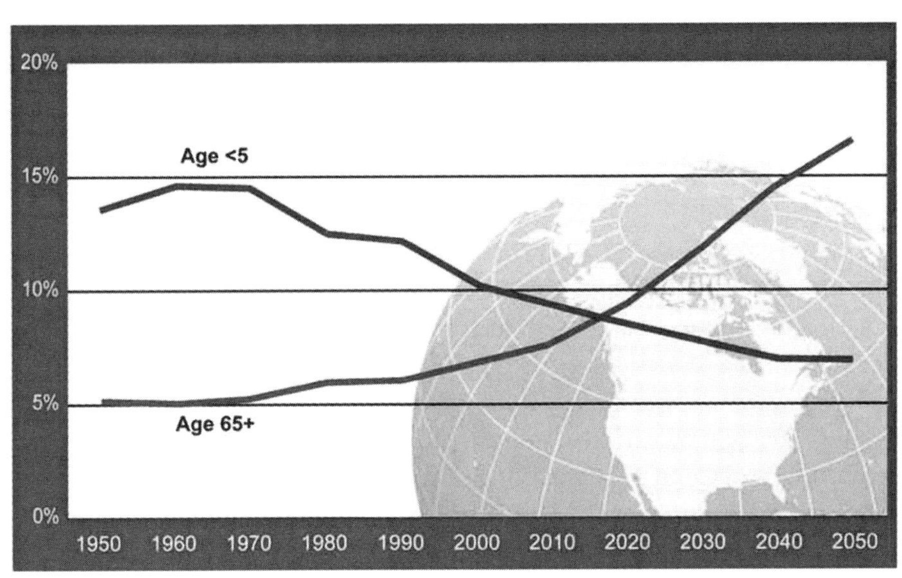

Source: United Nations. *World Population Prospects: The 2010 Revision.* Available at: http://esa.un.org/unpd/wpp.

adults and 90 percent of all persons aged 65 or older have at least one chronic condition with more than 22 percent of older people having diabetes (AARP 2017). Chronic diseases are estimated to account for more than 75 percent of US health expenditures (Centers for Disease Control and Prevention 2016a). Spending on healthcare is highly concentrated in specific population groups. Half of the US population accounts for only 3 percent of healthcare costs, while 1 percent spend 20 percent of healthcare expenditures (Schoenman and Chockley 2012).

Racial and ethnic minority groups also tend to use healthcare services differently and experience higher rates of disease. For instance, 12 percent of African Americans have diabetes and 8 percent have had a heart attack. The comparable figures for white people are 7 percent and 4 percent, respectively. African Americans are also 10 times more likely to be diagnosed with AIDS (Ubri and Artiga 2016). Likewise, American Indians suffer from diabetes twice as often as whites do.

Minority groups have less health insurance coverage and often lack a primary care provider; about one-third of Hispanics and American Indians and 20 percent of African Americans are uninsured versus 12.5 percent of whites. Similarly, half of Hispanics and one-fourth of African Americans do not have a regular doctor, compared to one-fifth of whites (Halle, Lewis, and Seshamani 2009). Furthermore, minority populations often express different cultural and lifestyle preferences—such as choice of foods, level of participation in sports, use of tobacco, and openness to discussing disease—that affect incidence of illness and rates of healthcare use. An understanding of healthcare utilization differences among segments of the population is critical to evaluating the external environment.

Consumption of healthcare varies by gender as well. Women use 32 percent more healthcare services, including visits to primary care providers, emergency and diagnostic services, and specialty care, than men do (Bertakis et al. 2000; Cylus et al. 2010). The number of females between ages 15 and 44 in the population affects birth rates; however, birth rates also are linked to economic and cultural factors. For instance, some have attributed the declining birth rate in the United States to the 2008 recession, and women are having babies significantly later in life. In 1990, mothers older than age 35 accounted for only 9 percent of all births, whereas in 2008 they accounted for 14 percent (Livingston and Cohn 2010). By 2016, the US national birth rate had dropped to an all-time historic low of 59.8 births per 1,000 women, less than half of its peak of 122.9 in 1957. The average age for a first birth was 26.3 years in 2016, as compared to 24.9 in the year 2000 (Park 2016).

To understand health issues in the external environment, healthcare organizations should identify their customers. Those planning should recognize the significant segments and concentrations and examine the relevant trends. Identifying where patients come from and where they go to for care is vital. Market knowledge helps hospitals understand and improve their competitive position, target their services, and better address community healthcare needs. Data or spatial (geographic) analysis, such as a patient origin study, can be used to locate the communities in which customers reside and provide important information to ensure that residents have appropriate access to healthcare services (Office of Statewide Health Planning and Development 2016; Ricketts et al. 1997). Exhibits 2.2 and 2.3 provide an example of this type of study. The proportion of patients residing in different zip codes can be determined and graphed to show primary and secondary service areas.

Patient origin study
Data that describe the proportion and number of an organization's customers (patients) who come from different geographic locations. These data can be arrayed and graphed to display the provider's primary and secondary service areas.

To create a **patient origin study**, divide the percentage of total admissions by zip code and sort them from the highest to the lowest percentages. In exhibit 2.2, the percentages arrayed on the map graphically show where patients originate. The zip codes that encompass 60 percent of total admissions are shaded differently in the second map to denote the organization's primary service area. As further discussed in chapter 10, populations can be segmented by many other characteristics, such as age, payer type, and race.

In healthcare, the identification of intermediate organizations—those between the patient and the provider—is likewise important. As shown in exhibit 2.4, patients may not have the freedom to select a provider of their choice. Physician practices and managed care contracts may significantly influence or

EXHIBIT 2.2
Use of Medical Geography and Patient Origin to Determine a Patient Service Area

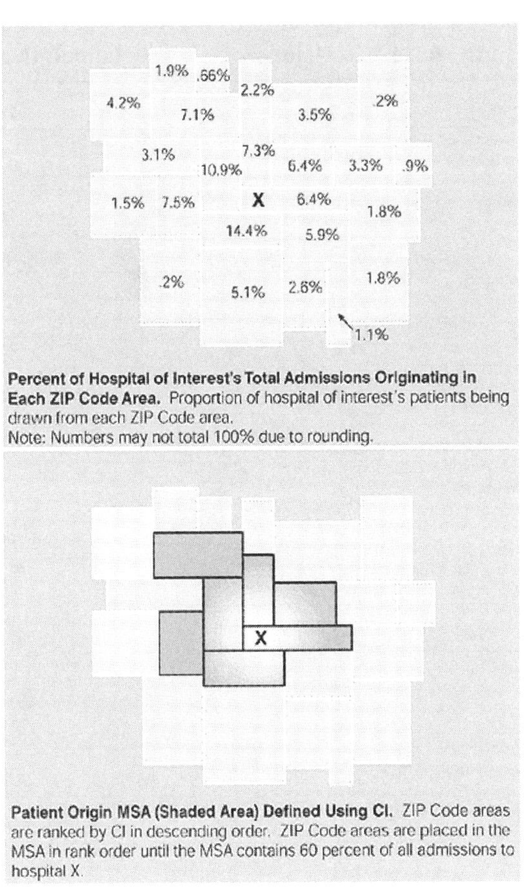

Percent of Hospital of Interest's Total Admissions Originating in Each ZIP Code Area. Proportion of hospital of interest's patients being drawn from each ZIP Code area.
Note: Numbers may not total 100% due to rounding.

Patient Origin MSA (Shaded Area) Defined Using CI. ZIP Code areas are ranked by CI in descending order. ZIP Code areas are placed in the MSA in rank order until the MSA contains 60 percent of all admissions to hospital X.

Source: Reprinted from Ricketts et al. (1997).

direct where a patient goes for care. Organizations should break out use patterns by important intermediaries to determine dependencies and trends. Such segmentation will enable an organization to better understand the location and type of customers it serves; both are important factors to consider when crafting strategic actions.

Governmental regulations highly influence the healthcare field. Regulations require licensure, training, inspection, and approval of physicians and nurses, healthcare institutions, healthcare financiers, drug and medical products, research bodies, and public health agencies. The US healthcare system is one of its most regulated sectors; almost every aspect of it is subject to federal or state scrutiny (Field 2007).

In most developed countries, the government pays for most of healthcare; in the United States, the government funds about two-thirds of overall

EXHIBIT 2.3 Percentage of Hospital Admissions by Zip Code

Zip Code	Percentage of Total Admissions	Cumulative Percentage
34237	14.4	14.4
34226	10.9	25.3
34240	7.5	32.8
34227	7.3	40.1
34225	7.1	47.2
34228	6.4	53.6
34229	6.4	60.0
34234	5.9	65.9
34238	5.1	71.0
34218	4.2	75.2
34222	3.5	78.7
34230	3.3	82.0
34224	3.1	85.1
34235	2.5	87.6
34221	2.2	89.8
34219	1.9	91.7
34232	1.8	93.5
34233	1.8	95.3
34241	1.5	96.8
34236	1.1	97.9
34231	0.9	98.8
34220	0.7	99.5
34239	0.2	99.7
34223	0.2	99.9

healthcare costs (CMS 2015). As a result, governments' legislation and resultant regulations that almost always influence funding and costs influence the demand for healthcare and the way it is provided. For example, the Patient Protection and Affordable Care Act of 2010 (ACA) significantly affected the healthcare field. The government forecast that the proposed expansion of insurance coverage would increase the demand for healthcare products and services while negatively affecting organizations' profitability and research efforts (Nexon

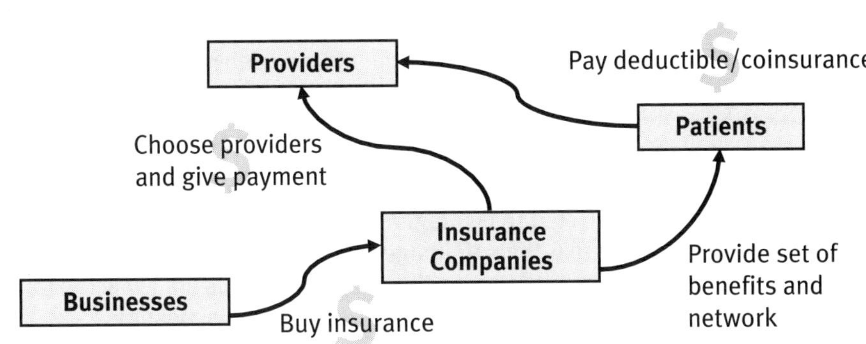

EXHIBIT 2.4
Intermediaries to Patients

and Ubi 2010). Likewise, Donald Trump's repeal of the ACA will alter the governmental rules and regulations on which US healthcare is organized to drastically alter Medicare, Medicaid, and private insurance (Wasik 2016).

Technology also has a significant influence on healthcare. Advances in technology, including prescription drugs, have been identified as a leading contributor to the increase in overall healthcare spending. **Medical technology** is broadly defined as the procedures, equipment, and processes used to deliver medical care. Examples are new medical and surgical procedures, such as implantation of cardiac defibrillators; new drugs; new medical devices; and new support systems. New technology can profoundly change the nature and process of care, which in turn may significantly influence organizations' strategies. Advances in cardiovascular treatment have reduced the rate of death from heart attack by almost half. Declining cardiovascular disease, although wonderful for the public, has a major impact on the number and type of providers required to care for this population. Similarly, the use of cardiac stents appears to have significantly reduced the number of coronary bypass surgeries performed in the United States—decreasing patient volume for surgeons but placing greater demand on cardiologists (Cayton et al. 2012). As shown in exhibit 2.5, new technology will continue to alter the provision of healthcare radically.

Medical technology
The procedures, equipment, and processes used to deliver medical care.

Market Structure

Organizations exist in **markets**—places, systems, and processes through which goods and services are exchanged. A basic knowledge of the concept of market structure is important. To understand the principles of market structure, one first should learn the difference between industries and markets. An **industry** is a particular category of business or economic activities. It is composed of groups of sellers whose products are close substitutes. For example, there is a pharmaceutical industry, a computer industry, and an aviation industry.

Markets
Places, systems, and processes through which buyers and sellers exchange goods and services.

Industry
A particular category of business or economic activity; an aggregation of sellers whose products are close substitutes.

EXHIBIT 2.5
Advancing Technology, Improving Healthcare

Healthcare technologies are advancing radically and will have far-reaching implications "in terms of diagnostics, treatments, and delivery of care in the future." Some of the major technologies predicted to disrupt healthcare by the year 2020 include the following:

- *Artificial intelligence* (AI). "By 2020, chronic conditions, such as cancer and diabetes, are expected to be diagnosed in minutes using cognitive systems that provide real-time 3D images by identifying typical physiological characteristics in the scans. By 2025, AI systems are expected to be implemented in 90% of the U.S. and 60% of the global hospitals and insurance companies."
- *Immunotherapies in cancer care*. "The market for check point inhibitors was valued at $3 billion in 2015 and is expected to reach $21.1 billion by 2020."
- *Liquid biopsy*. This innovation will noninvasively monitor for cancer cells, eliminating the need for physical biopsies.
- *CRISPR gene editing*. This technology will make targeted modifications to DNA. "It holds the promise of transforming the way R&D is conducted and products are developed across major sectors of the global life science economy."
- *3-D printing*. Medical practitioners will create customized "3D-printed scaffolds or prosthetics (orthopedic implants) and medical devices, such as dental implants and hearing aids. The game changer for 3D printing will be in human tissue printing: printed livers, hearts, ears, hands and eyes, or building the smallest functional units of tissues, which can lead to the fabrication of large tissues and organs."

Source: Das (2016).

However, no hard boundaries distinguish the industry in which a business belongs. For instance, one could argue that home health services should be considered distinct from the pharmaceutical drug and the nursing home sectors because they are not direct substitutes and complement, rather than compete with, each other. Yet in some situations they are substitutes; for example, drugs may reduce the demand for other healthcare services. Therefore, home health, prescription drugs, and nursing homes could be subsumed in a global industry that includes all aspects of healthcare.

The boundaries of nonhealthcare industries are similarly difficult to define, especially as technologies advance and competition changes. For instance, Nokia and Blackberry dominated the cell phone industry in the first decade of the twenty-first century, when simple texts and e-mail complemented phone services. With the advent of the iPhone (Apple), competition over apps ensued and the cell phone industry expanded. Today, the phone industry offers such features as cameras, global positioning systems, movie players, data storage, maps, and games in addition to voice and text transmission.

In markets, services and goods may be exchanged for other products and services (barter) or, more commonly, for money. Retail markets may be physical (e.g., shopping centers, malls) or electronic (e.g., eBay). People also sell their labor to companies. Stock markets exchange company shares. Illegal markets for illicit drugs and other unlawful products also exist. An established market facilitates trade by establishing rules and expectations to regulate distribution and pricing.

The number, concentration, and relative strength of organizations in an industry compose its **market structure**, and the market structure exerts a strategic influence on the intensity and form of competition in the industry. As a result, organizations vary their strategies according to the structure of the market in which they exist. Organizations most often seek market power—the ability to influence prices by exercising control over supply and demand—which is directly related to their market's structure and their relative position in that market (Hitt, Ireland, and Hoskisson 2016).

Market structure
The organizational characteristics of a market that exert a strategic influence on the intensity and form of competition.

There are four basic types of market structure, each of which reflects the number of organizations in the market and their degree of market influence:

1. Perfect competition
2. Monopolistic competition
3. Oligopoly
4. Monopoly

Exhibit 2.6 graphically displays the four market types and their relationship to the number of competitors and competitors' degree of market influence. Markets' structure rarely adheres strictly to one of the types but rather exhibits characteristics of the types to differing degrees. For example,

EXHIBIT 2.6
Market Structure by Degree of Control and Number of Competitors

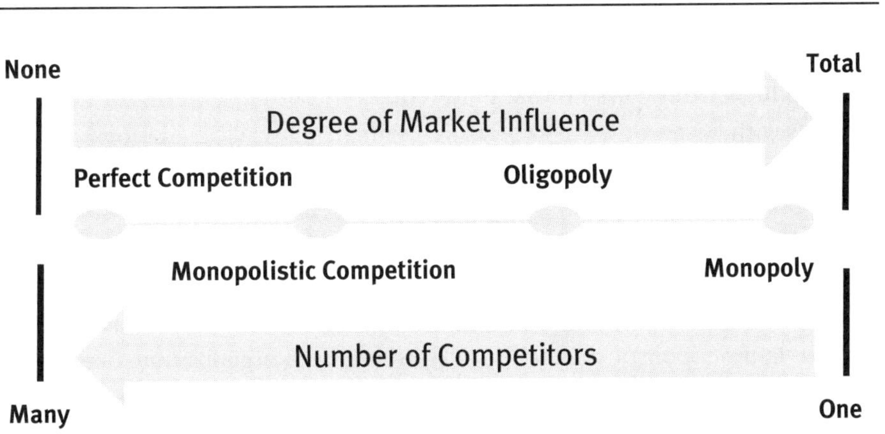

true perfect competition rarely exists, but some markets more closely resemble this structure than others do. Likewise, few markets are true monopolies; rather, they approach a monopolistic structure. The market for Microsoft's main products is one example of a near monopoly, with almost 90 percent of the operating system market in 2016. Android's dominant 80 percent global market share of smartphones is another (Dans 2016; Hruska 2016). In some states the health insurance market approaches monopolies in the individual healthcare insurance market, with about 90 percent controlled by one insurer in Alabama, New Hampshire, Vermont, and Rhode Island and approximately 80 percent in Arkansas, Maryland, North Carolina, and North Dakota (Kaiser Family Foundation 2014b).

Perfect Competition

Perfect competition
One of the four basic types of market structure. Perfect competition exists in markets composed of many small organizations that produce an undifferentiated, homogeneous product.

Exhibit 2.7 identifies characteristic differences among the market types. The first type, **perfect competition**, exists when many small organizations produce an undifferentiated, homogeneous product. Consumers may struggle to differentiate the products in such markets, so organizations compete on the basis of price and seek low-cost production solutions. There are few barriers or impediments to entering the market, so new competitors move in and incumbents move out frequently. In ideal perfect competition, consumers have enough information to make informed choices, and the prices they pay are close to production costs. Gasoline, generic drugs, currency markets, and agricultural commodities (e.g., wheat, rice, corn) are examples of markets that closely approach perfect competition. Because consumers often fail to distinguish companies' products in such markets, price often drives consumers' purchasing decisions. Therefore, low cost is the primary strategic focus in perfect competition.

Monopolistic Competition

Monopolistic competition
One of the four basic types of market structure. Monopolistic competition exists in markets composed of many organizations offering differentiated products.

Similar to perfect competition, **monopolistic competition** is a market involving many organizations. However, this structural type differentiates its products, so differentiation is the organizations' strategic focus; they seek to distinguish their products from competitors. Differentiation can be achieved by offering products with better or exclusive features, enhancing service, employing more helpful and friendly personnel, boosting distribution channel performance, creating attractive packaging, raising product quality, changing location, or improving the organization's image (McGuigan, Moyer, and Harris 2017). Many products are available to consumers, and competition increases as products and their perceived quality become more diversified. Competition is typically vigorous in monopolistic competition. However, each organization, depending on its degree of differentiation, has some control over the prices of its products. Organizations with greater product differentiation have more power to raise prices over those of their competitors.

EXHIBIT 2.7 Characteristic Differences Among the Four Types of Market Structure

	Industry Structure Type			
	Perfect Competition	**Monopolistic Competition**	**Oligopoly**	**Monopoly**
Number of organizations	Many	Many	Few	One
Type of product	Undifferentiated, homogeneous	Similar, but not identical; differentiated	Similar or identical	Homogeneous, limited options
Available substitutes	Many	Some	Some	None
Strategic focus	Price	Differentiation	Market share	Deterrence
Barriers to entry and exit	None	Limited	High	High
Ability to influence price	None	Some	Significant	Significant
Level of competition	Significant; based on price	Some; based on quality differences	Significant; not based on price	None
Consumer behavior	Consumers can easily find substitutes and have information to make informed choices.	Consumers often are influenced by advertising, perceived quality, or personal relationships.	Consumers have limited choices and usually make choices based on location or personal preference.	Consumers have few choices or substitutes and must pay higher prices.
Examples	Gasoline, generic drugs, currency markets, agricultural commodities	Restaurants, breakfast cereals, private physician services	Tertiary hospitals, drug companies, healthcare insurance companies, group purchasing organizations, airlines	Many rural hospitals, new drugs under patent, utility companies, National Football League

Entry into and exit from monopolistic competition is easy. Restaurants, manufacturers of breakfast cereals, and most private physician services in the United States operate in monopolistic competition structures. In the case of private physician services, for instance, physicians differentiate themselves by office location, specialization, and personal relationships with their patients. Because of these and other factors, price generally is not a major consideration when people are choosing physicians (Walston and Chou 2012).

Oligopoly

Oligopoly
One of the four basic types of market structure. Oligopolies exist in markets dominated by a few large organizations that offer similar or identical products.

Oligopolies are market structures dominated by a few large organizations that offer similar or identical products. Organizations in oligopolies focus their strategies on capturing market share, unless they can collude to increase profits by fixing prices or reducing supplies. A global example of collusion by organizations in an oligopoly is the formation of the Organization of Petroleum Exporting Countries (OPEC). In 1960, the large oil producers banded together to restrict the supply and raise the price of oil (Said 2015). Laws exist in many countries to prevent such anticompetitive behaviors (Hawk 2010).

Organizations seeking to enter or exit an oligopoly face substantial barriers. The cost of entry is often great, and the specialized nature of business in oligopolies makes leaving difficult. Consumers have limited choices because the producers of a product or service are limited in number, and buyers often choose services or products on the basis of location or personal preference. For instance, the construction of a new tertiary hospital may cost millions of dollars, require multiple permits, change referral patterns, and necessitate hiring a medical staff. Therefore, generally speaking, few tertiary hospitals compete in a market. Patients have limited choices for tertiary care. They may choose the tertiary hospital closest to their home, referred by their insurance company, or preferred by their personal physician. Examples of oligopolies in healthcare include tertiary hospitals, healthcare insurance companies, drug companies, and group purchasing organizations. Nonhealthcare oligopolies include airline, steel, aluminum, automobile, oil, tire, and beer companies.

Monopoly

Monopoly
One of the four basic types of market structure. Monopolies exist in markets that are dominated by a single organization.

A **monopoly**, on the other hand, involves just one organization. As a result, the monopolist has the power to control the type and quality of products and services provided. Competition is almost nonexistent, so the monopolist spends much of its time and strategic efforts creating and maintaining barriers to keep potential competitors out of its market. The service customers receive is often expensive and of marginal or poor quality. For example, as stated in the introduction to this chapter, hospital markets with monopolies charge more than 15 percent more than markets that have 4 or more hospitals.

Another example of monopolistic pricing in the United States is the high cost of pharmaceuticals allowed by the so-called monopoly rights given individual prescription drugs by governmental agencies. The monopoly and other factors make the US per capita spending on prescription drugs more than twice what other developed countries spend ($858 vs. $400) (Kesselheim, Avorn, and Sarpatwari 2016). Drug companies have greater ability to raise costs, with prices increasing at a rate eight times that of inflation. Patients with chronic diseases can spend more than $11,000 per year on prescription drugs. This situation sometimes results in clearly abusive business strategies—for example, when the cost of Daraprim, used to treat serious parasite infections, was raised 5,000 percent in 2015 (Tuttle 2016). Prices appear higher in monopolistic conditions in other healthcare sectors as well. Other examples of monopolies include utility companies, and the National Football League.

Because of the influence concentrated markets (monopolies and oligopolies) have on price and supply, the US government has passed antitrust laws and formed agencies such as the Federal Trade Commission (FTC) to restrict anticompetitive behavior and curb potential predation. (For more information, see the FTC's website at www.ftc.gov/tips-advice/competition-guidance/industry-guidance/health-care.)

Measuring Market Structure

A common measure of market concentration is the **Herfindahl-Hirschman Index** (HHI). Federal regulatory agencies examine the HHIs in markets where mergers and acquisitions are proposed. If a market is highly concentrated, the government may deny the merger or acquisition or apply restrictions.

Herfindahl-Hirschman Index (HHI)
A measure of market concentration calculated by squaring the market share percentage of each organization in a market and then summing the numbers.

The HHI is calculated by squaring the market share percentage of each organization in a market and then summing the numbers:

$$\text{HHI} = \sum_{i=1}^{n}(MS)^2 + (MS)^2 + (MS)^2 + \ldots (MS)^2$$

For example, if a market included six organizations—one with 50 percent market share, two with 20 percent, one with 6 percent, and two with 2 percent—the HHI would be calculated as follows:

$$\text{HHI} = (0.50)^2 + (0.20)^2 + (0.20)^2 + (0.06)^2 + (0.02)^2 + (0.02)^2 = 0.25 + 0.04 + 0.04 + 0.0036 + 0.0004 + 0.0004 = 0.3344.$$

The HHI approaches zero when many organizations of relatively small size compose a market. Conversely, the HHI for a monopoly is 1.0. The US government multiplies this number by 10,000, which changes the range from 0 (perfect competition) to 10,000 (monopoly). Using the latter conversion, the guidelines of the US Department of Justice states that HHIs lower than 1,000 denote unconcentrated markets; HHIs between 1,000 and 1,800 denote moderately concentrated markets; and HHIs higher than 1,800 identify markets that are highly concentrated and promote negative market behaviors (US Department of Justice 1997). On the basis of this index, the example in the previous paragraph would be considered a highly concentrated market (3,344).

The HHI examines organizations' market share only for a common product or service at only one point in time, so its usefulness is limited. Organizations may offer multiple products and services in distinct market areas. Likewise, technology and market share may shift radically over time, rendering point-in-time HHI analysis almost meaningless.

Markets in healthcare tend to be highly concentrated. Most urban hospital and healthcare insurance markets are oligopolies with HHIs greater than 4,000 (Luke, Walston, and Plummer 2004). Healthcare providers have often effectively implemented strategies to increase their market share and gain greater negotiating power to increase the prices paid by consumers and health insurance companies. Some believe that current legislative efforts to promote integrated care through accountable care organizations could lead to even greater market concentration in healthcare (Berenson, Ginsburg, and Kemper 2010).

Four-firm concentration ratio A measure of market concentration calculated by summing the market shares of the four largest firms in a market.

A simpler, less sophisticated measure of market concentration is the **four-firm concentration ratio** (FFCR). The FFCR is calculated by adding the market shares of the four largest organizations in a market to find their cumulative total output:

$$\text{FFCR} = \sum_{i=1}^{4}(\text{Firm}_1) + (\text{Firm}_2) + (\text{Firm}_3) + (\text{Firm}_4)$$

For example, the FFCR for the six-organization market used earlier in the HHI calculation would be

$$\text{FFCR} = (0.50) + (0.20) + (0.20) + (0.06) = 0.96, \text{ or 96 percent.}$$

A market with a four-firm ratio of 40 percent or less is considered unconcentrated, while markets with ratios greater than 90 percent are highly concentrated. Urban hospital markets and health insurers tend to be highly concentrated; urban hospital markets typically have FFCRs greater than 90 percent, and state insurance markets are generally dominated by one or two large insurance carriers (Cutler and Morton 2013; Furnas and Buckwalter-Poza 2010; Luke, Walston, and Plummer 2004). On the other hand, the top ten world pharmaceutical companies controlled only about 30 percent of the global pharmaceutical drug market in 2015 (Dezzani 2016).

The four-firm ratio does have drawbacks. The four-firm ratio's main limitation is that it considers only the four largest organizations in a market. Urban markets often include far more than four organizations.

Product Life Cycle

Markets also tend to go through cyclical changes. Most products and services go through phases or a life cycle that relates to the rate of sales, number of organizations in the market, and consumer demand. For decades managers and business researchers have seen the product life cycle as a useful framework for analyzing dynamic market conditions and applying more relevant, appropriate strategic alternatives (Day 1981). As shown in exhibit 2.8, it is typically depicted as four stages: emerging, growth, maturity, and decline. Product sales follow an S curve: They begin slowly in the emerging stage, rise precipitously in the growth period, flatten during the maturity stage, and decrease throughout the decline phase.

Emerging markets can be a difficult environment for organizational growth. Sales in emerging markets are limited because customers often lack adequate product knowledge and must be induced to try the merchandise.

EXHIBIT 2.8
The Product Life Cycle

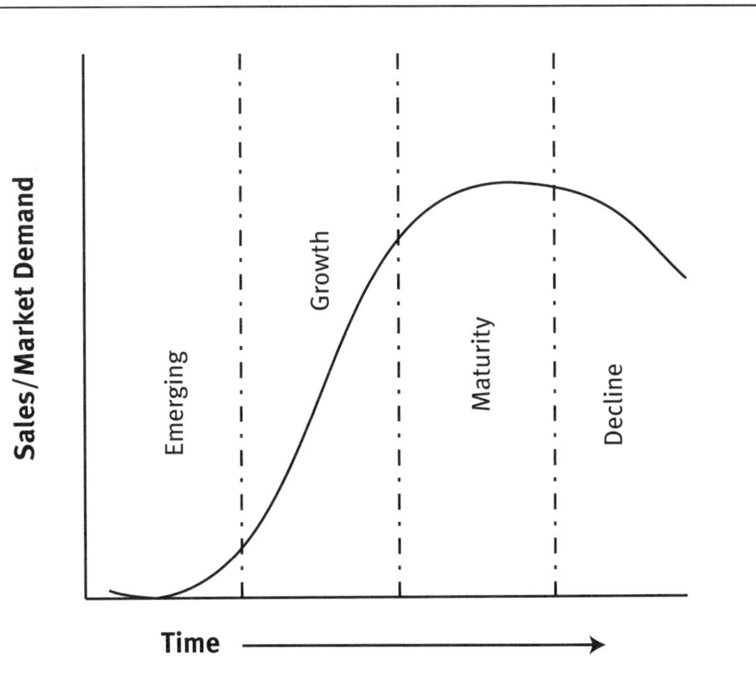

Few standards exist, and product quality can vary dramatically, further confusing potential buyers. The few companies initially present in an emerging market spend significant monies on research, advertising, and marketing. As a consequence, the sale of products in emerging markets produces little profit, and companies face a substantial risk of product failure.

Entry into emerging markets can be strategically important. Organizations in emerging markets anticipate the ultimate market structure and position themselves accordingly. Strategic risks are high in emerging markets, but—if the organization can find the correct strategic position—so is the potential for great rewards. Innovative organizations may participate in many emerging markets simultaneously, hoping for big returns in at least some of their ventures. One example is the company Google. Its top-secret laboratory, X, formally Google X, is pursuing "shoot-for-the-stars ideas," including drone delivery service and driverless cars (Dougherty 2016).

During the next stage—growth—sales increase rapidly. Overall, this stage is the best time for an organization to enter a new market. Competition is relatively low, customers are more forgiving, and businesses can obtain greater profits (Porter 1985). As more products sell, standards are set, customer acceptance increases, and the average cost of products drops because of economies of scale. At the same time, more competitors enter the market, eventually instigating greater price rivalry.

Rapid growth slows at some point, however, and a product enters the maturity stage. In this stage of market saturation, many organizations may consolidate and merge as profits decrease because of price competition and flat sales. Organizations increasingly compete for market share by differentiating their products and discounting their prices. Cost management becomes a critical competency, especially at the end of the maturity stage.

Ultimately, the demand for a product decreases because of changing consumer preferences, technological obsolescence, or availability of more effective substitutes. Many popular products have disappeared and faded into obscurity as the demand for them diminished. For example, the Sony Walkman, pagers, the PalmPilot, videocassette recorders, answering machines, and Atari game systems all were prominent products in the past. As consumers modified their preferences and technologies advanced, each product vanished and was supplanted by more effective substitutes (Grobart and Austen 2012). As demand drops, overcapacity leads organizations to exit the market or merge, leaving a smaller number of competitors. Again, cost and price competition dominate strategies in the decline stage.

The product life cycle, although helpful in strategic thinking, has some limitations as a framework for analysis. The S curve is not necessarily a sequential function. Some products skip stages or move back to a previous stage when new markets arise, new uses for the products are discovered, or technology advances.

In addition, the duration of each stage and of the transition to another stage is unpredictable. Fad products might grow rapidly, while durable products may experience extended, slow growth. For instance, the sales of Procter & Gamble's laundry detergent Tide grew consistently from its introduction in 1947 through 1976. Over that period, the company modified the formula 55 times to better match consumer preferences (Day 1981). On the other hand, product life cycles are extremely short in the semiconductor, computer, and telecommunication industries today as a result of constantly changing technologies and consumer demand (Goktan and Miles 2011).

Chapter Summary

The external environment of all organizations profoundly affects their ability to operate and prosper. An understanding of the context in which one operates is critical to strategic planning and strategic thinking.

The external environment consists of consumers, suppliers, buyers, competitors, and regulators. The powers and pressures emanating from these sources influence the strategic choices that organizations need to make. These components can be categorized as societal factors or market factors. The societal environment comprises general economic conditions, population demographics, cultural values, governmental regulations, and technology. Market factors include the number of organizations in a market and their degree of market influence. Common market structures include perfect competition, monopolistic competition, oligopoly, and monopoly. Oligopolies exist in many healthcare markets. The degree of market concentration can be determined by calculating the Herfindahl-Hirschman Index or the four-firm concentration ratio.

The product life cycle also is useful for analyzing markets. It identifies the stages through which products progress and illustrates the effects that changes in technology, markets, and consumer demand have on product growth.

Chapter Questions

1. How does a change in population demographics alter the use of healthcare?
2. Which components of population demographics have the most significant impact on healthcare?
3. What is a patient origin study, and how can it inform strategic thinking?
4. Which of the four market structures would be most preferable to consumers? To organizations' owners? To governments? Why?

5. What intermediaries exist between patients and their providers in the United States? What purpose do they serve?
6. How have technological advancements changed the provision of healthcare, and how might they affect healthcare in the future?
7. What are some of the exchanges that occur in the healthcare market?
8. What is the major difference between perfect competition and monopolistic competition?
9. Why do so many oligopolies exist in healthcare?
10. What are the main barriers to entering the healthcare market? Do they vary by type of organization? How?
11. What are two measures of market concentration? Why might one be preferred over the other?
12. How might healthcare services pass through the product life cycle? How do the size and number of organizations in a market affect the product life cycle?
13. What must a firm do to succeed in the declining product market stage?
14. How should the strategic actions of an organization whose product is in an emerging market stage differ from those of an organization whose product is in the mature stage?

Chapter Cases

Case Studies

Either "The Struggle of a Safety Net Hospital" or "The Battle in Boise," both found in the case studies section at the back of this book, can be used to explore concepts in this chapter.

Herman and Market Structures

Herman has been working in healthcare administration for ten years. He has finally taken a health strategy course and learned about different market structures. He wondered why different segments of healthcare respond differently in negotiations. One of his responsibilities is negotiating with physicians, insurance companies, and hospitals in his company's managed care unit. He has found that his ability to exact price concessions from different groups varies dramatically. Primary care physicians' market structure is a monopolistic competition, while prominent hospitals seem to hold monopoly power. Insurance markets, on the other hand, often are oligopolies. He now believes that the introduction of national quality standards for primary care physicians may make outcomes among physician offices easier to compare and thus reduce their differentiation. As a result, he may be able to gain greater price concessions from physicians in the future. Often, however, he almost has to beg prominent hospitals to join his system's network, and in turn he pays full prices. In insurance markets of only three or four major companies, each organization seems to offer the same terms. Herman thinks he now understands better what is happening with each group.

Questions

1. How are Herman's perceptions regarding his negotiations and market structure correct? Incorrect?
2. How would specialist physicians fit into the market structure, and how would Herman negotiate with them?
3. Could perfect competition exist in healthcare? How would one negotiate in this type of market?

Chapter Assignments

Identify the market shares for general acute care services, by organization, in a city of your choosing. Determine the HHI and the four-firm concentration ratio for this area. How much monopoly power exists in this market? Would the index vary significantly if you calculated it for a specialty, such as obstetrics or cardiovascular surgery? What if you expanded the area under evaluation to a larger region or state? How would the index change?

Write a one-page paper on the problems of monopolistic power in healthcare. How might the proposed changes in the ACA affect the market power of healthcare providers? What can the government and other stakeholders do to moderate monopoly power?

CHAPTER

3

BUSINESS MODELS AND COMMON STRATEGIES

> Five years from now," said a hospital CEO to his peers at a recent conference, "our organizations will look very different. They will operate with different incentives, different business models and different footprints." What does the future look like for community hospitals and health systems—and what are their marching orders?
>
> The hospital business model is under pressure. The costs of physicians, nurses, technology, compliance, and marketing are rising, while payments from all payer types are shrinking, as is inpatient utilization. We anticipate a 12 to 28 percent revenue decline over the next few years.
>
> Many community hospitals, already operating at razor-thin margins, soon may find themselves deep in the red. Although most hospital leaders realize this possibility, their responses to these pressures often betray a lack of focus. They react with across-the-board cuts, a race to acquire physicians, a superficial rebranding, or a search for elusive mergers and acquisitions. These incremental actions are unlikely to move the needle. What's needed is a new way of thinking about form and function.
>
> —Gary Ahlquist, "New Approaches for Community Hospitals and Health Systems," 2013

Learning Objectives

After reading this chapter, you will

- understand the concept and use of business models;
- be able to describe how business models vary in healthcare and how business models may provide a competitive advantage;
- comprehend generic strategies and their application to healthcare;
- be familiar with strategies for differentiation in healthcare, including focused factories; and
- recognize the advantages and disadvantages of first-mover strategy.

Organizations, even direct competitors, may form and pursue strategies in vastly different ways. This chapter discusses how organizations produce value for customers and how their structure, processes, and strategies influence their success. As discussed in chapter 6, success is relative to the values, mission, and vision of an organization. For for-profit organizations, sustained profits may signify competitive advantage and success. Not-for-profit organizations, however, may recognize other achievements as success. Therefore, the desired business outcome must dictate the business model of an organization.

Business Models

Whatever their definition of success, organizations constantly face the challenge of devising strategies that will enable them to enhance the value they provide to their key stakeholders. As stated in the introduction to the chapter, experts expect that healthcare and hospital business models will experience pressure to change. **Business models**, the underlying structure and function of organizations, build on the idea of value chains and value creation (Morris et al. 2006; Porter 1985). Although a common definition of *business model* has not been established, Walston and Chou (2012) define it as the core elements of an organization and how it is structured to deliver value to its customers and generate revenues. Business models encompass all aspects of organizations, including their economic, operational, and strategic domains, and successful organizations design their business models around their internal competencies (Morris et al. 2006). Appropriate, competitive business models often succeed when matched against organizations that have better ideas and better technology but a poor business model (Chesbrough 2007).

Business model
The underlying structure of an organization; the means through which an organization creates and delivers value to its customers and earns revenues.

Most established organizations in the same industry do not have distinct business models. Organizations that compete for the same set of customers frequently copy each other's structures and strategies. Over time, many organizations may come to offer similar sets of products and services. As discussed in chapter 7, barriers commonly restrict entry into an industry, and mobility barriers limit competition in strategic groups. With limited entry of new organizations and similar environmental conditions, incumbents become **isomorphic** over time, adopting homogenous forms and practices (DiMaggio and Powell 1983). As a result, pronounced differences in business models often emerge only when environmental shifts alter customer preferences, technology, and barriers to entry, thereby allowing new organizations to enter the industry.

Isomorphic
The tendency of organizations in a market to become similar in form and structure, offer similar products, and adopt similar practices over time.

New business models do not guarantee success and are often fraught with peril. For example, the US government has encouraged new organizations to experiment with distinct business models. Some experiments, like the Pioneer

Accountable Care Organization (ACO) Model program, created accountable care organizations that would provide savings (see exhibit 3.1). However, while many healthcare organizations initially welcomed the new approaches, most seemingly failed and abandoned the program.

Scholars often discuss business models as four interrelated components: value to customers, organizational inputs, organizational processes, and means of generating and obtaining revenues (see exhibit 3.2). The content and structure of these components should result from strategic decisions; their functions and interactions substantially contribute to the success or failure of an organization. As shown in exhibit 3.1, healthcare organizations moving to a new payment and business model may greatly struggle, and many may fail.

Customer Value

Organizations seek to produce what customers value. This perceived value consists of a range of products and services, a degree of customization, ease of availability and access, and the trade-off between cost and quality. Dissimilar business models may provide a different type of value to customers (e.g., Amazon vs. Walmart). Customers have differing desires and needs. Some may value ease of access and availability, others want low cost, yet others seek high quality. An innovative business model aims to address the needs and desires of

EXHIBIT 3.1
The Challenge of Business Model Change: ACOs

In December 2011, the Centers for Medicare & Medicaid Services (CMS) signed agreements with 32 organizations to participate in its Pioneer ACO Model. According to CMS, the model was "designed for health care organizations and providers that are already experienced in coordinating care for patients across care settings. It will allow these provider groups to move more rapidly from a shared savings payment model to a population-based payment model on a track consistent with, but separate from, the Medicare Shared Savings Program. And it is designed to work in coordination with private payers by aligning provider incentives, which will improve quality and health outcomes for patients across the ACO, and achieve cost savings for Medicare, employers and patients."

Moving to a new business model remains challenging. Five years later, only 9 of the 32 continued with the model program. The inability to accrue savings and increasing financial risk, coupled with the model's strategic, operational, and information technology challenges, were huge departures from these organizations' original business models, and few could successfully adapt. ACOs are much more complex and require significantly greater cooperation and coordination among healthcare facilities and professionals. CMS also required the health systems to track too many quality metrics, and organizations also found it difficult to attract and retain patients.

Source: CMS (2017a), Advisory Board (2014), Evans (2015), Leventhal (2015).

EXHIBIT 3.2
The Four Components of Business Models

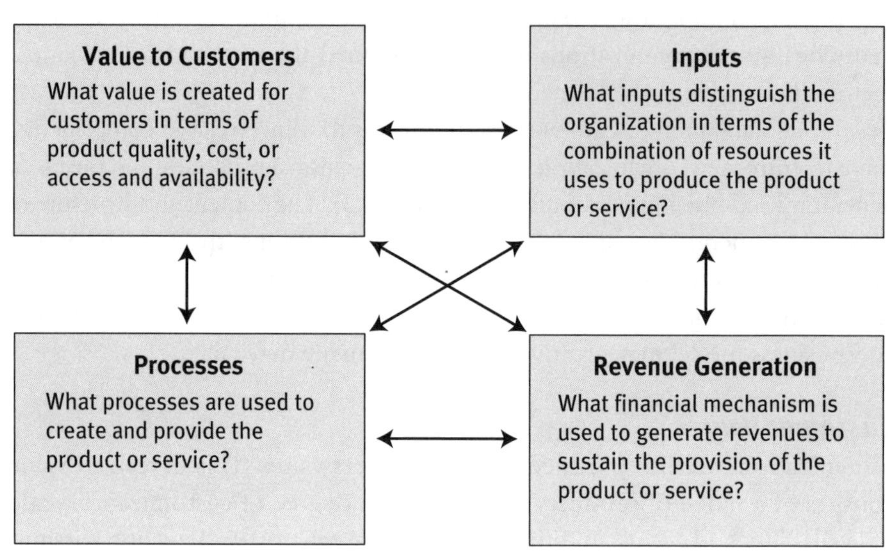

Value to Customers
What value is created for customers in terms of product quality, cost, or access and availability?
Inputs
What inputs distinguish the organization in terms of the combination of resources it uses to produce the product or service?
Processes
What processes are used to create and provide the product or service?
Revenue Generation
What financial mechanism is used to generate revenues to sustain the provision of the product or service?

Customer value
The perceived benefits of a product or service. Consumers may find value in many aspects of products and services, including range and type, degree of customization, ease of availability and access, and the trade-off between quality and cost.

Inputs
The combination, type, and mix of resources an organization uses to provide a product or service, such as personnel; materials; and strategic assets such as facilities, equipment, location, patents, networks, and partnerships.

all consumers or just a segment. The value provided by successful organizations reflects their mission and vision and differentiates them from competitors.

The following questions can be used to explore the **customer value** an organization provides:

- What value is provided to the customer segments served?
- What customer problems does the organization's product or service solve?
- What customer needs does the product or service satisfy? What needs are not satisfied?
- Does the value created by the organization support its mission and vision?
- How does this value distinguish the organization from competitors?

Inputs

The type and mix of resources organizations use to provide a product or service make up the **inputs** component of the business model. Resources include personnel, materials, and equipment. Organizations choose a mix of automated equipment and personal interaction and select types and quantities of materials and supplies according to the value they wish to deliver. Some businesses choose to hire personnel to answer phones and greet customers, while others automate customer interactions. Other inputs include organizational core competencies—a critical source of competitive advantage—and strategic assets, such as facilities, equipment, location, patents, networks, and partnerships. For instance, many hospitals have begun using hospitalists and intensivists as an input. An organization may change its inputs over time; for example, innovations in technology often trigger a change of inputs.

An organization can use the following questions to examine its inputs:

- What key inputs directly contribute to the value of the product or service?
- Are any inputs inconsequential? Could the organization lower costs or increase value if it changed any of its inputs?
- Are there new technologies that the organization should consider adding as new inputs?

Processes

A **process** is a series of steps that ultimately transforms inputs into customer-valued products and services. In addition to creating value, processes simplify decision making, increase efficiency, complete tasks, organize functions, and enable an organization to interface with external entities. A process sits between every input and resultant output. Processes are often formalized into policies and procedures and may be categorized as primary, support, or management processes (Rummler and Brache 1995). Each step in a process should add value. Organizations vary widely in their use of processes in their business models.

Process
A series of steps that transforms inputs into products or services (outputs). Processes usually are established to organize functions and interface with external entities.

The following questions can be used to examine processes:

- How do the organization's processes differ from those of its competitors?
- Which processes add value, and which do not?
- Could processes be redesigned to eliminate unneeded steps?
- Do processes unnecessarily delay final outputs?
- Can processes be automated?
- Is there new technology that could streamline existing processes?

Revenue Generation

All organizations must generate sufficient revenues to operate. To survive and prosper, even not-for-profit organizations must produce "profits" or take in more money than they expend. The ways in which funds are generated vary significantly. Organizations may obtain monies directly from consumers or through third parties. Payments for products and services can be made directly (e.g., fee-for-service), through bartering exchanges, via rebates from manufacturers, in advance (e.g., prepayments for a scope of services), and in other ways. Organizations can generate additional revenues indirectly from donations, grants, and taxation. To remain in business, however, its total direct and indirect income must exceed its expenses over time.

Profitability The degree to which the revenues generated by a product or service exceed the costs of producing that product or service.

Use the following questions to assess the **profitability** of a business model:

- In what ways does the organization generate revenues?
- If the organization generates revenues in multiple ways, which are the most important? Which will be the most important in the future?
- Could new technology significantly affect the ways the organization generates revenues?
- Does the organization generate enough revenues to achieve its mission? If not, what needs to occur?

Business Model Innovation and Adaptation

The four components of a business model constantly interact to execute an organization's strategies. To be successful, organizations must be willing to modify their business models as conditions change. However, organizations with established business models find them difficult to change because the four components are interlinked.

The innovative business models of new market entrants are often difficult for incumbents to imitate. For example, many of the major airlines have sought but failed to imitate Southwest's low-cost business model. The inability to copy new organizations' business models lies in the interconnectedness of the model components. Older organizations commonly try to compete with new organizations by changing only part of their business model, but this approach has consistently proved to be ineffective. For example, Continental Airlines established a no-frills, low-cost service in 1993, only to shut it down in 1995 after expending $140 million. Continental Lite mixed its business model by using its existing reservation system and employees, and even though it charged very low prices, few people flew with the airline (Bryant 1995; Hensel 2004). Recently, legacy airlines such as Delta and United have instituted lower-cost services, called basic economy. Passengers are not given frequent flier mileage points, they are not given the opportunity to select their seats, and small carry-on bags are only allowed under their seats. Many wonder if these changes can be sustained and successfully compete against low-cost airlines (Reed 2016).

Nonetheless, business models must change when the external environment substantially shifts and organizations must seek different ways to compete and survive. For example, most consider the traditional pharmaceutical business model unsustainable. It consists of large, vertically integrated organizations with large sales forces promoting drugs created from small-molecule compounds (Miller 2008; Tyson 2015). As detailed in exhibit 3.3, experts predict that by 2020, the business model of successful pharmaceutical companies will evolve

EXHIBIT 3.3
The Changing Pharmaceutical Business Model

Component	Traditional Pharmaceutical Business Model	Suggested 2020 Pharmaceutical Business Model
Value	Vendor of medicines to physicians and patients	Managing patient outcomes through pharmaceuticals
Inputs	Large, vertically integrated organizations, including research, clinical trials, marketing, and manufacturing based in Western countries	Nonownership agreements with universities, hospitals, technology providers, and organizations offering such services as compliance programs, stress management, nutrition, physiotherapy, exercise, and health screenings; more research to migrate to Asia
Processes	Discovery of small-molecule compounds, few of which are approved for sale; sales direct to primary care physicians and patients focused on primary care	Collaboration with many firms to provide offerings of medicine-plus packages; sale through insurance and regulated mechanisms
Profits	Profits generated for and by individual organizations; most profits obtained from sale of blockbuster drugs to pharmacies and physicians	Profits generated by joint company efforts to achieve health outcomes from sales through governmental payers, which will determine which medicines are prescribed

Source: Data from PricewaterhouseCoopers (2009).

into a collaborative network of firms that help manage patient outcomes through a so-called medicine-plus approach.

Some large pharmaceutical companies, such as Eli Lilly, are changing their business models and taking a more collaborative approach. For more than 130 years, Eli Lilly has functioned as a traditional, fully integrated pharmaceutical company. However, in response to skyrocketing discovery costs and other pressures, Eli Lilly instituted Chorus, a virtual network with nonowned companies that manage many discovery programs at a fraction of the in-house cost while significantly reducing the time of clinical trials (PricewaterhouseCoopers 2009).

The following excerpt from a company brochure further explains this new model (Chorus 2009, 3, 9, 10):

> Chorus is a small group of experienced drug developers focused on establishing clinical proof-of-concept (PoC) as quickly and inexpensively as possible. Chorus designs and manages drug development plans on new chemical entities. . . .

> The Chorus approach alters the balance of risk across the portfolio and enables clinical study of many more candidates at a fraction of the time and cost typically associated with traditional drug development. . . .
>
> Chorus teamed up with an external IT solutions partner to develop a custom, web-based enterprise management system called Voice. Voice enables small, virtual, global drug development teams to securely collaborate on all aspects of a project—including broad planning, detailed implementation, document development and approvals—and provides administrative solutions to numerous internal portfolio challenges. . . .
>
> The Chorus business model is built on the foundation of flexible outsource staffing through TPPs [third-party providers], offsetting fixed internal costs. Tactical outsourcing such as staff augmentation, functional outsourcing, and full-service outsourcing is an increasingly common method used by most pharmaceutical and biotech companies to reduce R&D fixed costs. Rather than dealing with inefficient outsource models, such as relying on a small exclusive group of providers, Chorus recognizes the need to leverage a wider group of external global implementation expertise to deliver multifaceted services. This external network provides Chorus with the flexibility to match each project's unique needs and strategic integration requirements to a wider array of global and niche TPPs. To support this more inclusive model, Chorus developed and maintains a large and growing network of providers to support each function. The Chorus external network continues to grow and currently consists of more than 200 global providers.

Since its inception, Chorus has demonstrated substantial productivity improvements in both time and cost compared to traditional pharmaceutical research and development (R&D). Lilly claims that Chorus helped it make decisions about 12 months earlier at around half the cost of comparable industry research. As a result of Chorus's successful track record and the increased demand for capacity, Lilly has expanded in Indianapolis, the United Kingdom, and India (Grogan 2011; Owens et al. 2015).

The principles and components of business models also can be used to examine macro business relationships, and they likewise apply to larger markets and industries. For example, many are calling for fundamental changes to the business model of the US healthcare system (Crean 2010; Lin 2008; Perkins 2010; Porter and Lee 2013).

US Healthcare Business Model

As illustrated in exhibit 3.4, healthcare in the United States conventionally has offered fragmented treatment of illness focused on acute care at the expense of primary and preventive care (Marvasti and Stafford 2012; Shih et al. 2008). Physicians and hospitals have been primarily engaged in curing disease on an

EXHIBIT 3.4
The Changing Healthcare Business Model

Component	Traditional Healthcare Business Model	Changing Healthcare Business Model
Value	Treatment of acute care problems; focus on curative outcomes	Improving population health; focus on preventive medicine and reduction of disease
Inputs	Fragmented system in which many different providers often compete with each other; separate ownership of physicians, insurance companies, and hospitals	Greater integration and communication among delivery systems focused on the health of a population; information systems needed to capture and manage key data
Processes	Insurance companies contract with businesses and individuals for healthcare services. Insurance companies negotiate with hospitals and physicians for services. Public health services are not integrated with traditional acute care. Focus on referrals to specialist physicians. Physicians obtain privileges to practice at independently owned hospitals.	Businesses and governments contract with systems to provide a wide scope of healthcare services. Public health services are integrated with acute care services. Focus is on treatment by primary care physicians.
Profits	Profits generated by fee-for-service: the more services provided, the more revenue produced	Profits generated by reducing disease and controlling expenses

individual basis. Little coordination has occurred among healthcare providers, instigating the delivery of duplicate services and driving up costs. American hospitals have become some of the most costly structures ever built and, as the hubs of healthcare provision, have promoted high-cost acute care medicine (Perkins 2010). Yet duplication and the high cost structure have increased hospitals' profits (Trinh, Begun, and Luke 2008). Insurance companies have taken the role of middleman, receiving monies from businesses and negotiating contracts with providers for healthcare services. The more services providers deliver, the more money they make.

From a public and consumer perspective, this business model has not produced consistent value. Despite spending more than double per capita on healthcare than any other system in the world, the US healthcare system performs relatively poorly in terms of mortality and morbidity outcomes. Despite the high spending, Americans had relatively poor health outcomes, with shorter life expectancy and more chronic disease. Consistently, the US healthcare system ranked last or next to last on quality, access, efficiency, equity, and health measures. Relative to global averages, the US government also invests little in social services that could potentially stem the tide of healthcare costs (Davis, Schoen, and Stremikis 2010; Squires and Anderson 2015).

The weaknesses inherent in the current US healthcare business model have created a fragmented, inefficient system (Shih et al. 2008, ix):

- Unassisted navigation by patients and families across different providers and care settings fosters frustrating, dangerous experiences.
- Poor communication and a lack of clear accountability for patients among providers lead to medical errors, waste, and duplication of services.
- The absence of peer accountability, a quality improvement infrastructure, and clinical information systems creates poor overall quality of care.

In addition, primary care practices' common structure consists of seven-minute visits in which the provider rapidly determines whether to prescribe a pill or refer the patient for a procedure or to another specialist. Little wonder primary care physicians are the most dissatisfied among physician specialties (Chase 2013). Some believe that various stakeholders will demand that the US healthcare business model be revised, moving to patient-centered, value-based, or population-based focus and requiring greater coordination of care and a greater attention to preventive and primary care (American Hospital Association 2017; CMS 2016; Friedman et al. 2016). As shown in exhibit 3.5, the largest payer of hospital services, CMS, has moved to a partially value-based payment system by setting aside 2 percent of overall monies for incentive awards based on clinical and service quality indicators. Improving the quality and value of healthcare has become an imperative for all.

To coordinate, manage, and control care more effectively, US healthcare delivery systems—whether owned companies or virtual networks—will need to implement comprehensive information systems capable of capturing both clinical and administrative data. In addition, methods of provider payment must change. Payers may contract directly with systems to establish a fixed rate covering the health of their discrete populations—for example, a fee per person per month or a global payment for a segment of the population. The new business model may leave out many insurance intermediaries. Finally, profits (called *surpluses* by not-for-profit organizations) will be generated by improving health outcomes, preventing disease, and controlling overall expenses more effectively rather than by providing more services.

One example of a health system that has transitioned to a new model is Western Maryland Health System in Cumberland, Maryland. In 2010, as

EXHIBIT 3.5
CMS Hospital Value-Based Purchasing

In September 2015, CMS published a document explaining its value-based purchasing, which provided incentive payments for more than 3,000 US acute care hospitals for the achievement of quality indicators related to their treatment of Medicare patients. The incentives are based on the following three primary factors:

1. The quality of care provided to Medicare patients
2. How closely best clinical practices are followed
3. How well hospitals enhance patients' experiences of care during hospital stays

Awards for 2018 are broken into four domains, with each receiving a quarter of the possible incentive payments. These areas are (1) patient- and caregiver-centered experience of care/care coordination, (2) safety, (3) clinical care, and (4) efficiency and cost reduction. Twenty-three indicators are tracked and performance is assessed by giving a hospital points for both achievement and improvement for each indicator against baselines and benchmarks. Hospitals must score in three out of the four domains to receive an incentive award. Incentives are funded by withholding 2 percent of hospital DRG payments.

Source: CMS (2015).

part of the state of Maryland's Total Patient Revenue System demonstration, this system moved to a fully value-based payment that resulted in inpatient admissions declining by 32 percent in four years. Yet the system is enjoying greater financial success. Changes included moving from a "a traditional delivery model, with the hospital and emergency department at the center" to "a continuum of care that elevates the importance of pre-acute services such as retail pharmacies and urgent care centers, and post-acute services, including rehabilitation and skilled nursing facilities, hospice, and palliative care" (Butcher 2014). Western Maryland Health System modified care delivery with resources set aside to manage patients with chronic diseases and high utilizers of services more effectively (Butcher 2014).

Disruptive innovations
Innovations that create new markets by discovering new categories of customers. They do this partly by harnessing new technologies but also by developing new business models and exploiting old technologies in new ways. (A. W. 2015)

The Threat of Disruptive Innovation

Popularized by Harvard professor Clayton Christensen, the concept of **disruptive innovations** suggests that disruption occurs when organizations successfully combine technological enablers and business model innovation (see exhibit 3.6) (Christensen 1997; Christensen and Mangelsdorf 2009). These factors can destroy existing organizational competencies and spur the rise of new, dominant organizations.

EXHIBIT 3.6 Components of Disruptive Innovation

Business Model Change	Type of Innovation: Radical	Type of Innovation: Sustaining
New	High potential for disruptive innovation; incumbents threatened	Low potential for disruptive innovation; innovation benefits incumbents
None	Low potential for disruptive innovation; new innovations change market relationships	No potential for disruptive innovation; incumbents strengthened

Technological enablers that have prompted radical innovation include the microprocessor, which helped personal computers overwhelm mainframes; the Internet, which gave rise to online news and the development of online retail stockbrokers, such as E*TRADE and Charles Schwab; and advancements in electronics, such as digital photography. As the quality of these new technologies improved, they overtook entrenched incumbents by offering better service and lower prices. Companies that previously controlled these markets, such as the *Los Angeles Times*, Merrill Lynch, and Kodak, are struggling to survive.

Novel business models that use disruptive technology enable organizations to better compete in the market and radically diminish incumbents' ability to generate profits. As a result, few dominant businesses ever survive disruptive innovation to remain the leading organizations in the new environment. For example, today's movie entertainment outlets used online technology and different business models to dominate the previous rental market king, Blockbuster. In the early 2000s, Blockbuster lost vast amounts of business to Netflix, Hulu, and Redbox and ultimately filed for bankruptcy in 2010 (Sherman 2010). For decades, Kodak produced excellent film for cameras and had expert competencies in chemical engineering. The advance to digital imaging destroyed the value and relative competence of the thousands of chemical engineers employed by Kodak. Electrical engineering skills were needed in the new world of digital imaging, and companies without these competencies failed to adapt to the new reality.

Healthcare has not generated many radical innovations—mostly sustaining discoveries that have benefited incumbents. However, many predict that future innovation, whether driven by legislative dictum (e.g., the Affordable Care Act) or scientific discovery, may disrupt existing healthcare relationships and the ways in which care is provided. It may also reconfigure service offerings to meet customer demand at lower prices (Nam 2016; Walsteijn 2012). Others suggest that the use of new midlevel providers (e.g., dental therapists) or retail clinics as alternatives for physician care might constitute disruptive innovation (Edelstein 2011; Pauly 2011). Advances in genomics, which plays a role in nine of the ten leading causes of disease in the United States, present great potential for disruptive innovation in the diagnoses, treatment, and prevention of disease (CDC 2017b). Clinical molecular testing, pharmacogenomics, and other medical genomics discoveries are rapidly expanding and helping physicians provide personalized medicine and make better prescribing and dosing decisions.

According to Hwang and Christensen (2008), healthcare is prone to fragmentation of care, coordination of care is difficult, consumers lack the proper incentives to shop for care, and many regulatory barriers exist. For these reasons, disruptive innovation does not easily take root in healthcare. Nevertheless, with steadily increasing costs and rampant inefficiencies, healthcare needs radical surgery, and strategists must recognize the possibility that new business models will emerge and bring about major change. "By coupling technological advances with appropriately matched business models, disruptive innovation has brought affordability and accessibility to industries ranging from steel making to personal finance, and it is the right prescription for the ailing U.S. health care system—a treatment that is desperately needed and long overdue" (Hwang and Christensen 2008, 1335).

Healthcare's unique structure, with intermediaries and ubiquitous governmental regulation, makes disruptive innovation more difficult. However, to be disruptive the innovation must do the following:

- *Cure disease.* Most innovations treat symptoms of disease. Disruptive innovation cures and resolves disease. For example, the introduction of the drug Sovaldi (and its successor Harvoni) was disruptive, as it cures 80 to 90 percent of those infected with hepatitis C.
- *Transform how medicine is practiced.* Disruptive innovation changes the practice of medicine. Examples include drug-eluting stents that made heart surgery less invasive and vaccines for polio and smallpox.
- *Take root deeply.* The effect (disruptive or sustaining) of a technology depends on how it is applied—many technologies, such as big data, sensors, and other tools have the potential to be disruptive, but only if applied to change radically the practice and cost of care (Nam 2016).

Generic Strategies

Generic strategies Commonly used strategies that combine a target market (e.g., a small segment of a population) and a type of differentiation (e.g., low cost).

Decades ago, Michael Porter (1980), professor of business administration at the Harvard Business School, proposed three **generic strategies** from which organizations may select. Others have since increased the number of generic categories to five (Bourgeois, Duhaime, and Stimpert 1999; Hill and Jones 1998; Thompson et. al 2016). Most authors define the generic types of strategy as combinations of a target market (a small, focused customer base vs. a large, general customer base) and the type of competitive advantage sought (low cost vs. differentiation). Exhibit 3.7 lists the possible combinations and provides examples of organizations that have adopted each type of strategy.

Broad Low-Cost Strategy

Broad low-cost strategy A type of strategy aimed at providing low-cost products to a broad customer segment.

An organization with a **broad low-cost strategy** targets a wide customer segment and seeks to achieve competitive advantage in the market by maintaining low costs and underpricing its competitors to earn higher profits. Low-cost positions can be gained by economies of scale; experience curves; efficient value chain management; effective bargaining; elimination of unnecessary features; and rock-bottom product costs through appropriate outsourcing, vertical integration, and information systems.

Use of the term *cost* frequently causes confusion because authors at times refer to cost as both the expense of producing a product or a service and the price charged for a product or a service. Although low-cost and low-price strategies ideally go together, organizations may adopt one but not the other. Low-cost strategies may be pursued concurrently with some aspect of differentiation to offer reasonable prices, coupled with some unique characteristic (e.g.,

EXHIBIT 3.7 Different Generic Strategies

Target Market	Type of Competitive Advantage	Example	
Broad segment	Low costs	Walmart, Dell	
Broad segment	Differentiation	Pepsi, Ford	
Moderate segment	Moderate costs and differentiation	Grocery stores, community hospitals	Middle strategy
Focused segment	Low costs	ALDI	
Focused segment	Differentiation	Rolls-Royce, Rolex, concierge medicine	

quality, service, access), while a true low-price strategy may need to offer the lowest price in the market (Yip and Johnson 2007). Although low production costs often do have a relationship with low prices, in this book *low cost* refers to the cost of production.

Broad low-cost strategies are most effective in markets where cost is more important than reputation or product characteristics or where large economies of scale exist. Firms producing commodities, such as wheat, oil, gold, and sugar, may more easily use a low-cost strategy. Likewise, companies that can exploit large economies of scale, such as manufacturers of computer chips, can compete on the basis of cost. As a result, organizations using a broad low-cost strategy strive to maximize their market share. However, low-cost products and services still must maintain a certain level of quality and differentiation. Consumers must perceive the lowest cost for the value received. Organizations often take one of the following approaches to create this perception:

- *Product line narrowed to standardized, no-frills goods.* Organizations pursuing a broad low-cost strategy may eliminate low-volume products and services from their offerings and retain only those that generate the greatest sales and profitability. They keep production costs low by using standard components, limiting the number of product models, and minimizing overhead and indirect costs. Noncore components may be outsourced. For example, specialty hospitals narrow the wide product line of general hospitals, standardize products and processes, and eliminate some services, thereby lowering their costs.
- *High asset turnover.* Organizations make optimal use of their assets and resources by managing large volumes efficiently and operating their facilities at full capacity. Examples include table turnover in restaurants, airlines' maximization of the time its planes are in flight, and maximization of actual surgical time in operating rooms.
- *Control of purchases and procurement.* Organizations seeking to keep costs low generally exercise control over their supply chain and purchases to minimize expenditures. Purchasing in bulk, consigning products (vendor-managed inventory), negotiating high discounts, and using just-in-time purchasing can significantly lower costs. Hospitals have often used consignment, especially for surgical implants (Crans 2009).
- *Low-cost distribution systems.* The logistics of the supply chain, including distribution, inventory management, sterilization, transportation, and so on are now the focus in the effort to lower costs in healthcare. Some systems, such as the University of Pittsburgh Medical Center, have established centralized, system-owned warehouses to limit costs, while others are working with medical and surgical distributors to distribute and store inventory more cost-effectively (Rubenfire 2016).

The costs of distribution are significant for many products and services. Low-cost strategies call for a wide distribution system at a minimal cost. Instead of using personal contact, organizations may use online sales and marketing tools to reach customers. Sophisticated software systems promote efficient distribution, and some organizations bypass distributors and sell directly to the consumer to reduce costs—for example, Dell and Apple. Customers order computers from low-cost-focused Dell via the Internet or phone. While Apple's customers may order computers these same ways, they also can visit one of Apple's many local stores and consult with service representatives. Likewise, manufacturers of generic drugs may market only to wholesalers, while brand-name drug companies have large, owned sales forces and market directly to consumers and physicians.

Focused Low-Cost Strategy

Focused low-cost strategy
A type of strategy aimed at providing low-cost products to a limited subset of the broad mass market.

An organization adopting a **focused low-cost strategy** competes on the basis of costs but targets only a subset of the mass market. This strategy refines the broad low-cost approach by narrowing its customer base and—possibly—undercutting the pricing of generalists. In highly competitive markets, smaller, low-cost organizations may find a niche in which the larger rivals cannot compete. For example, ALDI and Walmart are both large, international chains. Walmart employs a broad low-cost strategy, while ALDI employs a focused low-cost strategy. Yet their business models are similar in that both focus on cost and reasonable quality. ALDI, however, offers only a limited assortment of groceries and related items targeted to customers with low to moderate incomes and can often price these products almost 20 percent lower than Walmart (Pettypiece 2016). On ALDI's website, the company states that it "has been named the Low-Price Grocery Leader for the second straight year! . . . As a two-time low-price leader, we know that everything you buy should be of the highest quality. That's why all our products are backed by our Double Guarantee" (ALDI 2013).

As shown in exhibit 3.8, ALDI's strategy differs from Walmart's strategy mostly with regard to inputs and processes. Both offer low-cost groceries. However, Walmart sells dramatically more products and multiple brands, while ALDI sells relatively few products and only one brand of each product. ALDI also greatly minimizes personnel costs by having customers bag their own groceries and displaying products in cartons, among other techniques.

Low-Cost Strategies in Healthcare

Low-cost strategies succeed better in some segments of healthcare. The difficulty with a low-cost strategy in healthcare is the perception that low cost equates to low quality. Consumers want more than low cost in healthcare, especially if their health or the health of their family is in jeopardy. In such situations,

EXHIBIT 3.8
A Comparison of Focused Low-Cost and Broad Low-Cost Generic Grocery Store Strategies

Component	ALDI	Walmart
Value	Low-cost groceries	Low-cost groceries
Inputs	Stores carry about 700 mostly private-label products bought from independent producers and offer only one brand of each product. Products include a cluster of essential items and about 30 seasonal items. Store size is small, about one-tenth of the average Walmart, and use of information technology is minimal. Stores may function with only 4 or 5 employees.	Stores carry about 15,000 products, of which about 55% are food items. Only 15% of products are private label. The rest are national brands.
Processes	Customers pay 25 cents to use shopping carts. Stores do not accept checks and do not provide shopping bags. Goods are sold out of cartons. Customers bag their own groceries.	Food section looks like a normal grocery store. Checkout stands often are congested. A greeter welcomes customers at the door in many stores, and personnel help bag groceries.
Profits	Privately owned; expansion funded with cash; payment for products	Publicly owned; expansion funded with debt and stock; payment for products

Sources: Gerhard and Hahn (2005) and Pettypiece (2016).

quality almost always trumps cost. As Porter and Teisberg (2006, 98) state, "Minimizing costs is simply the wrong goal, and will lead to counterproductive results." Few would desire to have their loved ones undergo surgery in a hospital that promotes itself as the low-cost option. Likewise, patients generally prefer cutting-edge technology, even if the costs are higher.

Nevertheless, many ambulatory surgery centers (ASCs) and specialty hospitals and clinics promise to provide services at a unit cost lower than that charged by general hospitals. The lower costs have been attributed to reorganization into integrated practice units, breaking down silos with multidisciplinary teams that focus on patient outcomes and value (Porter and Lee 2013)

In segments where consumers are more price sensitive, low cost may help organizations achieve competitive advantage. For example, in obstetrics, plastic surgery, and the health insurance business, prices (costs) may have a greater influence on consumers' choices. Consumers with high out-of-pocket costs more often compare prices, choose lower-cost healthcare services, and select less expensive drugs and healthcare services (Buchmueller 2006; Penn Medicine News 2016; Ungar and O'Donnell 2015).

Broad Differentiation Strategy

Broad differentiation strategies
Strategies aimed at offering products that consumers perceive to be distinct from competitors' products and that appeal to a wide segment of a market.

Organizations using **broad differentiation strategies** offer products and services that have unique features and appeal to a wide segment of a market. Consumers purchase products and services that have singular characteristics or features they value, and they often will pay more for those valued features. Broad differentiation strategies tend to be most effective in large markets where

- buyer preferences and values are diverse,
- many organizations offer common products, and
- product innovation is rapid (Hitt, Ireland, and Hoskisson 2016).

Nearly all products and services can be effectively differentiated. Companies spend millions of dollars annually to differentiate both basic products, such as salt and soft drinks, and complex merchandise, such as microprocessors and automobiles. Differentiation can be based on characteristics of a product or service or on the attributes of an organization's personnel, distribution channels, and image.

Exhibit 3.9 lists many ways an organization may choose to differentiate its products and services. A pharmaceutical company might alter the size, texture, reliability, and duration of its medications; accelerate ordering and delivery; or improve the responsiveness and friendliness of its sales personnel. A radiological equipment manufacturer may elect to focus on ease of installation, customer training, maintenance and repair, and its personnel's credibility and reliability.

"Overall, a firm using the differentiation strategy seeks to be different from its competitors on as many dimensions as possible" (Hitt, Ireland, and Hoskisson 2016, 123). Porter (1980) suggests that an organization must have strong marketing capabilities and a perceived reputation for quality or another unique characteristic for a broad differentiation strategy to be effective. Organizations must understand and offer what buyers need and value to succeed through differentiation. Competitive advantage often is short lived and must be constantly renewed, so innovation and an ability to change are critical factors. An organization is using differentiation successfully if

- it can charge premium prices,
- sales are increasing, and
- customers become loyal to its brand (Thompson et al. 2016).

Certain hospitals have achieved a strong, broadly differentiated position and are able to use it to their competitive advantage. They have carved out "must-have" market positions that enable them to extract higher payments. A *must-have hospital* is one that insurance companies must have in their network;

EXHIBIT 3.9
Ways to Differentiate Products, Services, Personnel, Distribution, and Image

Products	
• Form: size, shape, and structure • Features: bundling or customization • Conformance/quality: consistency with specifications • Durability: expected useful life	• Reliability: probability of failure • Reparability: ease of fixing • Style: feel and look • Design: ease of operation and use
Services	
• Ordering: rapidity and ease of purchasing • Delivery: speed, accuracy, and attention to order • Installation: ease and cost of setup	• Customer training: quality and quantity of instruction • Customer assistance: level of responsiveness, quality of service • Maintenance/repair: speed and quality of problem solving
Personnel	
• Competence: knowledge and skill level • Courtesy: degree of respect and consideration shown • Credibility: promises and commitments kept	• Reliability: consistent, accurate performance • Responsiveness: rapidity of response to customers' needs • Communication: degree of interaction and clarity
Distribution	
• Coverage: extent of geographic area • Expertise: specialized knowledge	• Performance: efficiency and effectiveness of distribution
Image	
• Symbols: attractiveness • Prestige: Perceived status of users • Colors: desirability and variety • Slogans: meaningfulness • Atmosphere: attractiveness of the organization's environment and ambience	• Events: number of activities and events meaningful to customers (e.g., open houses, sales events, health screenings, grand openings)

else, they face the possibility of losing customers. These hospitals, such as Cedars-Sinai Medical Center in Los Angeles, have established excellent reputations and most often provide unique, specialized services. In negotiations with insurance companies, the must-have hospitals demand and frequently receive premium reimbursement rates (Berenson et al. 2012; Berenson, Ginsburg, and Kemper 2010).

On the other hand, there is some value to adopting strategies similar to those of competitors and not appearing different. Conformity sometimes enhances performance and promotes long-term survival. Customers see that the conforming organization's product is consistent with those of its competitors and may be more willing to try the new product. In fact, competitors quickly copy and imitate successful differentiation strategies to conform. An organization seeking to sustain a differentiation strategy must develop strong creativity and innovation by integrating its marketing and production and by hiring and retaining creative personnel (Shenkar 2012).

Focused Differentiation Strategy

Focused differentiation strategy A type of strategy aimed at offering products that consumers perceive to be distinct from competitors' products and that appeal to a limited industry niche or customer segment.

Focused factories A manufacturing strategy that concentrates on core (often single) products and a defined set of technologies and customers.

Focused differentiation strategy targets a narrow industry niche or customer segment. Companies can differentiate their product and services via the means listed in exhibit 3.8, but the differences are perceived as unique to a narrow group or population. For example, Rolls-Royce, Rolex, Saks Fifth Avenue, Harrods, Chanel, and Tiffany & Co. focus their products on the luxury market segment. They offer high-quality, prestigious products at high prices. Such organizations refrain from expanding into unrelated businesses and offer specialized products.

Some have long suggested that healthcare should be organized in a more specialized, focused way and should move away from its broad, unfocused strategies, which have led to quality and cost problems (Herzlinger 1997). A potential solution, **focused factories**, is a term that dates back to the 1970s and initially described a manufacturing strategy that concentrated on core (often single) products and a defined set of technologies and customers. Some scholars have suggested that this strategy was a major factor in the past revitalization of US business fortunes (Herzlinger 2000; Pesch 1996).

The creation of healthcare focused factories in the United States has been limited to separating common services, such as cardiology and surgery, from general hospitals and placing each service in its own facility. Examples include ASCs and specialty hospitals, both of which have rapidly increased in number. These focused healthcare organizations are often owned by physicians (in contrast to public ownership of most general hospitals), offer a relatively narrow line of services, and may attend to only one type of disease. For example, David Cook and colleagues found that the "focused factory model was appropriate for 67 percent of cardiac surgical patients." If implemented more widely, this system would reduce "resource use, length-of-stay, and cost," as well as variation (Cook et al. 2014, 746). Other possible focused factories may include diabetes clinics, cancer clinics, asthma clinics, and orthopedic surgery.

Focused differentiation has emerged in healthcare in other forms as well. As shown in exhibit 3.10, some physicians have devised a means of narrowing their customer focus and increasing their incomes by offering differentiated

EXHIBIT 3.10
Concierge Medicine

Primary care physicians often have a *patient panel*: a group of 2,000 to 3,000 patients they have seen in the past and would agree to see in the future. Under a fee-for-service payment model, physicians are reimbursed for each patient they see, creating an incentive to see many patients per day and minimize the amount of time spent with each patient, sometimes to less than ten minutes.

To increase their incomes and change their practice style, some physicians have adopted a focused differentiation strategy called **concierge medicine.** Under this arrangement, the physician restricts his patient panel to as few as 500 patients who are willing to pay an annual fee of, on average, $1,800 though it may be as high as $5,000—in addition to regular insurance payments for clinical services. For this additional fee, the patient receives longer, more immediate physician visits and house calls and greater coordination of care, along with other premium services. Typical patients tend to come from upper-middle-class families and earn between $125,000 and $250,000 per year.

Source: Chen (2010).

Concierge medicine
Also known as retainer medicine, a relationship between a patient and a primary care physician in which the patient pays an annual fee or a retainer for enhanced services.

primary care. In this arrangement, patients pay an annual fee in addition to regular clinic charges to obtain greater access to their physician and more personalized care. Similarly, various health systems and hospitals have sought to highlight their differentiation and specialties by establishing luxury services to attract wealthy domestic and foreign patients. Differentiating services include uniformed valets, professional greeters, 24-hour room service, and spas (Pourat 2016).

Although critics have raised ethical concerns about physician abandonment of patients who cannot pay the additional fee and the creation of a two-tiered system of care in which the more affluent receive better healthcare, the number of physicians entering concierge medicine has rapidly grown. By 2016, there were about 12,000 physicians practicing concierge medicine in the United States. Companies have been established to provide turnkey and franchise services for physicians desiring to convert to this practice style (Colwell 2016). Two journals, *Concierge Medicine Today* and *Concierge Medicine Journal*, have also been organized to promote the concept.

Middle Strategy

Middle strategy is also called *best-cost strategy* or *integrated cost leadership/differentiation strategy* because it intends to offer customers the optimal mix of distinctive value and attractive costs simultaneously. Middle strategies are more successful in markets where buyers desire a degree of product differentiation but at the same time are price sensitive (Hitt, Ireland, and Hoskisson 2016). A perennial example of a firm employing a middle strategy is Southwest Airlines, which combines low costs with measured differentiation. Porter (1980) initially

Middle strategy
A strategy that seeks to deliver low cost and differentiation simultaneously.

cautioned against this strategic position, believing efforts to achieve one facet would contradict the other and the organization would get "caught in the middle." He reasoned that efforts to lower costs would make differentiation more difficult and that greater differentiation would increase costs; as a result, businesses would alienate both high-volume customers demanding low prices and high-margin consumers desiring distinct products. Others have since noted that in some markets, a middle strategy may be effective, and recently, many large corporations have been employing it (Baroto, Madi Bin Abdullah, and Wan 2012; Luke, Walston, and Plummer 2004; Parnell and Lester 2008).

Middle strategy may in fact be the strongest position for many consumer product markets, including groceries, apparel, and hardware, and for many hospitals. Traditionally low margins—just 1.8 percent in 2008—force grocery stores to reduce costs. Yet they also seek to differentiate their services and products through coupons, unique ethnic products, in-store babysitters, fresh vegetables, cleanliness, and other features (Hiiemaa 2016). Many community hospitals selectively invest in sophisticated technology and offer "good enough" quality at generally lower prices than those charged by high-quality academic medical centers and tertiary referral hospitals (Luke, Walston, and Plummer 2004). Of course, the challenge for organizations with middle strategies lies in the difficulty of distinguishing themselves from competitors. Middle positions are copied more easily by competitors, and differences in cost and quality are often difficult to define to consumers clearly. For example, patients normally see little quality and cost differences among community hospitals.

The Dynamics of Competitive Strategies

Intense competitive and environmental pressures often encourage organizations to shift their competitive strategies. An organization with a low-cost strategy may add new features and products to increase its differentiation, while an organization with a middle strategy might provide a low-cost alternative.

For example, the ALDI grocery chain, which employs a low-cost strategy, now owns Trader Joe's. While Trader Joe's employs a more focused differentiation strategy, it also integrates many of ALDI's low-cost strategies. Trader Joe's offers specialty foods that have been described as "yuppie-friendly," exotic, affordable luxuries, such as Belgian butter waffle cookies and Thai lime-and-chili cashews (Farfan 2016; Kowitt 2010). As another example, high-cost academic medical centers may seek to develop low-cost clinics in large retail stores, such as Walmart.

As illustrated in exhibit 3.11, strategic positions may shift among the dimensions of cost and differentiation. Few organizations implement strategies

EXHIBIT 3.11
Shifting Strategies

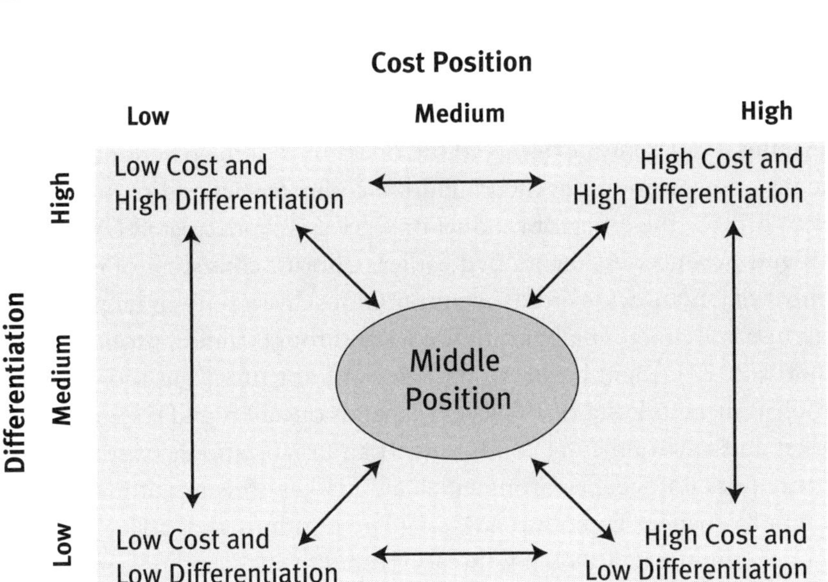

Source: Adapted from Luke, Walston, and Plummer (2004).

at the extremes, and most organizations, even those with low-cost strategies, proffer a degree of differentiation. Although any strategy may be difficult to achieve, some are much more difficult to develop and maintain. For example, sustaining a high-cost, low-differentiation position may be problematic. A successful firm must constantly be willing to examine and alter its position as required by competitive pressures (Luke, Walston, and Plummer 2004, 155): "In a competitive and turbulent environment . . . the requirements for occupying one or another position will change. . . . Therefore, organizations need to be vigilant about sustaining established positions and, in competitive market environments, work to improve those positions. Positioning threats can come from similarly positioned rivals; from rivals located in other, stronger positions . . . or from rivals that need to improve on weak positions."

Organizations usually shift their position only marginally, trying new products, pricing, and features to improve their business. Those that try to move from one extreme to another may not have the appropriate internal resources and competencies to transition successfully. For example, Tesla has faced immense challenges while shifting its cars from high-priced luxury vehicles to a more mass-produced, midrange, $35,000 product (DeBord 2016). Likewise, organizations moving from one strategic position to another must be careful not to abandon their mission. For instance, intense competitive pressures are moving many academic medical centers to develop integrated networks and reduce their costs to compete on price more effectively, which may distract them from their teaching and research missions.

Organizations desiring to try a radically different strategy may consider creating a separate organization (subunit) or a distinct brand name and managing it differently, external to the operations of the parent organization. The new organization can then build the competencies and resources necessary to provide the different product or service. Toyota created Lexus to offer high-end products. As mentioned earlier, Chorus, consisting of only a small number of employees, exists as an autonomous division of Eli Lilly to advance drug research more rapidly from discovery through clinical proof of concept (Chorus 2017). Rigid business strategies will not survive in today's volatile, turbulent market. Long-term success depends on agility and responsiveness to market and environmental conditions. If an organization's existing business strategy does not meet environmental and market pressures, it must be adept enough to change. Exploring new strategic positions with a view to exploiting opportunities and avoiding threats created by market conditions may be a pragmatic, realistic approach.

When an organization moves into a product market early, it is using a *first-mover strategy*. The speed with which organizations enter new markets greatly varies. **First movers** (also called *early entrants*) consistently search for innovation opportunities and attempt to gain first-mover advantages by being among the first to enter a new market. Others wait, watch, and analyze competitors' actions and move later into new markets.

First movers
Organizations that are the earliest to enter a market or an industry.

Although the first-mover advantage is a well-known strategy concept, authors have mixed opinions of its long-term benefits (Lieberman and Montgomery 1998; Suarez and Lanzolla 2005). Organizations seeking first-mover advantage move quickly into an unoccupied or uncrowded market segment or product space. First movers may enjoy durable advantages for many years, or the advantages may quickly fade as later entrants take over a market. One factor critical to the success of a first mover is its ability to establish barriers to entry by other organizations. First movers often can create entry barriers and sustainable advantage from

- technological advantage,
- acquisition and control of scarce assets, and
- reputation.

First, an early entrant can develop competitive advantages from having superior technologies. The technological advantage can come from patents, improved distribution channels, and learning. First movers may create innovative competencies that produce technical knowledge superior to that of competitors. Organizations learn by doing and not only develop innovation but also advance along a learning curve to better produce a product. When an organization first offers a new product or service, the unit price is generally high, especially in a new market where the processes for creating the product or service and necessary features are not well understood and the customer base is small. Over time, the organization can lower its unit price by developing more efficient processes and standardizing its products or services. Thus, first-mover organizations may gain technological and cost advantages over potential later entrants and discourage market entry.

A historical example of technological advantage is Richard Arkwright's invention of the modern factory system for spinning cotton. He developed original patents for spinning cotton in 1768, quickly built factories across England, and licensed his technology. By 1774, he employed 600 workers in 15 mills in England. Although he eventually lost control of his patents in 1785, he used the time before his patents expired to improve and position his mills, and competitors never caught up to him during his lifetime (Musson and Robinson 1960). Likewise, Xerox, Coca-Cola, and Nike leveraged their first-mover strategies into global leading companies.

Second, first movers may tie up critical, scarce resources, such as location, employees, and crucial partners, making it more difficult for new organizations to enter the market. Thus, speed alone is not sufficient to be successful as a first mover; such organizations must add the correct critical resources. The great Confederate general Nathan Bedford Forrest recognized the need to connect speed and resources when he responded to the question of what was key to his military success: The essence of his strategy was simply to "git thar first with the most men" (Catton 1971, 160).

Third, first movers often cultivate a base of loyal customers. One approach to retaining customers is to make it inconvenient or expensive to switch to later entrants' products. First movers should seek to gain a positive organizational image and reputation with customers and establish their product as the market standard. By raising the bar in terms of features and quality, first movers set a precedent that other organizations must surpass to enter the market successfully. All of these tactics, if executed appropriately, discourage other organizations from entering the market, which strengthens the first mover's advantage.

First movers often receive extensive free publicity and gain public name recognition and visibility. Sometimes the first mover becomes so prominent that the name of its product or service becomes the name used to describe all other products or services of the same type. For example, Twitter became the standard for micromessaging. It rapidly developed a large following and established the norm for this social networking medium. It has become so popular that *tweeting* is the term used to describe the action of sending a micromessage, regardless of the networking site used. As stated in 2011, "[Twitter was] among the most recognized brands on the Internet and a bona fide cultural phenomenon, with as many as 400 million monthly users" (*Colorado Springs Gazette* 2011).

On the other hand, as stated earlier, first movers may gain only temporary advantage or fail completely. Those that hurry to be the first in a market may not test their product designs and sell defective products or products with limited customer appeal as a result. Alternatively, some first-mover products may raise tremendous demand and overwhelm the organization's capacities. For example, although Twitter was initially highly successful, innovations from Facebook, Instagram, WhatsApp, Snapchat, and WeChat caused Twitter's growth to slow, and, given its executive turnover and financial struggles, many question its long-term viability (Topolsky 2016).

Some claim that subsequent entrants, or *fast followers*, succeed more often than do first movers because a level of demand already exists and consumers understand the benefits of the product (Shankar and Carpenter 2013). Secondary entrants may be able to imitate or "freeload" on first movers' research and initial investments. Later entrants also do not sustain the risk involved in creating a new customer base and are able to follow existing industry standards.

The success of the CT (computed tomography) scanner, a widely used radiological diagnostic tool, is a good example of how fast followers can succeed at the expense of a first mover. The sales and service of CT scanners generate huge profits. In 2007, healthcare organizations performed an estimated 72 million CT scans in the United States alone (Gonzalez et al. 2009). In the early 1970s, a British company, EMI, was the first to successfully develop and market a CT scanner. Primarily a music company, EMI had little experience in the medical equipment market. It estimated that it would sell up to 50 scanners in the product's first year and have three to four years to establish itself in that market before competitors arose. By 1977, the organization had achieved phenomenal success and had an order backlog of more than 300 units. However, rapid technological advances ensued and benefited later entrants, such as industry giants GE, Toshiba, and Siemens. In the early 1980s, EMI abandoned its investments in scanning technology and returned to its core music business (Alexander and Gunderman 2010).

Suarez and Lanzolla (2005) suggest that the relative short- and long-term success of a first mover may depend on two factors: the speed of technological advancement and the rate of market demand. As depicted in exhibit 3.12, first-mover advantage is sustained only in markets characterized by slow technological change. Rapid technological change poses serious challenges to first movers and enables new entrants to leap ahead of the quality and features of first movers' initial products.

In summary, being the first in a market does not necessarily translate into first-mover advantage. Sustained advantage depends on a combination of speed of entry, resources, speed of technological change, and market growth.

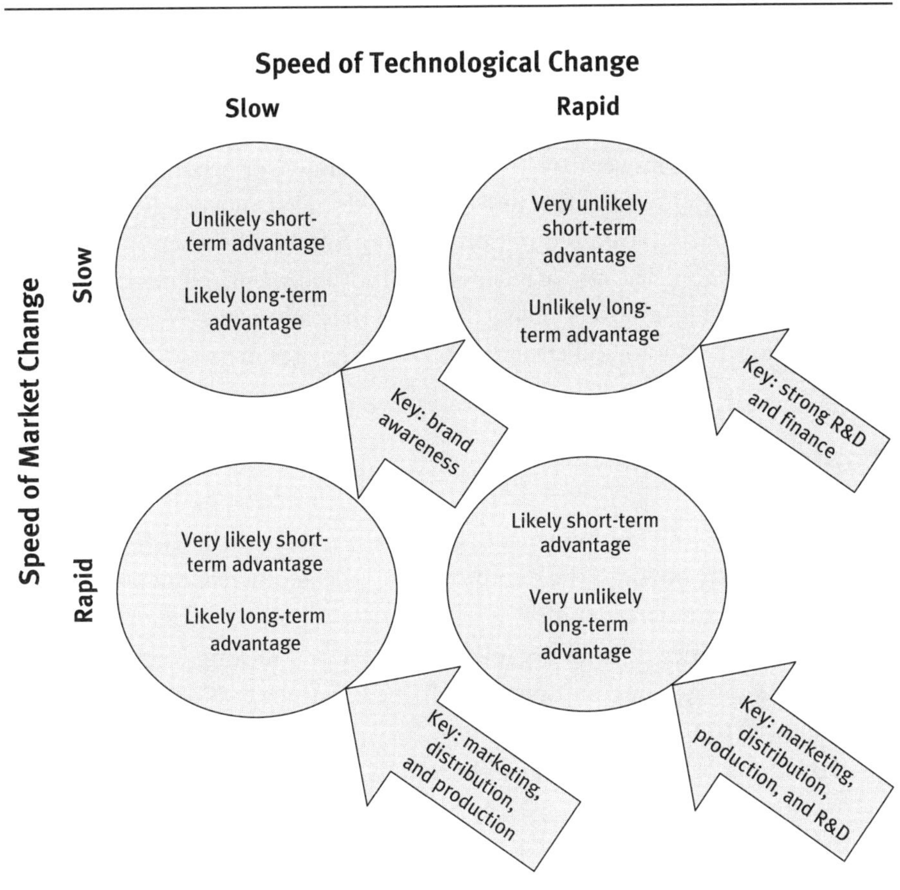

EXHIBIT 3.12
The Effect of Technology and Market Growth on First Movers' Success

Chapter Summary

This chapter examines the different ways organizations can strategize to achieve their missions. The underlying structures of an organization make up its business model. A business model includes the value produced for customers, the types and combinations of inputs, the processes used to create products, and the means for revenue generation. Changing business models may increase an organization's competitive advantage and enable it to distinguish itself from its rivals. An organization also must change its business model to compete effectively when its environment shifts.

Organizations use a variety of strategies to position themselves in different ways. Generic strategies include dimensions of either a focused or general market (customer base) and a dimension of cost (low vs. high) or quality (degree of differentiation). Low-cost strategies may succeed in some segments of healthcare. Differentiation strategies seek to provide unique features for which the consumer is willing to pay more. Differences may include product characteristics, service, distribution channels, reputation, and image. Concierge medicine is an example of focused differentiation in healthcare. Some organizations employ middle strategies, which offer a desired mix of distinctive value and attractive costs. Many general hospitals seem to use this type of strategy.

Many organizations seek to gain advantage by being the first to enter a market. Being a first mover may be a durable advantage or become a liability as later entrants learn from the first mover's mistakes. First-mover advantage may be gained from technology, acquisition and control of scarce assets, or superior customer reputation. The rate of technological advancement and market growth significantly affect first movers' ability to sustain their advantage. Markets characterized by slow technological change are positive environments for first movers.

Chapter Questions

1. How do the four components of a business model affect each other? For example, how can the depth of value to customers influence the means of revenue generation?
2. What difficulties does an organization face when seeking to change its business model? In your opinion, why have Barnes & Noble and Kodak struggled to shift their business models?
3. How can a new business model become a competitive advantage for an organization?
4. What changes could hospitals, physicians, pharmaceutical companies, and insurance companies make to their business models to position them more advantageously for the future?
5. Generic strategies' dimensions include type of competitive advantage and target market. In your opinion, how would a focused strategy differ from a broad strategy?
6. Are middle strategies most commonly used? Why or why not?
7. What actions can an organization take to offer a product at the lowest cost?
8. When is low cost a viable strategy in healthcare? When would it not be viable?
9. Which shift in strategy would be most difficult in your opinion: moving from low cost and high differentiation to high cost and high differentiation, or moving from high cost and high differentiation to low cost and high differentiation? Why?
10. A first mover can sustain its market advantage through technology, control of scarce resources, and reputation. Look at the first movers you are familiar with. Which of these approaches have they taken?
11. How does technological change affect a first mover?

Chapter Cases

Case Studies

"Move to a Concierge Model or a Direct Primary Care–Medicine Business Model?" "The Case of Humana and Vertical Integration," and "An Orthopedic Group Decides to Construct a Specialty Hospital" may be used to explore material in this chapter. They are found in the case studies section at the back of the book.

Integral Healthcare System and Proton Therapy

Integral Healthcare System (IHS), a not-for-profit organization with a strong, service-oriented mission, is one of the largest care systems in its region. Although highly profitable, it has seen its market share in certain specialties slip. The decline has been most prominent in oncology and cardiology because of the establishment of specialty hospitals and care centers by competitors. IHS's executives have attempted to differentiate the system and recoup its market share by setting up centers of excellence, recruiting physician specialists in these areas, and using extensive media advertising, but to date none of these strategies has reversed the market decline.

Recently IHS was approached by National For-profit Company (NFC) proposing a joint venture proton therapy center. In 2010, proton therapy became eligible for reimbursement by most insurance companies and Medicare. This service involves sending a beam of protons to irradiate diseased tissue, mostly cancers. The protons appear to effectively kill cancer cells and cause less collateral damage to normal tissue. However, medical professionals question whether it is any more effective than traditional radiation therapy. For this reason, only six proton therapy units exist in the United States, none of which are located in IHS's greater service area. The joint venture would be the first proton therapy unit in the region.

The problem with proton therapy is the facility cost; construction of a proton therapy unit could exceed $200 million. As a result, the cost per treatment often exceeds $100,000 per patient—two to three times the cost of traditional radiation therapy. Although state-of-the-art, the facility's massive cyclotron could be supplanted in the future by superconducting synchrocyclotrons, a newer technology that might cost less than half the proposed construction cost. Local insurance companies have also expressed concerns about paying for this service.

IHS has to decide whether it wants to pursue the partnership. By adding proton therapy, it may achieve the differentiation it desires. It might be able to distinguish itself in oncology and regain much of the market volume

(continued)

it has lost to competitors. Nevertheless, there are risks. The large capital cost would need to be financed or taken from IHS's limited capital reserves. NFC also has hinted that it may take its offer to one of IHS's competitors if IHS does not agree to the partnership. Moreover, the local university hospital has established oncology as one of its key competencies and has been seeking tax support to establish a proton therapy research and treatment center.

Questions

1. For IHS, what are the advantages and disadvantages of being the first mover into the proton therapy market?
2. How might IHS minimize the risk posed by the joint venture?
3. What additional actions would you propose IHS take to improve its chances for a successful partnership with NFC?
4. Would you recommend that IHS accept or decline the offer?

Deciding Between Innovative Options

A donor gave Major Boston Academic Medical Center (MBAMC) a large bequest to further its mission. Stakeholders were asked to come up with innovative proposals, which were narrowed down to two that were submitted to MBAMC's board. One proposed to use the funds to expand the existing tertiary services into more highly specialized quaternary services that would extend the "boundaries of its clinical excellence." The other created a unique nursing fellowship that would train nurses to provide services currently given by physicians, but at a much lower cost. After due deliberation the board chose the first option and all the donation was applied toward increasing the sophistication of MBAMC's services (Christensen et al. 2006).

Questions

1. Which proposal was a sustaining and which a disruptive innovation?
2. Why would an organization choose a sustaining innovation over a disruptive innovation?
3. Read the article the case comes from and discuss the impact disruptive innovation has on the social structure.

Chapter Assignments

1. Identify an innovation that is in the emerging stage of market development. Write a one-page paper describing how product standards and quality are established. Address how the rate of technological and

market change affects the product's potential for success during the emerging stage of market development.

2. How can a middle strategy be successful in healthcare? Write a one-page paper on what a healthcare organization must do to make this strategy successful. What problems might creating this type of strategy in healthcare present?
3. The MedCottage—sometimes called a *granny pod* or, more properly, an auxiliary dwelling unit (ADU)—is a portable hospital room that can be placed next to a private residence. The units are designed as a substitute for nursing homes and can keep elderly persons out of institutionalized care. The units are equipped with the latest biometric and communications technology, enabling physicians and nurses to monitor the occupant's vital signs directly, be alerted to emergencies, and even change the unit's temperature. ADUs run from $100,000 to $125,000. Read more about this innovation in the November 25, 2012, *Washington Post* article by Fredrick Kunkle titled "The Ultimate Care Package? 'Granny Pods' Help Keep Loved Ones Close." Write a one-page paper about how ADUs are disruptive innovation as described in this chapter and whether they present a first-mover opportunity.

CHAPTER

4

GROWTH AND INTEGRATION STRATEGIES

> Size does matter, but big doesn't. A hospital can be too small. And it can be too big. A hospital that's too small can't generate the proficiencies necessary to consistently deliver high-quality care or the volume necessary to effectively amortize the cost of technology.
>
> On the other hand, a hospital that's too big can become lumbering and ponderous. Organizational coherence, including consistency in care, becomes more difficult to orchestrate. Wayfinding becomes onerous not only for patients but for caregivers as well.
>
> There is a right size for a hospital—somewhere between 100 and 300 beds. Unfortunately, there's not much hope for the too-small hospital beyond government subsidies. The too-big hospital, on the other hand, can break itself up into a collection of smaller, focused hospitals. The big elephant may not be able to dance. But the little one can. Size is a choice.
>
> —Dan Beckham, "How to Make Strategic Planning Work for Your Health Care Organization," 2016a

Learning Objectives

After reading this chapter, you will

- understand how organizations use different growth strategies,
- perceive the advantages and disadvantages of the types of strategic expansion,
- grasp the strategic concepts of vertical integration,
- comprehend the issue of transfer pricing and its effect on vertical integration,
- recognize the difference between ownership and integration and the methods by which integration can be accomplished,
- know the strategic concepts of horizontal expansion, and
- be familiar with the concepts of related and unrelated diversification expansion.

Growth and *integration* are key organizational strategies. Growth can be generated by various means, including mergers and acquisitions, internal expansion, and networking. Organizations also may expand horizontally into similar products, diversify into new products, or extend vertically to own products and services offered by their suppliers or buyers. Integration is critical to achieving the potential benefits of growth.

Growth Strategies

Organizations have many motives for growth. It is an attractive prospect because it promises greater economies of scale, augmented reputation, swift entry into markets, achievement of synergies, increased market power, and higher salaries for top management. Expansion often energizes an organization by interjecting new ideas, people, and cultures. Growth can also help reposition an organization to take advantage of new opportunities and changing markets.

As the introduction to the chapter discusses, size can both help and hurt healthcare organizations. Too small may not allow the necessary volume for high quality and costs; too large can create many problems. As stated, size is a choice—a strategic choice.

As exhibit 4.1 shows, growth strategies sometimes go bad. Growth does not guarantee that an organization will realize any of the aforementioned

EXHIBIT 4.1
AHERF Bankruptcy

In July 1998, the Allegheny Health, Education, and Research Foundation (AHERF) filed for bankruptcy, revealing $1.3 billion in debt and 65,000 creditors. Up until this time, AHERF's bankruptcy was the largest nonprofit healthcare failure in the United States. A large part of AHERF's problems arose when it embarked on an ambitious strategy of horizontal and vertical expansion. AHERF began as a prosperous 670-bed facility, Allegheny General Hospital, in Pittsburgh in the early 1980s. With increasing competition and a new CEO, Sherif Abdelhak, the hospital rapidly expanded to create Pennsylvania's first statewide integrated delivery system. Between 1986 and 1997, AHERF grew from revenues of $195 million to $2.05 billion and employees from 4,000 to 31,000; where it once had one hospital, it eventually comprised 14. However, by 1998, because of financial irregularities, enormous debt, and general fiscal deterioration, AHERF was forced into bankruptcy.

Some observers have questioned the organization's growth strategy. Few payers in Pennsylvania appeared to want a statewide system with which to contract. The market share gained by AHERF's expansion was insufficient to increase its negotiating power. It was also unable to garner synergies and economies of scale through its rapid mergers. Overall, its growth strategy was a miserable failure, as "growing their business seems to have trumped fiscal restraint and responsible investment."

Source: Burns et al. (2000).

benefits. In fact, if significant synergies, market power, or economies of scale do not materialize, a growth strategy can seriously damage or destroy a firm.

Although an organization can grow in many ways, it usually accomplishes growth through three generally accepted methods:

1. Internal expansion
2. Acquisition or merger
3. Networks and alliances

Internal expansion
A method of business growth that builds on an organization's capabilities and resources and may include developing new products and services, launching marketing efforts to increase market share, or introducing existing products into new markets.

Internal Expansion

Internal expansion builds on an organization's own capabilities and resources to advance company activities, products, services, and revenues. Internal expansion may include developing new products and services, launching marketing efforts to increase market share, and entering existing products in new markets. As shown in exhibit 4.2, internal expansion is advantageous in many ways. It is less risky than other growth options, and internal funds and efforts can be engaged incrementally. Organizations can preserve—and expand—their culture

EXHIBIT 4.2
Advantages and Disadvantages of Different Growth Strategies

Growth Strategy	Advantages	Disadvantages
Internal	• Preserves organizational culture • More easily funded with internal resources • Builds on firm's strengths and reputation • Incremental growth rate • Generally less exposure to risk	• Slow growth and development of new products • Steep learning curve • May not be able to overcome established barriers to market entry
Acquisition/ merger	• Not subject to legal restrictions (e.g., certificate of need) • Rapid market entry • May become associated with the positive reputation of another organization • Purchasing a competitor reduces competition	• Culture and management structures of acquired organization may be incompatible, jeopardizing successful integration
Network/ alliance	• Lowest risk • Potential for rapid market entry • May obtain critical knowledge and market access	• Least control over outcomes • May easily dissolve • May lose technical and other key personnel

as they grow. This method also affords managers the greatest control over organizational growth and is generally less disruptive to existing operations. Internal expansion may work well when the product cycle is in the emerging stage and few product leaders exist.

Internal expansion may not be appropriate in all situations, however. Product development and market entry may be slow. If speed to market is critical, internal development may not be the best choice. Internally developed products may take time to acquire a positive market reputation. The organization also risks consumer rejection of its new products.

For example, many healthcare organizations have entered the retail clinic market. Retail clinics generally offer basic medical services for minor illnesses such as influenza, ear infections, back pain, sports physicals, or vaccinations and are often located in retail locations, such as drugstores and chain superstores. By 2016, there were about 2,000 such clinics across the United States, hosting more than 6 million visits per year. About half of visits occurred after most doctors' offices closed (Abelson 2016). Initially, large businesses such as pharmacy chains Rite Aid, Walgreens, and CVS, along with Kroger, Walmart, and Target, developed and staffed their own, in-house clinics. These companies owned about 93 percent of US clinics in 2016. However, more and more these chains are outsourcing the retail clinics to healthcare systems. For example, in 2016, Advocate Health Care took ownership of 56 Chicago-area Walgreens clinics, which allows for better-coordinated care (Hennessy 2016; RAND Corporation 2016).

Acquisition

Acquisition The purchase (or merger) of an existing organization. Through this method of growth, the acquiring organization gains an established product in the market and may also reduce competition by eliminating one of its competitors.

Acquisition can rapidly launch an organization into a market. By purchasing an existing business, an organization adds an established product to its market offerings; similarly, acquiring an existing business's research and development can expedite a product to market. The purchase of an existing organization (or the merger of two organizations) reduces competition by eliminating a market rival and can increase the combined organization's customer volume immediately.

Acquisition also may enable an organization to bypass regulators' restrictions on market entry. For example, in states that still have certificate of need (CON) laws, healthcare organizations must obtain permission to enter certain markets (the types of markets subject to restriction vary from state to state). In 2016, 37 states had some form of CON program, most restricting entry into the outpatient and long-term care markets. Permission to add new outpatient or long-term care capacity (internal expansion) could take months or years to obtain, and the state agency may deny the application (National Conference of State Legislatures 2017). In this case, acquisition of existing assets may be a better strategy—or the only option.

Nevertheless, acquisition has its drawbacks. Merged organizations sometimes have incompatible cultures and management systems, and this incongruity can inhibit success. One organization's culture may differ dramatically from the other's with regard to decision-making and managerial styles. The transfer of culture from one organization to another is often difficult, especially if the organizations do not have similar core values (Schraeder and Self 2003). A long line of failed acquisitions and mergers has been attributed to such differences.

A look at recent history reveals many examples of failed acquisitions. These include the failed mergers of Google and Motorola, Bank of America and Countrywide, and Kmart and Sears (CB Insights 2016). Culture incompatibility can be the "root cause of any merger's failure or success" (Bradt 2015).

For instance, the well-documented cultural clashes between Daimler and Chrysler ultimately led to operational problems and a $34 billion loss for Daimler when it sold Chrysler to a private equity firm in 2007 (Jacobsen 2012). Likewise, organizations may acquire products too late in the product cycle or find that the acquired product is inferior to that of the market leader. For instance, to enter the cell phone market more quickly, Microsoft acquired Nokia for $7.2 billion in 2008. But in 2010, less than two weeks after the official introduction of the new line of smartphones—the Kin One and Kin Two—Microsoft announced it was killing the products (Vance 2010). Then, in 2016, Microsoft sold its phone assets to Foxconn Technology for just $350 million (Kharpal 2016).

Hospitals have found that healthcare mergers are fraught with cultural and managerial problems. Many organizations ignored their differences until after the merger took place: "They devoted so much effort toward whether they could merge, they didn't stop to consider whether they should" (Andrews 2000, 52). Differing organizational personalities or cultures have been seen as a major factor in the failure of many healthcare mergers, as for the Henry Ford Health System and Beaumont Health System proposed merger that fell apart, less than a year after the announcement that they were "ideal partners," as a result of cultural and business differences (Gelineau 2015).

Networks and Alliances

Networks
Joint ventures and alliances between established organizations for growth purposes. By forming networks, organizations can enter a market more quickly and with minimal risk.

An organization can grow by linking with other established organizations through **networks** and alliances (e.g., joint ventures). As discussed in depth in chapter 5, these structures enable organizations to enter a market more quickly with minimal risk. However, organizations in these arrangements have less control over their business outcomes, and alliances can be difficult to manage. As a result, problems arise and many of these structures dissolve. Even though 85 percent of business leaders feel alliances are essential or important to their business, failure rates exceed 60 percent (Whitler 2014). Organizations also risk losing important proprietary knowledge. When a network dissolves, Partner

A can retain key technological information and perhaps even personnel from Partner B, potentially damaging Partner B's competitive position.

Vertical, Horizontal, and Diversified Expansion

Expansion also can occur vertically, horizontally, and through diversification. The literature often refers to vertical and horizontal expansion as vertical and horizontal integration. While in many cases the acquired organizations are not actually *integrated*, most of the benefits of these means of expansion accrue only if the organizations' operations are integrated.

Vertical expansion
Acquisition of a business that is a source of supplies for the acquiring organization (backward expansion) or that purchases from the acquiring organization (forward expansion).

Vertical expansion occurs when an organization acquires a business that is either a source of supplies (backward expansion) or an entity that may purchase from the organization (forward expansion). Thus, the organization buys stages of its industry value chain. For example, a paint manufacturer might own its own retail stores (e.g., Sherwin-Williams) or a hospital might employ physicians or own its own insurance company (e.g., a health maintenance organization [HMO], a preferred-provider organization).

Horizontal expansion
The acquisition or merger of two or more organizations that produce similar products or services.

Horizontal expansion occurs when similar organizations merge or are acquired—an organization grows by acquiring or merging with other businesses that offer comparable products. Many hospitals and physician groups have expanded horizontally to form multihospital systems and larger physician groups. In 2016, a total of 3,183 of 4,926 community hospitals belonged to a system (65 percent) (American Hospital Association [AHA] 2017). Health insurance companies also have merged; by 2015, the largest 10 insurance companies controlled more than half of the US market (Statista 2017b). Specialist physicians, especially cardiologists and orthopedists, are increasingly consolidating into larger, single-specialty groups (Kash and Tan 2016).

The third method of expansion is diversification, or the acquisition of organizations in different businesses. An organization may diversify into related or unrelated businesses. Related diversification leverages components of an organization's value chain to expand its customer or product base. For example, some of the largest health insurance companies, such as United Health Group, have related diversification into areas such as population health management, health information technology consulting, and pharmacy care services (United Health Group 2016) Unrelated diversification involves acquisition and expansion into markets that have little relationship with an organization's existing products and customers. A hospital acquiring a sports store, mall, or restaurant would be unrelated diversification.

Vertical integration
Assimilation of the vertical components of an organization through greater internal control and coordination.

Vertical Expansion and Vertical Integration

Vertical integration has long been known as "the combination or coordination of different stages of production" (Walston, Kimberly, and Burns 1996, 83).

In healthcare, vertically integrated structures include combinations of hospitals, physicians, insurance companies, nursing homes, durable medical equipment companies, educational programs, and home health care agencies in which one organization's products and services are inputs to or outputs from another organization's products and services. As depicted in exhibit 4.3, vertical integration in healthcare differs somewhat from vertical integration in traditional sectors. In the manufacturing industry, the value chain begins with raw materials, which are formed into components, fashioned into a product by a manufacturer, distributed, and finally sold to an end user. For instance, trees are grown, harvested, and used to make plywood. Distributors sell the plywood to local hardware stores, and then the hardware stores sell the plywood to homeowners. Some companies, such as Weyerhaeuser, grow trees, make wood products, and build homes.

Healthcare—a service field—does not have clear upstream and downstream product flows. The healthcare consumer—the patient—uses services at different levels of the value chain at different times. Generally, healthcare providers have sought to become vertically integrated by acquiring other types of providers (e.g., hospitals buy physician practices and nursing homes) and insurance companies. Merger with manufacturers of medical supplies and pharmaceuticals is less common.

Common ownership of healthcare's vertically related services promises to provide cost efficiencies through improved internal control and coordination and increased market power. Providers have been encouraged to organize integrated delivery systems—vertical integration of most patient care services into a single organization in order to advance to a population health focus (AHA 2014). Many administrators believe that ownership of services and employment of providers promote goal congruence, standardization of processes, and more efficient decision making, enabling conflict resolution and quick adjustment to market conditions (Luke, Walston, and Plummer 2004).

EXHIBIT 4.3 Contrasting Traditional and Healthcare Vertical Integration

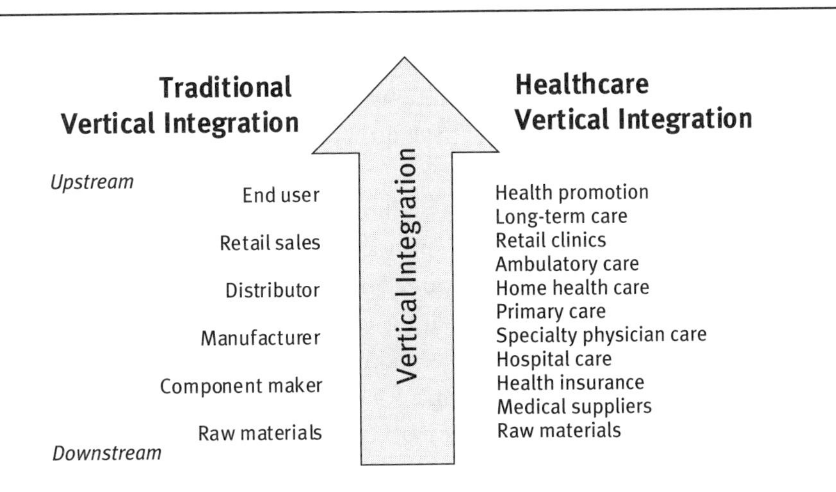

Many have assumed that these benefits and synergies would emerge on their own, especially from common ownership of hospitals, physicians, and health insurance plans. However, research has demonstrated that the benefits of vertical ownership do not simply materialize—they are achieved only when the organization's vertical components are proactively integrated though appropriate management structures, protocols, processes, and incentives that can be difficult to implement. In fact, rather than create a more efficient structure, vertically integrating hospital and physician practices can lead to higher prices and spending (Baker, Bundorf, and Kessler 2014). Lawton R. Burns and Mark V. Pauly (2002, 132) have noted: "All too often, however, they [vertical-owned healthcare organizations] failed to develop a common, standardized set of activities across the different IDN [integrated delivery network] components to closely link the new structures with the new organizational processes of providing incentives to physicians, managing medical staffs, and developing leadership. Thus, the structural integration was not accompanied by a processual approach to integration. All too often the structural and processual activities were only loosely linked together, with some disregard for day-to-day operations."

Transaction cost economics
A theory that suggests that organizational boundaries influence organizations' efforts to mitigate the costs of the transactions and contractual hazards incurred by buying and selling assets and services.

The theory of **transaction cost economics** articulates a rationale for pursuing vertical integration, suggesting that organizational boundaries are influenced by organizations' efforts to mitigate the costs of transactions and contractual hazards. All organizations buy and sell resources and services to others. Each exchange has some cost. Transaction costs might include shipping and handling fees; the markup added to a good's price; and the costs of writing, monitoring, and enforcing contracts. Any inefficiencies that arise from the exchange are another form of transaction cost (Joskow 2010). When transaction costs are high, an organization may choose to acquire the supplier or the distributor.

The cost of transactions increases when there are few critical suppliers or buyers and a high frequency of exchange, as well as when information is not freely shared and trust is low. If an organization requires a critical product and there are few sources from which to buy it, the vendor may unreasonably increase the product's price. This opportunistic behavior intensifies when production information is not shared between buyer and seller and the organizations involved in the exchange have little trust in the fairness and honesty of each other's behavior.

This lack of trust is characteristic of many relationships between major organizations in healthcare. Hospitals, insurance companies, and physicians have intense and often conflicting exchange relationships. Hospitals need contracts with insurance companies to obtain admissions from physicians. When a health insurer or an HMO controls a large percentage of the local insurance market, it becomes a critical, frequent supplier for a hospital. However, transparent information exchange often does not occur. Insurance companies generally have much better information regarding the healthcare costs and utilization of their customers and commonly do not share it with hospitals. As a result, little trust exists between the parties, and opportunistic behavior becomes the norm. The relationship between Texas Health Resources and Blue Cross Blue Shield of Texas described in exhibit 4.4 illustrates how these factors may lead to bitter negotiations, threats, and potential increased costs to both parties.

Because of perceived high transaction costs, hospitals and insurance companies have acquired ownership of vertically related organizations. Some believe that the most successful vertically integrated healthcare system is Kaiser Permanente. As of September 2016, this not-for-profit organization served more than 10.6 million people, employed more than 18,600 physicians, and owned 38 hospitals across the United States (Kaiser Permanente 2017). Other successful provider ventures that have expanded vertically into HMOs include Carle, Marshfield Clinic, Geisinger, Scott & White, and Mayo Clinic. However, many attempts to expand vertically have been unsuccessful because of low capitalization, medical loss ratios, conflicting capital needs, and lack of actuarial science applications. Rather than lowering costs, vertical integration may increase them (Goldsmith et al. 2015). For example, as mentioned in chapter 7, FHP, an HMO, attempted to expand vertically by constructing a hospital in Utah, but the hospital later became economically unsustainable (Jones 1999).

Vertical integration of hospitals and physicians has similarly been a difficult prospect. Many hospital systems have professed a desire for closer alignment with their affiliated physicians to improve quality and lower costs. However,

EXHIBIT 4.4
Blue Cross Blue Shield May Drop Texas Health from Its Network

Blue Cross Blue Shield of Texas (BCBSTX), the largest insurance provider in Texas, threatened to terminate its contract with Texas Health Resources, one of the state's largest hospital systems, on December 31, 2016. In early December, negotiations had acrimoniously ended. Texas Health Resources CEO Barclay Berdan stated that BCBSTX's "continued delays place patients, their employers, and their physicians in the middle of this and may ultimately and significantly disrupt care."

Texas Health Resources had asked for a 4 percent increase in rates in the contract extension. BCBSTX offered 2 percent, which Texas Health Resources rejected. The insurer noted that the difference could potentially cost it $57 million, an increase that it deemed "unacceptable." BCBSTX added, "Texas Health rejected our proposed extension and countered by proposing new short-term contracts with egregious rate increases that would cause our members to bear the burden of additional unnecessary and unwarranted costs with no guarantee of better health outcomes." As the "defender for low cost care in Texas," BCBSTX felt it necessary to reject Texas Health Resources' demand.

In response, a Texas Health Resources spokesperson said that any numbers that BCBSTX provided "should be taken with a truckload of salt" and that "any figures BCBSTX uses is [*sic*] an effort to grab headlines."

Source: Hoye (2016).

because of conflicting incentives and priorities and a lack of physician leadership, many have failed (Burns 2015).

Transfer Pricing

Transfer pricing The price charged for intraorganization trade (i.e., the sale or transfer of goods and services within an organization).

Another factor that causes conflicts in vertically owned structures is **transfer pricing**—the "price" charged for a transaction of goods or services between two divisions of an organization (Business Dictionary 2017). For example, Company XYZ's manufacturing division obtains raw materials from its supplier division and pays an intracompany price. In a vertically integrated healthcare organization, the organization's insurance unit would pay the organization's hospitals and physicians a price for their services. This disbursement might occur via an actual cash transfer or intracompany credit. Transfer prices should be established to encourage goal congruence across units of a vertically integrated healthcare organization—that is, the organization's insurance unit, hospitals, and physicians should use transfer pricing methods that further the organization's mission, whether it be community benefit or profit maximization. Despite these recommendations, however, experts have long considered transfer pricing to be one of the most difficult management control problems, often creating organizational disruption and conflict (Finkler and Ward 1999).

Transfer pricing is set through one of three common methods, each of which poses potential problems:

1. Cost-based prices: Prices are based on actual fixed and variable costs or just variable costs.
2. Full market prices: Prices are based on actual market prices.
3. Discounted prices: Prices reflect some discount from actual market prices.

As do most businesses, healthcare organizations frequently reward their managers for their units' operational successes. For instance, if an organization's hospitals and physicians charge the organization's insurance unit cost-based prices, the insurance unit will be pleased; it will enjoy higher profits and in turn can charge its customers lower rates. The organization will reward the manager of the insurance unit for the unit's success.

However, the organization's physicians and hospitals also want rewards for their operational success, so they may resist setting cost-based prices for intraorganization transactions, especially if they can attract patients from outside insurance companies and operate at full or close to full capacity. Prices charged to outside customers are substantially higher than cost-based prices and would markedly increase their profits. If they have capacity constraints (i.e., they are operating at full or almost full capacity), the organization's physicians and hospitals may choose to treat higher-paying outside patients rather than lower-paying system patients.

On the other hand, if the organization's physicians and hospitals charge the organization's insurance unit full market prices, the insurance unit may be able to find outside hospitals and physicians who charge lower prices and may direct patients to outside providers, even if the organization's providers have unused capacity, such as empty beds. Humana's choice of transfer pricing between its insurance company and hospitals in the 1980s and early 1990s demonstrates one of the major reasons for the eventual divestiture of its hospitals. Humana had set the transfer prices for its owned hospitals higher than the market prices for its competitor hospitals. As a consequence, Humana's insurance company preferred to refer its patients to non-Humana hospitals. (See "The Case of Humana and Vertical Integration" located in the case studies section of this book.)

Competition with Existing Customers

Another issue with vertical integration is that it foments competition with existing customers. For instance, a typical hospital relies on referrals from multiple insurance companies and physicians, who could be considered its key stakeholders. A hospital's owned insurance company or employed physicians generally account for only a small fraction of its total patient volumes. The major referral entities remain nonowned insurance companies and independent physicians with whom the hospital-owned insurance company and employed physicians compete. This dynamic can cause the nonowned physicians and insurance companies either to seek prices that are lower than the prices of the owned entities or, potentially, to move patients to other hospitals that do not compete with them.

This situation can be especially problematic when an existing insurance company has a **most-favored-nation clause** in its contracts. This clause guarantees that a nonowned insurance company, often a Blue Cross entity, receives the lowest prices of any contract. The financial arrangement with the owned insurance company sets the floor for the most-favored-nation contract, which can severely damage the competitive ability of the owned entity. As a result of this and other issues, providers claim that this clause imposes an unfair advantage and discourages innovation. Given the US Justice Department's lawsuits against insurers with most-favored-nation agreements, many US states, including Michigan, Indiana, and Connecticut, have prohibited or restricted most-favored-nation clauses, and other actions are pending (Becker 2011; Schencker 2016).

Most-favored-nation clause
A clause in a contract between a provider and an insurance company that guarantees that the provider will charge the insurance company prices that are lower than the prices the provider charges all other insurance companies it does business with.

Unmatched Services and Incentives

Two additional problems with vertical integration in healthcare are unmatched service areas and incentives. As illustrated in exhibit 4.5, the components of vertically integrated healthcare systems—insurance companies, hospitals, and physicians—attract customers from vastly different markets. Insurance companies compete in expansive markets with large populations, often statewide. General hospitals compete regionally, and primary care physicians compete locally (specialists have wider service areas). To be successful, insurance companies must

EXHIBIT 4.5
Differences in Service Areas for Vertically Integrated Healthcare Systems' Components

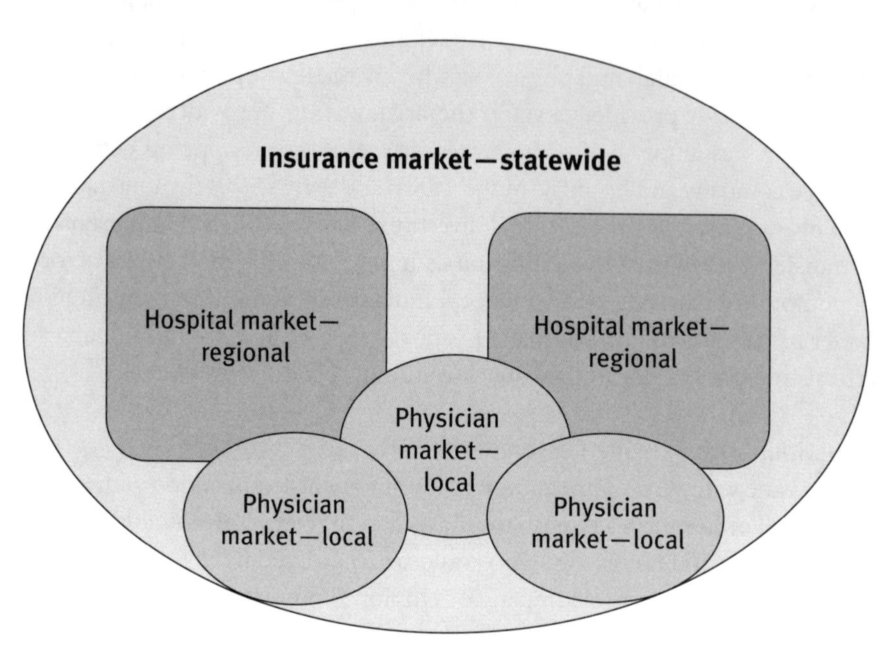

contract for services across a large population base. In many cases, vertically integrated healthcare systems' insurance companies have customers in areas where the systems do not own hospitals and employ physicians, making contracting with nonsystem providers necessary. As a result, systems sacrifice many potential economies of scale. In these situations, vertical integration tends to increase overhead costs because it adds new administrative functions and required competencies to manage the expanded base of operations. Overall, the clinical competencies required to deliver healthcare are rather distinct from health insurance organizations that focus on network development and risk (Robinson 1999).

Likewise, the incentives of insurance companies and providers differ. An insurance company's profitability increases as its customers' use of healthcare services decreases. On the other hand, hospitals in the United States are still generally paid on a fee-for-service basis, and they increase their finances through additional admissions. Providers are rewarded by a fee-for-service payment system that promotes intensive use of services and frequent use of technology to increase billings. Scholars have identified this conflict as a major barrier to system integration and the improvement of healthcare delivery (Porter and Kaplan 2016).

Integration of Vertically Owned Structures

Many suggestions have been made regarding what needs to be accomplished to integrate vertically structured systems. Ownership is relatively easy to achieve. However, the benefits of ownership cannot be achieved without integration. Ghoshal and Gratton (2002) identify four essential areas of integration:

1. Operational integration: standardization of the technology and infrastructure
2. Intellectual integration: development of a shared knowledge base
3. Social integration: creation of cultural bonds that drive collective performance
4. Emotional integration: establishment of a common identity and purpose

Integrating all of these aspects can be challenging and take a great deal of time. Given the challenges these four areas present in healthcare, many vertically owned structures have long recognized the difficulty of realizing the promises of vertical integration.

Yet the allure of vertically integrated structures still draws healthcare organizations. At the end of 2010, vertically integrated structures called **accountable care organizations (ACOs)** were promoted as a means of improving the quality of care and lowering costs. However, although the concept is very appealing, results have not lived up to the hype. Many feel that patients, providers, and payers must work more closely together before ACOs can become successful (Schroeder 2015).

Accountable care organization (ACO) A payment and healthcare delivery model in which a group of healthcare providers work together to coordinate a patient's care, improve quality, and reduce costs.

Some believe that only capitation—a system that offers a fixed amount per person—will incentivize organizations to refocus efforts to a population-based system, requiring vertical integration across providers and services to lower total healthcare costs (James and Poulsen 2016). The challenge for healthcare organizations lies in designing the processes, structures, and mix of personnel needed to integrate vertically owned organizations effectively. As Peter P. Budetti and colleagues (2002, 209) state: "Newer approaches emphasize outcomes of care and would hold health systems to a new level of accountability. It is unlikely that either health systems or physicians will be able to meet these challenges without closer integration and cooperation in redesigning how health care is delivered and measured. The new accountability demands could push physicians and health systems closer together but could also pull them farther apart. Physicians are unlikely to cooperate with heightened accountability requirements if health systems cannot provide clinically relevant feedback."

Recent studies confirm that much still needs to be done to integrate vertically owned health systems. Scholars have reported that physician employment by systems may improve quality through better clinical integration but also increase overall healthcare costs. Hospitals appear to have used employed physicians more often to gain market share in lucrative service line strategies than to lower costs through integration (Baker, Bundorf, and Kessler 2014; O'Malley, Bond, and Berenson 2011). Many predict that healthcare systems will continue to employ more physicians to enlarge and further develop clinically integrated networks to promote population health and value-based models (Jacobs 2016).

Insurance companies also are slowly buying healthcare providers or engaging in cooperative deals and payment models to share risk. Although many predicted health insurance companies would rapidly expand their purchase of physician practices, the progress has been measured. For instance, only a few prominent US health insurance companies have made large acquisitions. In 2010, Humana purchased Concentra, a provider of occupational medicine, urgent care, physical therapy, and wellness services, for $790 million, though its business activities and services did not align with Humana's strategies and core competencies. Concentra was later sold to a specialty hospital chain and a private equity firm for nearly $1.1 billion. Humana still owns 22 primary care centers, mostly in Florida. In 2011, WellPoint, Inc., paid about $800 million to acquire CareMore, a provider of preventive services that is structured to lower costs for patients with chronic diseases. Also in 2011, UnitedHealth Group Inc. bought Monarch HealthCare, an association of 2,300 physicians in a range of specialties. However, by 2016, only about 2 percent of all primary care physicians worked for insurance companies (Herman 2015; Matthews 2011). Exhibit 4.6 describes some of the dynamic integration efforts in Pennsylvania.

Virtual Vertical Integration

Virtual integration Coordination of intraorganization processes, flows, and outcomes through contractual, nonowned mechanisms.

An alternative to vertically owned, integrated systems is virtual vertical integration. **Virtual integration** can be achieved with contractual, nonowned mechanisms that provide more flexible means of coordinating cost-effective patient care but do not incur the costs of ownership. In the mid-1990s, Richard A. D'Aveni and David A. Ravenscraft (1994, 1196) suggested, "True competitive advantage may be gained by replacing vertical integration [ownership] with vertical relationships." These interorganizational alliances may rely on a mix of exclusive long-term contracts and operating agreements that align the organizations' purposes and integrate stages of care.

Most insurance companies take the role of the virtual integrator of healthcare—the intermediary coordinator of care for patients across a spectrum of providers. These entities exist in many forms, as open-panel HMO networks, independent practitioner associations, third-party administrators, or traditional insurance plans.

The integration of hospitals and post-acute care providers has experienced both virtual and ownership vertical integration. Many health systems are integrating with skilled nursing organizations, home health agencies, inpatient rehabilitation facilities, behavioral health, paramedic and ambulance systems, and others through acquisitions or partnerships. Linking acute care with post-acute care organizations promises to permit a greater continuum of care, leading to better outcomes. For instance, Granville Health System, located in Oxford, North Carolina, offers a transitional care program that reaches out to post-acute providers. For example, it partners "with a local pharmacy to ensure home medications

EXHIBIT 4.6
Continued Attempts at Vertical Integration in Pennsylvania: The Proposed Merger of Highmark and West Penn Allegheny Health System

Highmark was created in 1996 by the merger of two of Pennsylvania's Blue Cross companies. Centered in Pittsburgh, it had become one of the largest health insurers in the United States by 2010, covering almost five million members and posting revenues of $14.6 billion. Highmark dominated the health insurance market in western Pennsylvania, controlling 65 percent.

Highmark dealt with all providers in its area but was having increasing difficulty negotiating with the dominant provider, UPMC, a vertically integrated, ten-hospital system with its own health plan. UPMC, which generated $8 billion in revenues in 2010 and provided services to about 34 percent of patients in western Pennsylvania, was using its market power to demand higher payments from Highmark.

In a surprising strategic move, Highmark broke off negotiations with UPMC in June 2011 and announced an agreement to acquire West Penn Allegheny, the second-largest health system in western Pennsylvania, making it one of the few insurers to purchase a healthcare system. West Penn reported $1.6 billion in revenues in 2010 but had suffered losses for a number of years. With this strategic vertical integration, Highmark believed it would be able to compete directly in all stages with UPMC.

As a result of the pending merger, UPMC announced that it was working to enhance and expand its contracts with other insurers, including Aetna, Cigna, HealthAmerica, and UnitedHealthcare, and proposing to offer more choice and competition in health insurance in a market long dominated by Highmark.

After more than a year of extensive negotiations and turmoil, Highmark and West Penn announced in January 2013 that the merger would take place. In the meantime, the acrimony between Highmark and UPMC escalated to such an extent that the governor of Pennsylvania had to intercede to encourage the feuding groups to find a compromise. The agreement they eventually reached extended through 2014. UPMC announced that it looked forward to competing with Highmark's new integrated system but would not renew or extend the contract with Highmark on expiration. These two dominant, vertically integrated systems appear to be changing the nature and degree of competition in western Pennsylvania's healthcare market.

Sources: Evans (2013), Herman (2013), Langley et al. (2012), Lee (2011).

are delivered to the patient's bedside prior to discharge" (Buell 2017, 15). The system is also collaborating with physician practices with a chronic care management program that will embed the system's nurses in key primary care practices.

Owned systems may be more effective in stable environments, whereas virtual arrangements may perform relatively better in unstable environments (Walston, Kimberly, and Burns 1996). Virtual structures reduce the massive capital expenditures needed to form an owned system. Virtual organizations have greater flexibility and higher capital reserves and preserve the option of investing in critical services as an environment shifts. Chapter 5 discusses alternative forms of alliances, partnerships, and networks.

Affordable Care Act (ACA)
A law passed by the federal government in 2010 that sought to decrease the number of uninsured to improve health outcomes and streamline the delivery of healthcare.

Many predict that healthcare reform efforts in the United States will bring about the formation of more vertically integrated healthcare systems. By proposing to change the current form of federal reimbursement to some form of capitated payment in 2015, the **Affordable Care Act (ACA)** encourages the formation of ACOs. Although the actual composition of ACOs may vary, they will comprise vertically organized components, and they will receive payments from and distribute payments to different stages of healthcare provision. The Centers for Medicare & Medicaid Services (CMS) defines ACOs as follows (CMS 2017a): "Accountable Care Organizations (ACOs) are groups of doctors, hospitals, and other health care providers, who come together voluntarily to give coordinated high quality care to the Medicare patients they serve. Coordinated care helps ensure that patients, especially the chronically ill, get the right care at the right time, with the goal of avoiding unnecessary duplication of services and preventing medical errors. When an ACO succeeds in both delivering high-quality care and spending health care dollars more wisely, it will share in the savings it achieves for the Medicare program."

Although Congress may repeal the ACA, pressures to expand access to healthcare while controlling costs will encourage a shift toward structures similar to ACOs. Such structures may contain costs by establishing vertically integrated relationships with the intent to lower costs and improve quality. These goals may be accomplished by either ownership or virtual relationships.

Horizontal Expansion

Horizontal expansion involves the merger of two or more organizations that produce the same product or service. Significant horizontal expansion has occurred in healthcare since the 1970s. Physician practices have merged to form group practices, insurance companies have expanded to have national presences, and hospitals have merged to create multihospital systems.

Throughout most of the last century, a majority of US physicians practiced alone or in small group practices. This situation began to change significantly in the 1980s and 1990s. In 1983, 60 percent of physicians worked in group practices (Burns 2000). By 2016, only 17 percent of physicians were in solo practices and one-third operated independent practices. Group practices and physician employment have been the fastest-growing segments in healthcare, prompted by the move toward a population health–management model and ACOs or other integrated systems. Some observers have suggested that the shift is motivated primarily by the need to gain negotiating leverage with health insurance plans, lower costs, and spread financial risk under capitated arrangements (Berry 2011; Boukus, Cassil, and O'Malley 2009; Casalino, Pham, and Bazzoli 2004; Physicians Foundation 2016).

Likewise, healthcare insurance companies have rapidly expanded to become large, horizontal entities. Many of these mergers resulted from acquisitions made by former regionally based Blue Cross plans. By 2012, WellPoint posted $60.7 billion in revenues and profits of $3.6 billion (Anthem 2013). Originally a Blue Cross plan in California that converted to for-profit status, WellPoint expanded by frequent mergers and now operates in 14 states (Anthem 2017). Other Blue Cross plans have maintained their not-for-profit status but also have rapidly expanded. One example is the Health Care Service Corporation, the former Blue Cross plan in Illinois, which has grown to include Texas, Oklahoma, and New Mexico (Benko 2007).

By 2015, the health insurance market was dominated by five huge national companies—United Healthcare, Anthem, Aetna, Humana, and Cigna. The number of major competitors was proposed to drop to three when, in 2015, Aetna and Humana announced their intent to merge; shortly thereafter Anthem and Cigna agreed to do the same.

Concerns arose because of the market power of the proposed mergers. For example, if the merger had occurred, Humana and Aetna would have controlled 43 percent of the Florida Medicare Advantage market. Given these concerns, the US Department of Justice has sued to block the mergers. As a result, Aetna and Humana called theirs off in early 2017. In mid-2017, Anthem appealed to the US Supreme Court to overturn the rejection (Garcia 2016; Hersher 2017; Laszewski 2015; Radelat 2017).

Since the 1970s, hospitals also have merged to form broader horizontal systems. As mentioned before, by 2016 about two-thirds of US hospitals belonged to a health system (AHA 2017). For-profit and religious systems have become the largest healthcare systems in the US. The ten largest nongovernmental hospital systems in 2015 include

1. Hospital Corporation of America (HCA), a for-profit system with $39.7 billion in revenue;
2. Community Health Systems, a for-profit system with $19.4 billion in revenue;
3. Ascension Health, a Catholic-owned system with $18.8 billion in revenue;
4. Tenet Healthcare Corporation, a for-profit system with $18.6 billion in revenue;
5. Catholic Health Initiatives, a Catholic-owned system with $13.3 billion in revenue;
6. Trinity Health, a Catholic-owned system with $12.5 billion in revenue;
7. Providence Health & Services, a Catholic-owned system with $11.8 billion in revenue;
8. Dignity Health, formally Catholic Healthcare West, with $11.4 billion in revenue;
9. University of California Health system, a governmental system with $10 billion in revenue; and
10. Sutter Health, a not-for-profit system with $9.6 billion in revenue (*Modern Healthcare* 2016).

Like vertical expansion, horizontal expansion has the potential to yield benefits if horizontal integration occurs. As shown in exhibit 4.7, the rationale given by healthcare organizations for horizontal mergers highlights possible economies of scale or cost efficiencies and improved access or expansion of the delivery network (Burns and Pauly 2002). However, greater market power and the ability to negotiate better payments are also primary reasons for horizontal expansion (Weil 2010).

Horizontal integration has the potential to reduce costs by eliminating duplicative equipment and services. Healthcare organizations can also reduce administrative and purchasing costs by spreading fixed expenses over a larger volume of business. For example, horizontally expanded healthcare insurance companies may spread administrative overhead, such as product development, finance, quality management, information systems, and utilization management, across a larger number of enrollees to achieve lower costs per enrollee. Organizations can also share marketing costs, spreading them across a larger customer base—especially for regional and local mergers. In addition, many horizontal systems apply organizational competencies obtained in one market to others to attain economies of learning (Robinson 1999).

However, achieving the promised savings can be very difficult. Many horizontal mergers have struggled to achieve their anticipated efficiencies (Evans 2016). In fact, rather than lowering prices through efficiency, mergers can concentrate an organization's power to increase prices in local markets, as mentioned in chapter 2. With the exception of some for-profit hospital systems, consolidation and horizontal expansion have occurred mostly in local markets. When such mergers are proposed, they may be subject to review by the US Department of Justice and Federal Trade Commission (FTC) to ensure they do not affect consumers negatively. For instance, in 2013, the FTC challenged the merger of Capella Healthcare and Mercy Hot Springs , claiming the merger would injure competition and increase prices. The systems withdrew their proposal (Miles 2016).

A number of studies indicate that completed hospital consolidations do increase market power and enable facilities to raise inpatient prices, especially if the consolidated hospitals were in contiguous markets (Capps and Dranove

EXHIBIT 4.7 Theoretical Benefits of Horizontal Integration

Economies of Scale	Market Power	Access
• Merged/consolidated services • Lower administrative costs per consumer • Shared marketing costs	• Ability to charge higher prices	• Greater utilization • Easier entry to system • Increased customer use across markets

2004; Evans 2015; Vogt and Town 2006; Weil 2010). On the other hand, research also suggests that many horizontal mergers and consolidations do not achieve their predicted efficiencies and cost savings (Burns and Pauly 2002; Evans 2016; Weil 2010). As described in exhibit 4.8, legislators commonly believe that, in most cases, horizontal consolidation in healthcare only occasions higher prices.

EXHIBIT 4.8
Minutes from Hearing on Healthcare Consolidation Before Subcommittee on Health of US House Committee on Ways and Means, September 9, 2011

Representative Wally Herger, Republican from California and subcommittee chair, called the meeting to order. He then made the statement excerpted in the following section.

> Today we're going to hear from a panel of witnesses regarding consolidation in the health care industry.
>
> Consolidation among hospitals, doctors, and insurance plans has occurred for some time. I recognize that, at least in theory, consolidation can lead to greater efficiencies and improved outcomes. Unfortunately, research has shown that higher prices are more often the result.
>
> Consolidation allows providers to command higher private insurance payment rates. As one official at an Ohio hospital that is seeking to merge with another hospital stated in an internal document obtained by the Federal Trade Commission, such a partnership would allow them to, quote, "Stick it to employers; that is, to continue forcing high rates on employers and insurance companies," close quote. Research has repeatedly shown that after hospitals merge, the prices they charge to those with private health insurance increase significantly. Unfortunately, research has not shown that such consolidation leads to greater efficiencies or improved quality.
>
> In my own state, a 2010 report conducted by the *Sacramento Bee* concluded that one California hospital system's large market share has allowed them to obtain reimbursement rates with markups more than double what it costs them to provide services.
>
> Consolidation also enables providers to receive higher Medicare reimbursements by simply changing their designation on paper. While this increases provider revenue, it results in higher cost for beneficiaries and an increased burden on taxpayers with no discernible community benefit.
>
> When hospitals purchase physician groups, hospitals are able to further increase revenue by controlling referral patterns and creating a situation in which they could pressure their physicians to perform more procedures. Similarly, insurance plan consolidation leaves consumers with fewer coverage options and providers with fewer carriers paying claims.

Source: Subcommittee on Health of the Committee on Ways and Means, US House of Representatives (2012).

The concentration and dispersion of horizontal expansion strategies tend to differ by organizational purpose or mission. As illustrated in exhibit 4.9, horizontal systems can be widely dispersed or highly concentrated. Healthcare generally is a local business, and the benefits of horizontal integration become more difficult to achieve when the distances between facilities are large. For-profit organizations initially expanded into states whose laws facilitated higher profits through less regulation and lower wages (e.g., no or weak CON laws and limited or no unionization), creating horizontal companies across the United States. Catholic hospitals, whose missions generally focus on serving the disadvantaged, expanded into poor areas across the United States. In contrast, most not-for-profit hospitals, whose missions emphasize caring for the health of a local or regional population, expand into adjoining markets. For-profit have tended to be dispersed, while not-for-profit hospital systems usually are concentrated in one region. For example, HCA operates 168 hospitals in 20 states, while Texas Health Resources has 24 hospitals, mostly in North Texas. HCA has fewer than 10 hospitals in 16 of the 20 states (HCA 2016). Exhibit 4.9 illustrates dispersed and concentrated systems.

Evidence suggests that for-profit organizations have recognized the difficulty of achieving horizontal integration across a widely dispersed system. For instance, HCA has begun to cluster its hospitals in regions to achieve greater efficiencies and better integrate its facilities (Barkholz 2016). TriStar Health System, one of these regional groups, includes 13 hospitals, 57 medical group

EXHIBIT 4.9
Dispersed Versus Concentrated Health Systems

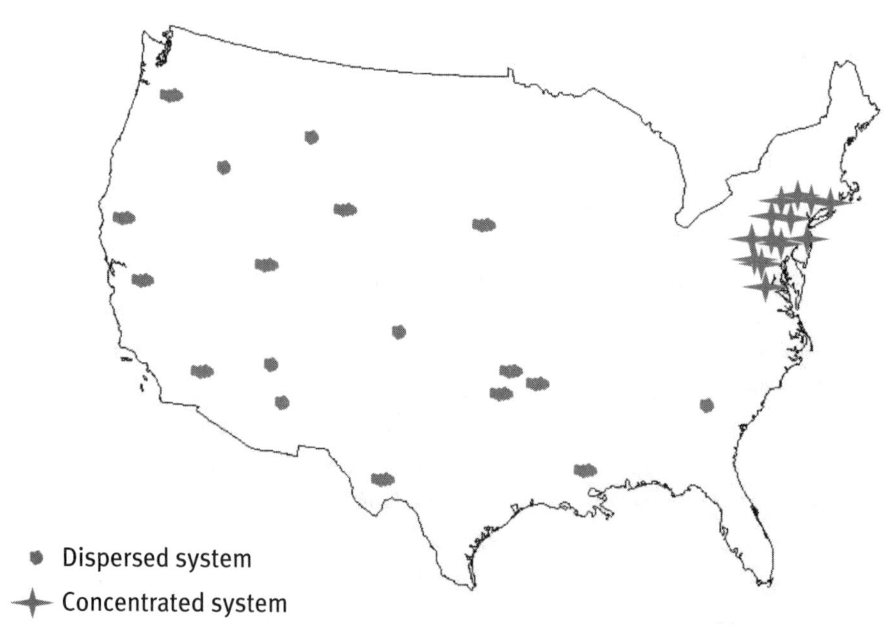

offices, 10 urgent care centers, and 1,600 physicians in middle Tennessee and southern Kentucky. (TriStar Health 2017):

> **What's the advantage of being part of Tristar Health System?**
> Across the country, there is a continuing increase in the cost and complexity associated with healthcare delivery. The benefits of a number of hospitals and medical centers working together, sharing the best practices in quality care and focusing on reducing costs, far outweigh the costs of working alone or independently.
>
> **Is Tristar a part of HCA?**
> HCA is a national healthcare system, and its markets have their own identity separate from the corporate office. We are one of their markets. This is *not* a break from HCA, but merely an opportunity to position ourselves across Tennessee and Southern Kentucky as a comprehensive healthcare delivery system. Through shared strengths, knowledge, resources and support we are the most comprehensive healthcare system in the entire region. This reinforces the company's strategy and strengthens individual decision making.

Mergers and expansion are expected to continue. Merger talks began in late 2016 with Dignity Health and Catholic Health Initiatives. If consummated, the merger will create the US's largest not-for-profit hospital company, with combined revenues of $27.6 billion. In addition, Ardent Health and LHP Hospital Group, both for-profit companies, announced their proposed merger, which occurred in 2017 and created the second-largest privately owned system in the Unites States, comprising 19 hospitals in six states and producing $3 billion in revenues (Livingston 2016; Rege 2017; Taylor 2016).

Diversification
Strategic expansion into different businesses.

Diversified Expansion

Another expansion strategy is to diversify into other types of business. **Diversification** may be related or unrelated. **Related diversification** occurs when an organization (1) enters a different business that uses similar technologies (sometimes called *concentric diversification*) or (2) adds new products or services to its current offerings (also called *horizontal diversification*). For example, a manufacturer of pharmaceuticals for humans might diversify into veterinary drugs. This approach uses the company's existing technologies and opens up a new customer base. Pharmaceutical companies also might diversify into new products for their existing customers—for example, by offering diagnostic equipment and nutritional supplements.

Related diversification
Expansion into a different business that uses similar technologies (also called *concentric diversification*) or adds new products or services to an organization's existing offerings (also called *horizontal diversification*).

Related diversification engages new business activities—such as manufacturing, marketing, and technological development—in one or more components of an organization's value chain (Hitt, Ireland, and Hoskisson 2016). This strategy seeks to leverage an organization's assets and expand its markets or products to achieve greater competitive advantage. Related diversification also pursues economies of scale by combining manufacturing, distribution, advertising, and other costs.

Related diversification generally poses fewer risks than those presented by unrelated diversification because the expansion involves comparatively similar businesses of which their leaders may have relevant knowledge. Related diversification allows the potential for transference of core competencies and increased market power. For instance, hospitals have expanded into providing dental care for the disabled, drug detoxification and counseling, bariatric weight loss surgery, sleep disorder clinics, long-term care, and health promotion (Eastaugh 2014). These diversification efforts are relatively similar to providing hospital care, and hospital managers' knowledge and competencies may be transferable to these areas.

Unrelated (conglomerate or lateral) diversification
The addition of new products or services that have little or no overlap with an organization's current products or services and assets.

Unrelated diversification (also called **conglomerate** or **lateral diversification**) occurs when an organization adds new products or services that have little or no overlap with its current products and assets. Some of the most famous companies in the world practice unrelated diversification. The Walt Disney Company, General Electric (GE), Kraft Foods, and Phillip Morris all are conglomerates that own dissimilar products and services. For example, Disney owns movies, parks and resorts, and consumer products, while GE offers financial services, energy, industrial manufacturing, and healthcare products and consulting services.

Unrelated diversification has been the role of venture capitalists, such as Bain Capital, a prominent venture capital fund. For example, Bain Capital and Kohlherg Kravis Roberts & Company (KKR) invested about $1.2 billion and assisted in the 2006 buyout of the hospital chain HCA. At that time, HCA was a publicly traded healthcare company. The buyout enabled the company to become privately owned. Bain and KKR partners served on the HCA board of trustees, and after five years of restructuring, the company was taken public again and the private equity firms recouped about three and a half times their investment (Creswell and Abelson 2012b).

Likewise, the acquisition of Surgical Care for $2.3 billion by UnitedHealth Group Inc., one of the largest health insurance companies in the United States, could be considered an unrelated diversification, even though both are in healthcare. UnitedHealth will pare the acquisition to its urgent care business and place the company in the outpatient surgical business (Tracer 2017).

An organization may gain a number of benefits by expanding through diversification. Some organizations seek to acquire poorly run companies and restructure them to improve their efficiencies and increase their resultant value. These improvements may be achieved by transferring management talent or sharing assets and competencies. On the other hand, diversification expansion also has the potential to impose additional costs on an organization and depress its profitability. Both related and unrelated diversification can increase the levels of management and control structures required to administer an organization. As an organization's businesses increase in number, the difficulty and bureaucratic costs of running them also increase. Although success often appears easier to achieve via related diversification than by unrelated diversification, both pose similar challenges, and organizations that become extensively diversified tend to be less successful (Hitt, Ireland, and Hoskisson 2016).

Diversified organizations more often succeed when they maintain a common business model across their corporations. As discussed in chapter 3, business models are the core operational structures of organizations, encompassing their processes, inputs, revenues, and value to customers. For example, Britain's Virgin Group owns a wide array of products and services, including records, airlines, trains, cinemas, and finance, yet the company's business model is common across all of its units. Virgin's approach to all of its products and services is "low cost, flair, strong reliance on its brand and an appeal to younger customers" (Yip and Johnson 2007).

To diversify successfully, the central organization must recognize that its distinct services may require diverse technological, managerial, and cultural competencies to operate and that it may need to give each service sufficient autonomy to meet local needs. Although provided decades ago, the advice of Shortell, Morrison, and Hughes (1989, 485) is applicable today: "You cannot manage this kind of activity [a primary care center] as you do the hospital's radiology department. . . . The needs are different—different markets, different kinds of staff, different technologies. We found that they didn't even want to use our purchasing system because they [the primary care center] felt they could build good will by purchasing from a local vendor."

Chapter Summary

Organizations may position themselves through growth and integration. Growth may occur through mergers, acquisitions, internal growth, and networks and alliances. Each growth option presents unique challenges and opportunities for organizations seeking to become more efficient and gain market power. Internal expansion preserves organizational culture but can take much longer. Acquisition facilitates more rapid market entry, but culture and existing organizational structures may impede integration. Networks and alliances may also enable rapid entry, but organizations may have difficulty sustaining them and obtaining the value they desire from these arrangements.

Firm expansion can occur vertically, horizontally, and through diversification. Vertical expansion occurs when an organization acquires one or more of its suppliers (i.e., backward expansion) or companies to which it sells its products (i.e., forward expansion). Vertical integration promises increased cost efficiencies through greater internal control and coordination and market power. Organizations often have difficulty integrating vertical structures, although some organizations—such as Kaiser Permanente—have done so successfully. The ability to structure transfer pricing properly affects the success of vertically integrated organizations.

Ownership does not equate to integration. To achieve many of the benefits of expansion, an organization must integrate its functions. An organization's operations, knowledge, social interactions, and culture should all be integrated. Many organizations find this endeavor difficult, and studies demonstrate that the promises of integration often are not realized. However, these difficulties have not discouraged healthcare organizations from pursuing both vertical and horizontal expansion strategies.

Horizontal expansion is the merger of organizations that produce the same product or provide the same service. Healthcare organizations continue to grow larger through horizontal expansion. Like vertical integration, horizontal integration promises greater cost efficiencies and market power, but many organizations struggle to realize these benefits. Research suggests that mergers often do not achieve efficiencies but do enable organizations to raise prices. To guard against excessive market power, the federal government—through the Federal Trade Commission and state agencies—regulates merger activity.

Diversification expansion includes related diversification (entering a business that uses similar technologies or adds distinct products to an organization's offerings) and unrelated diversification (adding products that have little or no overlap with an organization's current products and assets). Organizations using the latter strategy are also known as conglomerates.

Chapter Questions

1. Why do organizations repeatedly use growth as a key strategy?
2. What are the benefits and challenges of growing through internal expansion? Acquisition? Networks and alliances?
3. What are the main differences between upstream and downstream vertical structures in a manufacturing organization and those in a healthcare organization?
4. How do transaction costs influence the need for vertical integration?
5. What is transfer pricing, and how might it affect an organization's ability to achieve vertical integration?
6. Other than transfer pricing, what are potential barriers and challenges to successful vertical integration?

7. What is virtual vertical integration? How might this strategy lower healthcare costs and improve quality?
8. The promises of horizontal integration include improved efficiencies and greater market power. Which of these benefits is most easily achieved? Why?
9. In your opinion, would horizontal expansion across a large geographic area or concentrated expansion more effectively increase an organization's market power and improve its efficiencies? Why?
10. Which existing assets of an organization does related diversification leverage?
11. Why would an organization seeking to expand through diversification succeed more often by entering similar businesses?
12. What are the major challenges of unrelated diversification expansion? Identify some healthcare conglomerates.

Chapter Cases

Case Studies

1. Read "The Case of Humana and Vertical Integration" in the case studies section at the end of this book. How does the history of Humana demonstrate both vertical and horizontal integration? What problems did Humana encounter? What could Humana have done to prevent some of these problems?
2. Read "The Battle in Boise" in the case studies section at the end of this book, and answer the questions that follow the case.

Deciding on Where to Focus

Sarah was appointed the director of development for Carston Healthcare System two years ago. She has recently been assigned the management of Carston's merger with a smaller system in an adjacent state. Their combined system will include 19 hospitals, 5 of them critical-access, generating revenues of $12.2 billion. The system also include 15 nursing homes, 3 home health agencies, 55 physician clinics, and 23 outpatient or urgent care centers. They have a joint venture health plan with a local Blue Cross company that has been moderately successful.

Leaders anticipate some rough spots during integration but want most of the critical problems resolved and strategies decided within the next six months. The CEOs indicate a willingness to approve consolidation

(continued)

of numerous corporate functions and overlapping services (e.g., duplication of obstetrics in two cities).

Leaders from both systems sold the merger to their communities based on projected savings of at least 10 percent and a commitment not to raise rates for two years. Sarah has been charged with finding the savings and recommending changes to meet the promised objectives. She is working diligently to achieve this but has found the task daunting. To help herself and her colleagues understand the challenge, she has provided the following cost drivers:

1. Labor costs: 35 percent
2. Prescription drugs: 5 percent
3. Professional fees: 5 percent
4. Professional liability insurance: 2 percent
5. Rising demand of care: 34 percent
   a. Population growth: 15 percent
   b. Use rate increases: 19 percent
6. Increased hospital intensity: 2 percent
7. All other: 17 percent

Sarah notes that the merger provides greater opportunities for savings in some of these categories than others. She needs to decide which she should focus on and what strategies might best help reduce costs in these selected areas.

Questions

1. Which of these areas would be affected (both positively and negatively) by horizontal integration? Vertical integration?
2. Which areas should Sarah concentrate on? Why?
3. What types of strategies may reduce costs for the new combined system? Why?

Chapter Assignments

1. Research one large healthcare system, and note its core business and any diversified organizations. Is the system practicing related or unrelated diversification? How does this strategy reflect its mission and vision?
2. Read the 2002 article "Integrated Delivery Networks: A Detour on the Road to Integrated Care?" by Lawton R. Burns and Mark V. Pauly in *Health Affairs*, volume 21, issue 4, pages 128–43. What are the authors' findings and recommendations regarding vertical integration in healthcare?

CHAPTER

5

STRATEGIC ALLIANCES

Join the Premier Alliance

Today you have a greater need than ever to lower costs, improve outcomes and assume more risk, knowing that pressures have only increased with healthcare reform provisions. As a member of Premier, you'll be prepared for the future of healthcare and will actually help transform it. Our members come in all shapes and sizes. The Premier alliance could be a good fit for you too.

You'd be in good company with approximately:

- 3,750 U.S. hospitals
- more than 130,000 other provider organizations

Plus, our supplier partners are critical to the success of our alliance. Approximately 1,100 suppliers are part of our alliance, with 2,000 contracts, helping our members reduce costs and improve quality of care.

Through the collaborative power of the alliance, you will:

- Improve outcomes and lower costs
- Reveal key opportunities for improvement
- Join the ranks of top performers in the nation
- Share in the latest clinical best practices, cost reduction strategies, safety measures and more
- Influence policy that shapes the future of healthcare

It's easy to join. Whether you want to lower your supply spend by participating in our group purchasing organization, increase your quality and safety with our healthcare informatics solutions, or improve care delivery by joining one of our collaboratives, we welcome you!

And all members get access to our state-of-the-art technology platform, PremierConnect®—connecting you with actionable information, knowledge and communities of your peers across the country.

Bottom line: If you want to join a group of passionate, forward-thinking healthcare organizations that are committed to transforming healthcare, we welcome you!

—Premier, "Who It Benefits," 2017

Learning Objectives

After reading this chapter, you will

- understand why strategic alliances are more frequently used in healthcare than in other fields,
- be aware of the pitfalls alliances may encounter as well as their potential benefits,
- be able to distinguish the different forms of strategic alliance,
- comprehend how organizational mission should relate to alliance structure, and
- recognize alliance structures that appear to work in healthcare and those that have been problematic.

As discussed in chapter 4, healthcare organizations are using increasingly diverse interorganizational strategies to better fulfill their missions and expand their capabilities, ranging from loose alliances, partnerships, joint ventures, networks, consortia, and trade associations to interlocking directorates referred to as *virtual organizations* (Luke, Walston, and Plummer 2004). Strategic alliances have also been called "quasi firms" and "hybrid arrangements" (Kaluzny, Zuckerman, and Ricketts 2002).

Strategic alliance A mutually beneficial, long-term, formal relationship formed between two or more parties to pursue a set of common goals or to meet a critical business need while remaining independent organizations. Also called *quasi-firm* and *hybrid arrangement.*

Strategic alliances may be defined as "a mutually beneficial long-term formal relationship formed between two or more parties to pursue a set of agreed upon goals or to meet a critical business need while remaining independent organizations" (McSweeney-Feld, Discenza, and DeFeis 2010, 13). Thus, strategic alliances establish interorganizational linkages to help member organizations achieve their missions and strategic objectives.

Relative to acquisitions, alliances are "cooperative, negotiated, and not so risky" (Dyer, Kale, and Singh 2004, 110). As the invitation from Premier in the introduction of this chapter suggests, organizations establish strategic alliances to gain joint competitive and collaborative advantage and share each other's resources and capabilities. As environmental demands change, new resources and skills may become critically important. As suggested by prominent strategy authors, "Strategic alliances are an important source of resources, learning, and thereby competitive advantage . . . few firms have all the resources needed to compete effectively in the current dynamic landscape" (Ireland, Hitt, and Vaidyanath 2002, 413). Organizations across the world continue to engage in numerous strategic alliances. A 2016 survey by PricewaterhouseCoopers, a prominent international consulting firm, found that almost half of global CEOs and two-thirds of healthcare company CEOs planned to make a strategic alliance in the following year (PricewaterhouseCoopers 2016).

Strategic alliances differ from coalitions and professional and trade associations by their partner selectivity. Strategic alliance partners should bring complementary resources, skills, and personnel, while coalitions and associations often encourage as many organizations or parties in an industry or profession as possible to join (Judge and Ryman 2001).

Potential Benefits of Strategic Alliances

Today there are many reasons that companies form alliances. Exhibit 5.1 illustrates traditional reasons for alliance creation, as well as new drivers. Note that most benefits involve access to a resource or market, plus sharing the risk of a strategic effort.

However, alliances often do not produce immediate, tangible benefits. Their outcomes are perceivable only over the long term and may be intangible. Because of this lag of benefits, organizations must consider opportunity costs when assessing the value of an alliance. Participants in an alliance must weigh the costs and risks of membership against alternative strategies and not just consider potential return on investment. Value emerges when organizations couple their resources with those of others and all participants benefit over time.

The benefits of strategic alliances can be seen in some recent ventures. For example, General Motors (GM) recently entered into an alliance with the car-share company Lyft, investing $500 million. GM benefits by becoming the preferred provider of vehicles to Lyft drivers and by promoting its electric car, the Chevy Bolt; it also gains a seat on Lyft's board. Moreover, GM has positioned itself to strengthen Maven, its personal mobility car-sharing service launched in January 2016, through the development of a network of on-demand autonomous vehicles in the United States. GM plans to help Lyft grow and position itself as a leader in self-driving cars (Welch and Newcomer 2016).

EXHIBIT 5.1
New and Traditional Drivers for Strategic Alliances

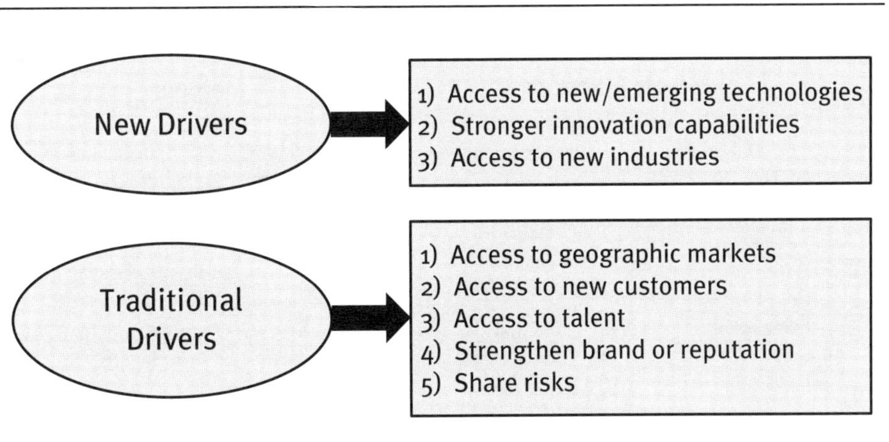

Source: Adapted from PriceWaterhouseCoopers (2016).

Organizations often need to cooperate with other organizations that have profoundly different missions, cultures, and strategic intents. Such differences commonly arise in healthcare. As shown in exhibit 5.2, the alignment or misalignment of missions and cultures highly affects the success of mergers and strategic alliances. Clearly, organizations that have aligned missions and cultures find cooperation and coordination much easier, and mergers and strategic alliances among organizations with conflicting missions are more likely to fail. For example, mergers and alliances among Catholic healthcare providers are more likely to be successful because they share similar missions and cultures. Nonetheless, strategic alliances in lieu of ownership can buffer organizations that have significantly different cultures—they may separate cultures enough to allow goals to be met.

Sadly, most alliances fail. Prashant Kale and Harbir Singh (2009) suggest that between 30 and 70 percent of alliances fail to meet the goals of the alliance and do not deliver the anticipated operational or strategic benefits. Others suggest that the rate of failure could be as high as 80 percent (Zajac, D'Aunno, and Burns 2012). In many cases, members withdraw and join competing alliances. Nevertheless, strategic alliances in all industries continue to grow by 25 percent annually, and many consider them to be a significantly better option than traditional ownership (Judge and Ryman 2001).

Organizations also form strategic alliances in times of heightened environmental uncertainty. As discussed in chapter 1, environmental uncertainty significantly affects an organization's strategies. As uncertainty increases, so does risk. In an environment of sustained uncertainty and change, entry barriers deteriorate and new knowledge and technologies are required for success. Rather than purchase assets and commit significant funds, organizations seek less costly opportunities to place smaller bets through alliances. Although alliances create interdependencies, members retain substantial independence

EXHIBIT 5.2
Influence of Alignment and Misalignment of Mission and Culture on the Success of Strategic Alliances and Mergers

Strategic Alliances

Cultures	Missions: Aligned	Missions: Misaligned
Misaligned	Higher potential for success	Reasonable potential for failure
Aligned	Reasonable potential for success	High potential for failure

Mergers

Cultures	Missions: Aligned	Missions: Misaligned
Misaligned	Higher potential for success	Reasonable potential for failure
Aligned	Reasonable potential for success	High potential for failure

and autonomy, much more so than do organizations in owned vertical and horizontal structures. Fewer interdependencies and less investment give organizations more flexibility during high environmental uncertainty, and they can easily withdraw from alliances if they bet incorrectly.

Healthcare organizations have long experienced heightened environmental uncertainty and have engaged in strategic alliances to address their insecurities and competitive risks. Not-for-profit hospitals formed many of the first strategic alliances in healthcare in response to the emerging threat of for-profit systems (Zuckerman and Kaluzny 1991). Following early experimentation, the formation of strategic alliances exploded during the 1990s, and by 1997 more than two-thirds of healthcare organizations were involved in one or more strategic alliances (Judge and Ryman 2001). Some research suggests that organizations' interest in alliances declined somewhat following this explosion. In 1996, 33 percent of hospitals participated in a **physician–hospital organization (PHO)**, but this percentage decreased to 26 percent by 2000 (Burns and Pauly 2002). Nevertheless, many of today's successful managed care organizations operate and share risk in alliances. Past sector leaders, such as Oxford Health Plans, PacifiCare, and US Healthcare, traditionally did not hire their physicians but ran virtual networks (Morrison 1998). Many organizations perceive virtual networks as a way to position themselves strategically for the future (Bolch 2012; Carlson 2012).

Physician–hospital organization (PHO)
A strategic alliance between a hospital and its medical staff established to develop new services and compete effectively for managed care business.

Healthcare organizations are finding that alliances and partnerships can greatly assist in moving toward patient centered services and preparing a transition toward a population health model. Partnering quickly expands the data undergirding diverse population health programs that may come from affiliations with "community health centers, school districts, local public health departments, chambers of commerce, and faith organizations." For instance, alliances with school districts could make "physical exams, screenings, and diagnosis and treatment" more available to pediatric populations, which would reduce the use of more expensive health services (Lasser 2016).

Similar to all interorganizational structures, the outcomes of strategic alliances may be positive or negative. On the positive side, strategic alliances encourage cooperation, trust, commitment, and shared risk among participating organizations. They address organizational inertia by creating novel relationships and engendering new knowledge and practices. Unlike organizations in horizontal and vertical mergers, alliance members retain their autonomy and independence and have greater strategic flexibility.

On the negative side, strategic alliances can divert an organization from its mission. As discussed earlier, alignment of participating organizations' missions is critical to the success of the alliance. If an alliance focuses on something outside or even tangential to its members' core missions, members will accrue few real benefits and may become sidetracked. Relative to ownership, alliances are much more difficult to establish and unity of purpose and organizational cohesion are more difficult to maintain. Furthermore, setting up such structures can be costly and time consuming. Strategic alliances often demand top leaders' time and involve significant legal fees. If handled improperly, participation in strategic alliances can create antitrust problems. Organizations should be certain that their agreements meet legal conditions in order to avoid collusion (Zajac, D'Aunno, and Burns 2012).

Alliances may be a better option than ownership if the key assets involved in the collaboration are softer in nature—for example, human resources and knowledge. Research has shown that key personnel often depart following mergers, taking key company knowledge with them. Key personnel may be more likely to remain with organizations that participate in alliances, particularly equity alliances (DePamphilis 2014; Dyer, Kale, and Singh 2004).

As shown in exhibit 5.3, strategic alliances in healthcare take many forms. Manufacturers of healthcare goods have entered into numerous alliances with other manufacturers to spur research, development, and commercialization of their products. Pharmaceutical and biotechnology companies have entered strategic alliances to accelerate drug discovery and time to market. When valuing stock, market analysts recognize organizations participating in strong alliances.

One past example of a highly successful strategic alliance between two pharmaceutical companies was the pairing of Pfizer and Warner-Lambert to develop and market Lipitor, a cholesterol-reducing drug. The market was saturated with four similar drugs, and Warner-Lambert—the developer of Lipitor—did not have the marketing abilities and access to the distribution channels the company needed to quickly break in. The first six months of a drug launch generally make or break sales, so timing was critical. The patent

EXHIBIT 5.3 Different Strategic Alliance Arrangements by Organization Type

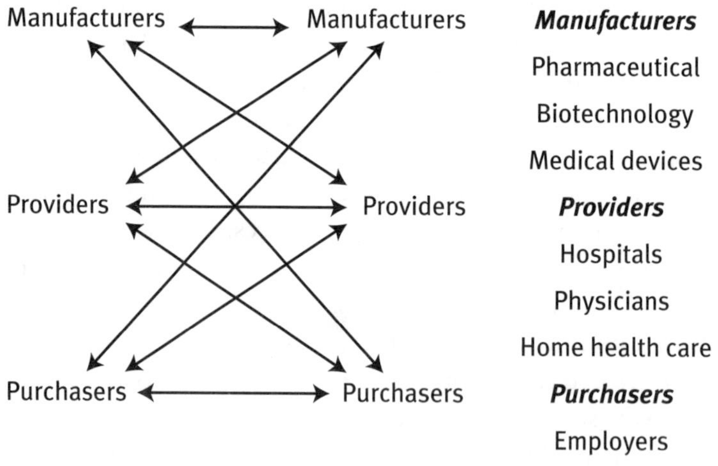

for Merck's cholesterol drug was set to expire in 2001, leaving only a narrow window of time before a lower-priced generic drug would enter the market. Pfizer, one of the few large pharmaceutical companies without a cholesterol-fighting drug, was interested in Warner-Lambert's proposal. Pfizer agreed to pay Warner-Lambert $205 million and other milestone payments and to split marketing and clinical trial costs. In return, Pfizer would receive about half of all net sales. Together, the companies fielded an army of more than 2,200 sales representatives to sell Lipitor during its launch in the United States and distribute 7.3 million samples of the drug to physicians. The strategic alliance was extremely successful. In its first year, Lipitor sales totaled $1 billion, and the drug went on to become the market leader among cholesterol-fighting drugs (University of Michigan Business School 1999).

Examples of Healthcare Alliances

The following section provides four healthcare alliances. The first involves United Healthcare, a large for-profit insurance company allying with a large not-for-profit integrated provider system. The second includes two major healthcare providers, a multinational for-profit system and a regional not-for-profit academic medical center in Connecticut. The third is an alliance between a religious provider, St. Dominic, and a retailer, Walmart, formed to deliver primary healthcare in Walmart stores. The last is an alliance between a large regional provider and a small rural facility.

For-profit Insurer and Not-for-profit Provider

United Healthcare, the largest for-profit US healthcare insurance company, teamed with the largest integrated system in New York, the North Shore-LIJ Health System (now known as Northwell Health). North Shore-LIJ comprises 21 hospitals, along with rehabilitation and skilled nursing facilities, a home care network, 9,000 physicians, a hospice network, and progressive care centers offering a range of outpatient services.

The alliance introduces a new suite of tiered health benefit plans that include accountable care concepts built around physicians and hospitals affiliated with the North Shore-LIJ Health System. UnitedHealthcare began offering the health plans to Nassau, Suffolk, and Queens Counties employers for January 1, 2013, enrollment. The new health plan suite, called UnitedHealthcare North Shore-LIJ Advantage Plans, is part of UnitedHealthcare's ongoing emphasis on increased collaboration, outcome-based payment, and new benefit designs that are transforming how healthcare is paid for and delivered.

"UnitedHealthcare and North Shore-LIJ are working together to improve the local delivery of care and lower costs for our customers," said Bill Golden, the CEO of UnitedHealthcare Employer and Individual of New

York. "Thanks to North Shore-LIJ's leadership and willingness to innovate with us, new benefit designs like the Advantage Plans will help enhance the quality and cost efficiency of care provided through a focused, easy-to-access provider network" (Business Wire 2012b).

As part of the collaboration with UnitedHealthcare, the North Shore-LIJ Health System has the opportunity to earn financial incentives based on quality health outcomes and medical cost reductions in both office and hospital settings among fully insured individuals enrolled in the United Healthcare North Shore-LIJ Advantage plans (Business Wire 2012b).

For-profit Provider and Not-for-profit Provider

Tenet Health, a large multinational healthcare provider with 83 US hospitals, has allied with Yale New Haven Health System—the largest healthcare system in Connecticut—to build new clinical networks in the Northeast. The two systems' alliance may be unlikely; Yale New Haven Health is a respected regional academic medical center, while Tenet is a for-profit hospital system with national and international operations. The systems state that the alliance members complement each other—Yale New Haven Health provides clinical expertise, while Tenet brings its financial strength to help fund potential acquisitions. The relationship allows Tenet to enter the clinical network market (for-profit organizations are not legally allowed to develop clinical networks in Connecticut).

A similar strategic alliance previously occurred in North Carolina, where Duke University Health System and LifePoint—a for-profit group of 60 facilities in 20 states—formed a joint venture (Diamond 2014).

Religious Provider–Retailer

On November 8, 2010, St. Dominic Hospital in Jackson, Mississippi, opened a primary care clinic at the Walmart in the neighboring town of Pearl through a strategic arrangement. "The Clinic" encourages walk-in visits, and referrals for additional care are made to St. Dominic's providers. The Clinic also is connected to St. Dominic's electronic health record system. Kevin Flynn, vice president of network administration for St. Dominic, stated, "Our mission is to serve the community, and the Walmart Pearl location is one more way we can fulfill that mission" (Chandler 2010, 4).

"Walmart is dedicated to serving our customers and our communities, and this type of clinic helps expand their access to quality healthcare," said Bruce Shepard, Walmart's director of healthcare innovations (at the time). "St. Dominic is a well-known and respected healthcare provider in this area, so our customers will receive quality care from people they know and trust" (Chandler 2010, 4). As of 2013, 118 clinics operate in Walmart store locations in 22 states through alliances with independent healthcare providers (Walmart 2017).

Urban Provider–Rural Provider

Formed in 2012, a strategic alliance between PMH Medical Center in Prosser, Washington, and Kadlec Regional Medical Center in nearby Richland made medical specialists available in Prosser. The alliance enables PMH to use Kadlec's new electronic medical record system, facilitating referrals and patient care. Prior to the alliance, Julie Peterson, PMH's CEO, stated, "This is not an acquisition, a merger or some kind of takeover. We will remain a public hospital district with an elected board." PMH Medical Center is a small community hospital with 62 licensed beds. Kadlec Regional Medical Center, a 215-bed facility, is located approximately 30 miles from PMH (Von Lunen 2011).

Interdependencies and Strategic Alliances

The type and extent of organizations' resources also influence their decision to form an alliance rather than expand through ownership. Organizations combine resources in different ways to achieve desired outcomes. These combinations create **resource interdependence**. As shown in exhibit 5.4, the degree of organizations' interdependence depends on whether they have a pooled, sequential, or reciprocal relationship. **Pooled interdependence** exists when organizations' resources are modular in nature—that is, the organizations share limited common assets, and management of those resources needs little coordination (Thompson 1967). For example, a group of primary care clinics might have pooled interdependence. The clinics can function independently and share only resources that benefit all of them, such as billing and information systems.

Resource interdependence
The relationships, dependencies, and interactions among organizational resources.

Pooled interdependence
An arrangement in which organizational subunits group their resources but mostly have their own separate processes and require little coordination.

EXHIBIT 5.4
Interdependency and Alliances

Degree of Interdependence

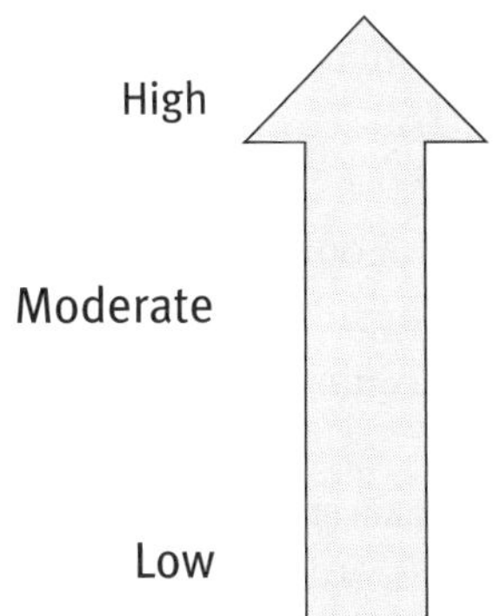

Reciprocal: Resources are interactive; high degree of coordination is needed.

Sequential: Resources are handed off from one unit to another; moderate degree of coordination is needed.

Pooled: Resources are modular; low degree of coordination is needed.

Sequential interdependence An arrangement in which resources or tasks are handed off from one organization or organizational subunit to another. Information, materials, products, and resources must be highly coordinated among organizational subunits because these exchanges occur in a particular order.

Reciprocal interdependence An arrangement in which organizational subunits have multiple interactions and make multiple exchanges of outputs or products among organizational subunits prior to producing a final outcome. Complex products that necessitate constant learning and communication are developed through reciprocal interdependence.

In a relationship of **sequential interdependence**, one organization produces a product and hands it off to the other. This type of interdependence is greater than pooled interdependence. Increased coordination is required to ensure that the transferred products meet both parties' requirements. Drug discovery and the governmental approval process are an example of sequential interdependence. A pharmaceutical company can fully focus on discovery and then hand its discoveries to another organization for approval. As a result, companies can conduct clinical trials more efficiently and bring drugs to market more quickly.

Reciprocal interdependence involves multiple interactions and integration of participants' knowledge. For example, the physicians and other healthcare professionals who deliver medical care in an intensive care unit have reciprocal interdependence. In a hospital, physicians, nurses, respiratory therapists, dietitians, and others are mutually dependent, continuously interacting and transferring knowledge among one another to adjust patient treatment. Coordination is much more complex and difficult.

Another factor influencing organizations' decision to participate in an alliance is the nature of the resources among them. This factor is more important when excess capacity exists. If organizations seek to combine hard resources, such as factories, hospitals, and other costly assets that produce products and services, a merger or an acquisition may be best. Such assets are easier to price than knowledge-related resources, and if combined, managers may substantially eliminate excess capacity.

Although many alliances fail, some have been successful for a number of years. One enduring example is Centura Health System, headquartered in Colorado. In 1996, two faith-based groups—Adventist Health System (sponsored by the Seventh-Day Adventist Church) and Catholic Health Initiatives (sponsored by the Catholic Church)—joined forces as a not-for-profit healthcare network to manage and strengthen their hospitals and services in Colorado and Western Kansas. The system—composed of 17 acute care hospitals, 14 ambulatory surgery centers, senior communities, diagnostic imaging centers, home health care services, hospice services, and physician clinics—serves more than a million outpatients annually (Centura Health 2016). The religious groups' common mission is to "extend the healing ministry of Christ by caring for those who are ill and by nurturing the health of the people in our communities" (Centura Health 2016). The two sponsoring organizations continue to coordinate their assets and skills to leverage their combined position in the Colorado and Kansas healthcare markets.

Given the continued uncertainty regarding market and governmental reform in healthcare, the role of strategic alliances probably will continue to grow. This shift has been especially been true in the development of accountable care organizations (ACOs) and the push toward a population health focus. For example, in 2014, six Wisconsin health systems, which in total provide care to about 90 percent of their state, created a nonequity strategic partnership to develop a low-cost, high-quality ACO. Patient data will be shared among partner organizations to facilitate and streamline patient care (Herman 2014).

Types of Alliances

Alliances can be categorized by the degree of control and equity that members have in the arrangement. Exhibit 5.5 shows where different types of alliances lie on the control–equity continuum. Learning and purchasing alliances, such as professional associations and group purchasing organizations (GPOs), generally involve little capital investment (often just participation fees), and members have minimal control over the direction and activities of the alliance. On the other end of the continuum, joint ventures involve shared ownership and investments, and members have greater control.

Strategic alliances and participants' relationships change over time. As alliances mature, their purposes and value may change. For example, many of today's large GPOs originated to benefit a select group of providers and required large capital contributions from their founding organizations. As the GPOs grew and matured, their memberships greatly expanded and the influence and money required to participate decreased.

For example, a strategic alliance between Roche Diagnostics, an international diagnostics testing firm, and Cedars-Sinai Medical Center, a large healthcare provider in Los Angeles, is an example of a low-equity, low-control relationship. The organizations share knowledge and the results of molecular diagnostics testing with intent to "collaborate and capitalize on scientific

EXHIBIT 5.5 Types of Strategic Alliance by Degree of Control

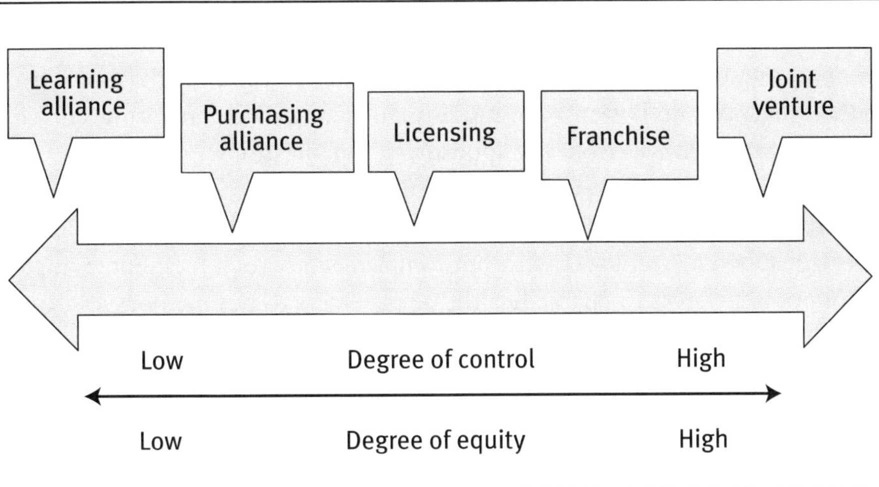

knowledge in molecular testing and, in turn, accelerate the advancement of new test methods and technology" (Roche Diagnostics 2011). Except for their personnel and knowledge, the parties contribute little capital, and the effort depends on cooperation and trust. Neither party can dictate or control the joint work.

Large pharmaceutical companies, such as Eli Lilly, have used alliances effectively to foster research and development. In this way, it can draw on a wide range of external resources. Its cooperative agreements with universities, hospitals, and other drug companies allow much greater flexibility and also speed drugs to market (see chapter 3). A few drug firms, such as Shire Pharmaceuticals, have gone so far as to outsource such functions as discovery, medical monitoring, data management, statistics, and medical writing via alliance-type contracts (Garguilo 2016).

Some have categorized strategic alliances according to membership size, governance structure, and whether they pool or trade resources (Zajac, D'Aunno, and Burns 2012). By nature, low-control, low-equity strategic alliances often have large memberships. GPOs, more fully described in chapter 7, have thousands of members. For example, Novation, established in 1998 with the merger of the VHA and UHC purchasing programs, had 5,200 health system members and 118,000 non-acute health system affiliates from which members purchased more than $50 billion goods and products in 2015 (Dietsche 2015).This GPO continues to grow with the acquisition of MedAssets in 2015 and a change of name to Vizient (Rubenfire 2015).

Although size diminishes each member's control, it can create significantly more overall power and synergies. Healthcare GPOs can demand large price and delivery concessions from suppliers as a result of their size. Larger coalitions can also wield more clout when dealing with governmental agencies, regulations, and legislation (Walston and Khaliq 2012).

An alliance's governance structure often is proportional to the size and equity position of the alliance. Large alliances tend to have larger governance boards. Vizient's board of directors, for example, consists of 22 members from its supporting organizations (Vizient 2017). Joint ventures, which involve two or three participants, often have much smaller boards or operating entities consisting of executives from the sponsoring organizations.

Pooled-service alliance
An arrangement in which the resources of a large number of organizations are grouped to produce value for member organizations. Group purchasing organizations are an example of this type of alliance.

Alliances, moreover, can be distinguished by the type of resources members bring together. In some alliances, members pool similar resources, while in others, members contribute distinct but complementary resources. For example, GPOs pool resources to enable healthcare providers to buy supplies jointly at a discount, while Tenet Health and Yale New Haven each contributes a different resource—Tenet Health shares capital resources; and Yale New Haven provides clinical expertise and reputation.

Exhibit 5.6 illustrates the three types of alliances discussed in this chapter: the pooled-service alliance, the joint-venture alliance, and the network outsource alliance. A **pooled-service alliance** combines resources from a relatively

EXHIBIT 5.6
Types and Functions of Strategic Alliances

Pooled-Service Alliance

Member organization

Member organization | Pooled-service alliance | Member organization

Member organization

Function: Pooled alliances and leverages resources to return value to its members.

Example: GPOs negotiate prices for supplies and equipment for their large memberships.

Joint-Venture Alliance

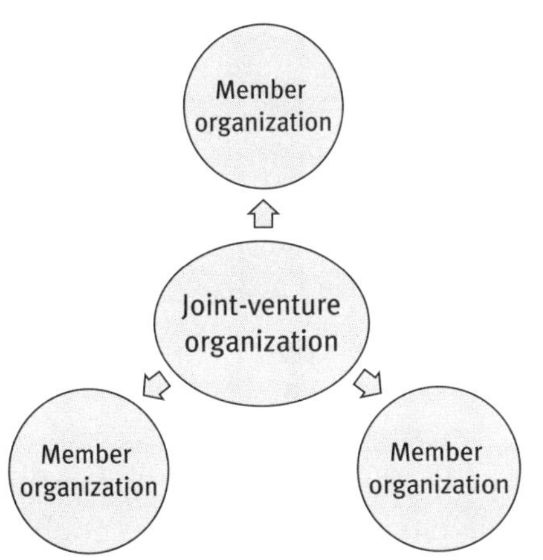

Function: Members contribute resources to co-own a separate organization. The joint-venture organization produces value for its members.

Example: A hospital and physicians create a medical services organization to produce value for its member—and in some cases nonmember—organizations.

Network Outsource Alliance

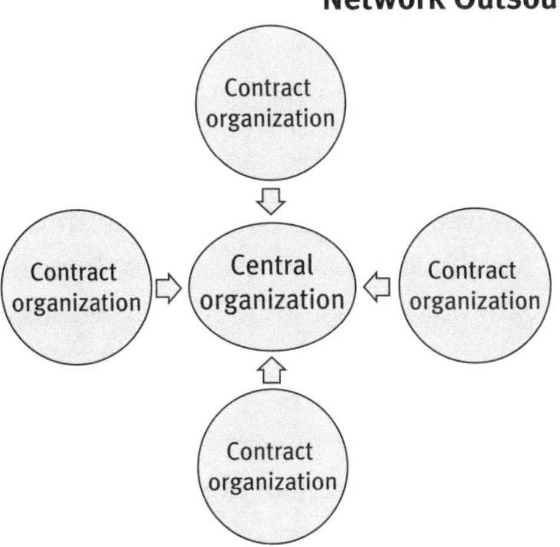

Function: A central organization contracts out components of its functions. The contract organizations return value to the central organization.

Example: A pharmaceutical company contracts out research and development or clinical trials.

Joint-venture alliance
A partnership between a small number of organizations in which each member has a direct ownership position in a shared investment and directional authority over the investment.

Network outsource alliance
An arrangement in which a core organization outsources functions to contract organizations. For example, some pharmaceutical companies use this type of alliance for drug discovery and clinical trials.

large number of members. The alliance leverages the resources to benefit its members. Member organizations often contract with the alliance for services. Again, GPOs, which combine members' purchase volumes to engender greater price concessions from suppliers, are an example of a pooled-service alliance.

A **joint-venture alliance** is similar to a pooled-service alliance in that participants pool resources but differs in that it generally has fewer members, and members have a direct ownership position and greater directional authority. Many medical services organizations began as joint ventures between a hospital and its associated medical staffs. All parties contribute capital and jointly hold equity in a company that can furnish needed administrative services to its members.

A **network outsource alliance** revolves around a core organization that contracts out critical products and services. The core organization facilitates activities through an initial capital infusion, licensure, or some other means. The strategic alliances that large pharmaceutical companies have created with universities, biopharmaceutical companies, and other organizations are fashioned on this model.

Management of Alliances

As stated earlier in this chapter, the majority of strategic alliances fail to achieve their objectives, often as a result of poor preparation and management. An alliance's governance function relies on consensus among member organizations. However, unanticipated conflicts almost always arise and make consensual governance exceptionally difficult.

Before a strategic alliance is established, a statement of the agreement's purpose or mission must be in place. Too often this critical factor has not been addressed. "The lack of an articulated mission statement is often cited as the root of many failures in organizational strategy. The same is equally if not more true for strategic alliances" (Zajac, D'Aunno, and Burns 2012, 327). Many alliances have collapsed because of a lack of well-understood objectives and expectations. To be successful, a strategic alliance must have a mission that delineates the reasons for the collaboration.

As discussed in chapter 6, if its purposes are ill-defined, a strategic alliance can quickly become a liability for all parties involved. Some, such as previously popular PHOs, have had a history of ambiguous motives. Hospitals can bring various motivations to the alliance; they may be seeking to increase their revenues by attracting physician outpatient markets, grow their market power to negotiate better managed care contracts, or improve physician loyalty. On the other side, physicians' motives may contradict their hospital partner's purposes; physicians may desire capital, technology, greater control, and higher incomes. It is no wonder that studies on PHO efforts have demonstrated few significant economic benefits.

All parties need to understand the goals of the alliance, and their actions should reflect those aims. New alliances have been found to have rather "broadly stated goals that do not necessarily coincide with their activities" (Zajac, D'Aunno, and Burns 2012, 333). Specific goals are easier to establish when an alliance includes only a few members. A narrow set of goals tends to appeal to select, homogeneous parties with common interests. Broader goals make the management and direction of an alliance more uncertain but can draw a wider range of participants. Shared expectations facilitate commitment and success.

Alliances must have a management structure that has the authority, responsibility, and resources to accomplish the goals that members have set. Uniquely, strategic alliances "involve two or more leaders who have relatively expansive power [in their own organization] . . . but relatively constrained power and authority over a strategic alliance" (Judge and Ryman 2001, 73). Top leaders often struggle with the ambiguous alliance governance structure because they are accustomed to exercising a high degree of control in their organizations. Those that succeed realize this difference and adjust to the cooperative nature of an alliance. Cooperation means sharing commitments, not controlling them. As suggested by Ohmae (1989), "Good partnerships, like good marriages, don't work on the basis of ownership or control. It takes effort and commitment and enthusiasm. . . . You cannot own a successful partner any more than you can own a husband or wife." Cooperation drives success. Attempts to control bring failure.

A lack of sustained commitment and compromise among partners also disposes an alliance to failure. In many cases, members fully engage in an alliance initially, but over time their enthusiasm wanes and they tacitly withdraw their support. Top executives commonly set up alliances but limit their interaction to indirect activities once the agreements are in place.

Participants are more likely to remain engaged if they perceive they are benefitting from the alliance. Milestones (key performance indicators) should be set and achieved. Alliances' goals in healthcare need to address what constitutes critical, contemporary value for alliance participants. Key stakeholders, such as board members and physicians, need to buy into the alliance. Outcomes such as improved quality, lower costs, and increased access should be identified, tracked, and evaluated. Healthcare alliances that have not addressed these important outcomes increasingly fail (Hoffman 2014).

Trust is a critical element of interorganizational relationships. As discussed in chapter 4, lack of trust encourages opportunistic behavior and conflict among the parties involved. Strategic alliances are fragile and can quickly be destroyed if participants distrust each other. Trust develops if values and goals are explicit and shared, processes are transparent, and outcomes are achieved.

Sadly, trust does not emerge on its own. As stated by Judge and Ryman (2001, 75), "Trust is an essential glue that holds strategic alliances together, but it is very difficult to develop and maintain in the healthcare industry." If relationships and trust break down, alliances will almost always end. Building strong relationships and trust can be the only things that can sustain an alliance, especially when conflict arises (Steinhilber 2008).

Conflict ensues even in the best of circumstances, however, and one way of promoting trust is to establish conflict resolution mechanisms. Many alliances fail to do so. Pharmaceutical companies report that almost 70 percent of their alliances failed because the members ignored festering problems that early conflict resolution might have corrected. Only 40 percent had an internal alliance management group responsible for resolving conflict and maintaining lines of communication between partners (PR Newswire 2006). The more successful pharmaceutical strategic alliances employ project managers, who "proactively identify conflict and facilitate resolution" (Eager 2010).

The fragmented yet dependent nature of the healthcare field makes conflict resolution exceptionally important. Top executives often are rewarded for decisive decision making and not for collaborative behavior, and only through continuous cooperation can alliances be successfully managed and trust built. Uncoordinated priorities and uncooperative behavior can quickly lead to poor outcomes. Collaboration results when all partners consider both their own and others' benefits. When the benefits of others are ignored, cooperation diminishes and the strategic alliance can easily fail. Scholars have found that win–win collaborations that lead to shared decision-making processes and build trust are essential to alliances' success (Judge and Ryman 2001).

Collaboration can be difficult to achieve in healthcare, especially among providers and managed care (insurance) companies, whose incentives, backgrounds, and perspectives greatly differ. Problems include "high levels of naiveté and mistrust between hospitals, doctors and health plans. Partners speak different workplace languages, view health care through different lenses, and typically have given little thought to wider perspectives" (Bilchik 1997).

Another factor is personnel's commitment to the alliance. Commitment can be formed by dedicating capable managers exclusively to the alliance effort (Zajac, D'Aunno, and Burns 2012). Because much of the commitment comes from the personal relationships between top executives, the turnover rate of CEOs and other key leaders can directly affect the alliance. Although turnover is unavoidable, succession planning should be part of an alliance's strategic thinking. Alliances that do not plan for turnover may fail when an executive departs.

Leaders of alliances cannot mandate commitment and compliance. Direct control conflicts with the goals of an alliance, and leaders face the difficult task of seeking commitment through a loosely coupled structure. Some organizations, including GPOs, encourage commitment by tiering their prices on the basis of members' level of commitment. Alliance members that purchase all of a contracted product (e.g., all of their orthopedic products) through the GPO receive larger discounts than do those that buy only a portion.

As strategic alliances mature and environmental conditions change, alliances may need to reassess their structure and purpose. Partners need to recognize the changes and be willing to reexamine fundamental features such as membership, geographic presence, and desired outcomes. Alliances that make such alterations are more likely to survive over time.

Some organizations use alliances to reduce the risks of acquisition and intend many of their alliances to mature to ownership. Technology firms, such as Cisco, use alliances extensively in highly uncertain environments and then seek to acquire their partners when their joint products become more established. As of 2004, almost 25 percent of Cisco's acquisitions had begun as strategic alliances (Dyer, Kale, and Singh 2004).

Chapter Summary

Organizations create alliances with other industry players to fulfill their missions and strategic objectives more fully. During environmental uncertainty, alliances enable organizations to share the risk of developing and exploring new products, gain market power, and learn new skills. Many alliances fail because of a lack of commitment among members, misunderstandings of the alliance's purpose, and a deficit of leadership and resources. Successful alliances work diligently to develop trust, commitment, and cooperation; resolve conflict; and achieve explicit outcomes that return value to their members.

The role of strategic alliances in healthcare will continue to increase. Pooled-service alliances have been successful at negotiating lower supply and capital prices. Numerous pharmaceutical companies are forming network outsource alliances, and many predict that this strategy will be the future of drug development. Different alliances require different approaches. Some involve significant capital investment, while members in other alliances simply share data and knowledge. Regardless of approach, the success of all alliances depends on dedicated effort and cooperation.

Chapter Questions

1. How might alliances be less risky than ownership?
2. When should an organization consider an alliance rather than ownership?

3. What major benefits do alliances seek?
4. What major factors can cause an alliance to fail? What components are key to an alliance's success?
5. Which type of alliance might work best for a not-for-profit organization? For a for-profit organization? Why?
6. How does the use of alliances for research and development help drug companies improve their efficiencies?
7. How does interdependence determine the type of alliance organizations should form?
8. Why does members' degree of control often correlate closely with their degree of equity in an alliance?
9. How can trust affect the success of an alliance? Why is trust more important in an alliance than in a solely owned firm?
10. What can occur as an alliance matures? Why?
11. What are the trade-offs of having a larger versus a smaller alliance membership? When would a smaller number of participants be preferable?

Chapter Cases

Case Studies

Read and discuss one of the following cases: "Response to St. Kilda's ACO Offer," "Build a New Service Because of a Large Donation?", or "Dissolving a Long-Standing Affiliation and Moving On" in the case studies section at the end of the book. Answer the questions at the end of the case.

Read "An Orthopedic Group Decides to Construct a Specialty Hospital" in the case studies section at the end of this book. How could the other hospitals in the area have used the concepts of alliances to prevent the construction of an independent orthopedic hospital?

A New Clinically Integrated Network

Jackie serves as the vice president for network development for a large, midwestern healthcare system. She has worked with many rural and semirural hospitals to improve efficiency by offering shared services, consulting, and purchasing. She also develops in-house hospital management abilities, and her system currently provides contracted management services for three rural hospitals.

As part of her network development, she invites 15–20 rural and semirural hospitals quarterly to a network dinner and brainstorming session.

Generally, 8–10 attend, but the information and suggestions they made were always helpful.

In an earlier meeting, most of the attendees wanted Jackie to explore the possibility of setting up a clinically integrated network (CIN) that could encompass the smaller, networked hospitals. Her hospital had been working on establishing aspects of a CIN within its own system, and she knew that it had spent many years and significant resources on the project. However, given the interest expressed by the attendees, she agreed to present more information at the next meeting.

When the next quarter arrived, Jackie presented how CINs work and what their desired outcomes are. CINs seek to improve patient care while reducing costs and existing redundancies. These networks should develop a team of primary care and specialty physicians to work together to streamline their care delivery model. CINs also allow both employed and affiliated physicians to partner and negotiate with insurers for contracts. Generally, a CIN should do the following:

- Establish a network of providers that enhances coordination of care.
- Create a partnership model with hospitals and their employed and independent physicians.
- Define roles for physician leadership.
- Clearly establish performance improvement initiatives to provide demonstrated value.
- Provide a structure for joint contracting to support care redesign and performance improvement initiatives.
- Negotiate with businesses and insurers for risk-based contracts.
- Implement consistent clinical protocols across the network to achieve patient care.
- Collectively own a reporting system.

Health systems have used many structures to implement CINs. Jackie presented various options that would work best in different circumstances. These ranged from a joint venture to a pooled-service alliance to a network outsource alliance.

During the subsequent discussion, almost all attendees concurred that they would like to pursue this together. They felt that critical aspects included involving their physicians, improving patient care, lowering costs, and providing a mechanism to negotiate joint contracts.

(continued)

Questions

1. Given what the leaders want to accomplish, what structure would you suggest? Why?
2. What are the advantages and disadvantages of using each of the three structures to establish a CIN?
3. What other structures could they use?

Chapter Assignments

1. Select a GPO. Identify its locations, services, facilities, and sites, and determine the criteria for membership.
2. Search the Internet for strategic alliances. Find one example of each of the three types shown in exhibit 5.6. In a one-page paper, identify the strengths and potential weaknesses of each alliance.

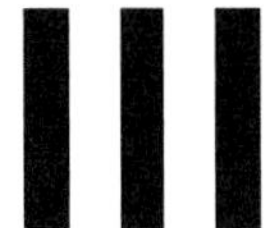

PART III

ORGANIZATIONAL PURPOSE

An organization's purpose and core reason for existence are critical, foundational components of strategy. Strategies should be informed, formulated, and directed by organizational purpose. Chapter 6 transitions from previous chapters' discussion of possible strategies and theories to an examination of values, mission, and vision; their role as the basis of strategy selection; and their relationship to organizational stakeholders.

CHAPTER

6

STAKEHOLDERS, VALUES, MISSION, AND VISION

ACHE's vision, mission and values provide the basis for organizational direction and decision making in service to the organization and profession. ACHE's fundamental purpose (mission) and the essential core values of the profession form the foundation for our strategy. Creating the desired long-term future (vision) is a fundamental guiding principle for ACHE's strategic direction.

Vision: To be the preeminent professional society for healthcare executives dedicated to improving health.

Mission: To advance our members and healthcare management excellence.

Core Values: As members of the American College of Healthcare Executives, we are committed to:

- *Integrity*: We advocate and demonstrate high ethical conduct in all we do.
- *Lifelong Learning*: We recognize lifelong learning is essential to our ability to innovate and continually improve ourselves, our organizations and our profession.
- *Leadership*: We lead through example and mentoring, and recognize caring must be a cornerstone of our professional interactions.
- *Diversity and Inclusion*: We advocate inclusion and embrace the differences of those with whom we work and the communities we serve.

— American College of Healthcare Executives,
"Strategic Plan, 2017–2019," 2017

Learning Objectives

After reading this chapter, you will

- understand who organizational stakeholders are and their importance in creating the company's strategic intent;
- comprehend that strategic intent consists of three components: mission, vision, and values;
- know the importance of values to a company and how they can be identified; and
- recognize the differences between mission and vision statements and be able to describe how they are created.

Stakeholders and Organizational Purpose

Stakeholders
Persons who have a claim to or obtain some benefit from an organization.

Organizations are created to accomplish some aim or output for a group(s) of stakeholders efficiently and effectively. **Stakeholders** are individuals and groups that have some investment in an organization or obtain some benefit from it. Ultimately, organizations exist for the benefit of their stakeholders. For instance, the values, mission, and vision of the American College of Healthcare Executives (ACHE) define healthcare professionals as ACHE's stakeholders and its purpose as advancing members and healthcare management excellence. Other organizations' outputs might be the manufacture of cars or prescription drugs or the provision of community benefits or healthcare services, to name a few.

Types of stakeholders range extensively, but major classifications include internal groups and external groups. Internal stakeholders have connections inside an organization. Employees, investors, stockholders (of publicly held companies), and board members are internal stakeholders. External stakeholders may include customers, suppliers, governments, local communities, and the general public. As shown in exhibit 6.1, a reciprocal relationship exists between an organization and its stakeholders; as the Agency for Healthcare Research and Quality (AHRQ) states, stakeholders are "persons or groups that have a vested interest. . . . Stakeholders may be patients, caregivers, clinicians, researchers, advocacy groups, professional societies, businesses, policymakers, or others. Each group has a unique and valuable perspective" (AHRQ 2014). For example, organizations seek to attract customers by offering products or services that benefit the consumer and at the same time seek benefits in the form of payments or other types of support (e.g., reputation, regulatory approval). The number of stakeholders can appear immense for a healthcare organization and may include

- program managers and staff;
- local, state, and regional coalitions;
- advocacy partners;
- state education agencies, schools, and other educational groups;
- universities and educational institutions;
- local government, state legislators, and state governors;
- privately owned businesses and business associations;
- healthcare systems and the medical community;
- religious organizations;
- community organizations; and
- private citizens (Sharfstein 2016).

An organization must consider both its stakeholders' needs and the support it requires when formulating and implementing its strategies. If the organization fails to consider one or both of these interests, stakeholders may withdraw their contributions, and the organization may incur serious negative consequences as a result. For example, key governmental entities might refuse to grant crucial approvals, investors may withdraw critical capital funds, or customers may seek services and products from other organizations. Neglecting to attend to the interests of key stakeholders can contribute to poor implementation of strategic decisions and subsequent failure. Integration and an understanding of key stakeholders are important in all organizations but can

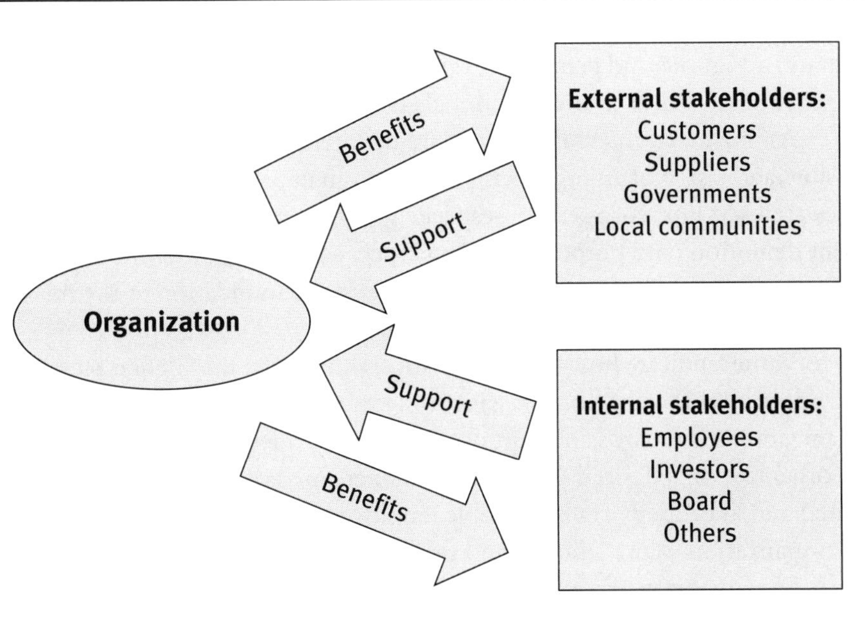

EXHIBIT 6.1 Relationship Between Stakeholders and Organization

be especially critical in public organizations, many of which are healthcare providers (Bryson 2004; Huotari and Havrdova 2016).

Strategic Intent

Strategic intent Statements, including mission, vision, and values, that describe an organization's perception of its purpose, its direction, and acceptable conduct.

One of leaders' key functions is to craft their organization's strategic intent in order to signal where the organization needs to go. For example, ACHE aims to be the preeminent professional society for healthcare executives. **Strategic intent** is a key gauge of an organization's relationship with its stakeholders. It identifies stakeholders most important to the organization and the benefits they are to receive. It also should be a statement of commitment to stakeholders and the basis on which the organization defines its successes and failures. Strategic intent should aim to fulfill the organization's mission and should express the organization's values and the stakeholders' values. It defines what an organization does, how the organization accomplishes it, and what the desired outcomes are.

Strategic intent informs all of an organization's decisions about its future. Organizations that are unclear on their strategic intent or base their activities on multiple strategic intents set conflicting priorities, waste resources, suffer from indecision, and frustrate their workforce (Ice 2007). Strategic intent should be realistic and unambiguous and directly reflect the beliefs and desires of senior managers. A statement meeting these criteria often is difficult to establish. Even if an organization has taken the time to craft a written document defining its strategic intent, it may not be tied to the organization's actions (Pitt 2001). Properly constructing and communicating strategic intent "in ways that are both unambiguous and persuasive, setting forward what is to be sought in the longer run" is critical to organizational success (Useem 2016).

Values Statements expressing the ethics that guide an organization's actions and processes and standards for behavior among its staff.

As illustrated in exhibit 6.2, strategic intent is composed of the values, mission, and vision of an organization. Although in practice these terms sometimes are used interchangeably—especially *mission* and *vision*—they have different definitions and purposes. Strategy texts commonly order these terms as mission, vision, and values; however, values are the foundation of the mission and vision and therefore should precede them.

Mission A statement of an organization's purpose, aims, and values.

Vision A statement of the desired future state of an organization.

Values indicate how the organization should act; they define acceptable and unacceptable behavior. **Mission** reflects these values by expressing the organization's standards and purpose. **Vision** provides direction by depicting the organization's desired future state. Values, mission, and vision are interrelated and, if properly crafted, enable employees to understand and articulate the organization's core strategy and priorities.

For organizations to enjoy sustainable prosperity, they must be driven by their mission and vision and be committed to practicing a set of values. Values need to be incorporated into all organizational operations and processes,

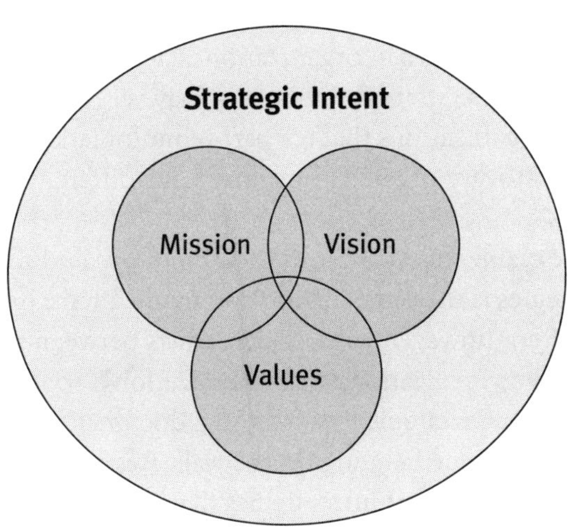

EXHIBIT 6.2 Relationship Between Strategic Intent and Mission, Vision, and Values

including hiring, performance review, promotion, reward, and dismissal (Nelson and Gardent 2011; Regan 2012).

As stated in chapter 1, organizations' diverse strategic intents drive widely different strategies. Diverse organizational intents engender dissimilar values, missions, and visions as well as different approaches to strategy, especially in the healthcare sector, where different segments consist of a dissimilar mix of for-profit and not-for-profit organizations. Exhibit 6.3 shows that the percentage of for-profit organizations in different healthcare service segments varies from only 21 percent among acute care hospitals to almost 100 percent

EXHIBIT 6.3 Percentage of US Healthcare Organizations That Are For-Profit, by Type

	Percentage for Profit
Acute care hospitals[1]	21
Hospice programs[2]	63
Psychiatric hospitals[3]	69
Home health agencies[2]	80
Nursing homes[4]	70
Dialysis centers[5]	86
Medical device companies*	≈ 100
Pharmaceutical companies*	≈ 100
Physician practices*	≈ 100

Source: American Hospital Association (2017);[1] Kaiser Family Foundation (2014a);[2] Span (2014);[3] CDC (2016c);[4] Johnson (2014).[5]

*Estimated.

among pharmaceutical companies, physicians, and medical device companies. In addition, strategic intent differs among academic medical centers; community-owned facilities; rural and urban organizations; large corporations; and small, family-owned companies. Strategic intent also may vary between single-market organizations and organizations that are part of multimarket systems. Furthermore, different healthcare organizations may have different stakeholders and different purposes.

Although organizations differ in their emphasis and focus, the basis of all successful strategies is the organization's strategic intent: its values, mission, and vision. Too often, however, a disconnect exists between the writing of the strategic intent and its inculcation in an organization's strategies and actions. The components of the strategic intent sit in a document on the CEO's desk or are inscribed on a plaque hanging on the wall. Researchers have noted that executives often compose beautiful strategies that are never implemented. Staff members do not internalize the written documents or use them as guides to making difficult decisions (Walston 2017).

When managers write the strategic intent and seek to communicate it to stakeholders, yet the intent does not inform and drive strategic actions, serious damage can result. Organizations create problems for themselves when they espouse wonderful-sounding values, missions, and visions and then act contrarily to these dictates. They find themselves at odds with their stakeholders and may face civil and criminal penalties. The indictments and fines they suffer can lower their stock prices, tarnish their public image, and damage their employees' morale.

Values

As stated earlier, *values* are the foundation of an organization's mission and vision. They express the ethics that guide an organization's actions and processes. Values should be the final metric by which an organization determines whether it has succeeded or failed. If an organization achieves its goals or benchmarks, especially financial ones, but does so by violating its values, it has failed. Likewise, if an organization with a culture and embedded values that promote innovation makes an honest but unprofitable investment or if it fails to achieve a written strategy because of changing market conditions, it still could be deemed a success.

As exhibit 6.4 shows, Thomas J. Watson, Jr., past CEO of IBM, believed that following organizational values is more important than organizational outcomes. The ultimate criteria for evaluation should not be bad investments and untoward results but rather the application of organizational values, which, in this case, were innovation, trust, and respect.

Many organizations set aside their value statements and fail to ingrain them into their culture. Too often statements are used only as marketing slogans, or organizations fixate on financial results and profits. When managers

EXHIBIT 6.4
Interpreting Results on the Basis of Organizational Values

Thomas J. Watson Jr., CEO of IBM between 1956 and 1971, was a key figure in the information revolution. Watson embedded in IBM the values of innovation and creativity. In one case, a young executive had made some investments that did not work out, and the decision cost IBM several million dollars. He was summoned to Watson's office, fully expecting to be fired. As he entered, he asked Watson whether he wished him to resign. Watson is said to have replied that he had just spent a couple of million dollars educating the junior executive, so why should he be fired?

Source: Schein (2010).

stress financial outcomes and ignore other stated values, ultimately a company's culture, reputation, and long-term viability suffer.

Emphasis on short-term profits is a common mantra of for-profit firms seeking to maximize shareholder value. Scholar have long suggested that this single-minded focus is flawed at its core and not sustainable over the long term (Drucker 1959). A primary value of maximizing profits cannot motivate large groups of employees to deliver exceptional performance, and organizations driven by profits lose their direction over time (Sabria 2016). They are ships without a real rudder to direct their actions. Leaders may practice contingent ethics, changing their values from situation to situation, and make opportunistic short-term decisions that have disastrous long-term consequences.

If adhered to appropriately, values can be essential principles guiding all of an organization's actions and the basis of its culture. Values should create the ethical environment in which all employees function. They should inform organizational decisions and be used to resolve conflicts. For values to function as a guide, all internal stakeholders should be aware of them, accept them, and integrate them daily into their organizational decisions and actions (Nelson and Gardent 2011). Authors have suggested that ingrained values in hospitals contribute significantly to lower patient mortality rates (Curry et al. 2011).

Values should endure across time. Strategies will (and should) change, but values should not. Values must be deeply embedded in an organization's culture and in the hearts and minds of its employees, not just written and hung on a wall.

Values should be based on the core beliefs and expectations of key shareholders. The following guidelines describe one method for understanding and establishing an organization's values (Walston and Chou 2012):

- *Obtain key stakeholders' expectations for the organization.* In some organizations, the owners might be the only group deemed to be truly important. In others, multiple groups—including owners, customers, employees, and suppliers—might be powerful enough to be included. As discussed in chapter 8, one way to identify key stakeholders is to ascertain who would suffer the most if the organization ceased to exist.

Once key stakeholders are identified, the organization can conduct surveys or interviews to determine which values stakeholders believe to be important. Questions might focus on what employees want the organization to be known for; what makes employees proud to be affiliated with the organization; who the organization's heroes are, and why; and, among the organization's ethical values, which five are most important.

- *Identify common values among stakeholders.* Commonly expressed values should be identified and related values merged to establish the ethical base of an organization's purpose. Managers should place an emphasis on values that distinguish the organization from its competitors.
- *Make values visible and tangible to employees.* Make organizational values visible and tied to performance. Clearly incorporate the values into employees' (including the CEO's) evaluations to assess how well they live these ideals. Link values to measurable strategic outcomes, such as satisfaction scores or error rates.
- *Keep values memorable.* Express values in terms that stakeholders understand and can remember. As a rule of thumb, organizations should establish no more than seven values. The best values statements consist of more than just a word or a phrase; they also include a brief description.

Organizations can also use written values to shape employees' attitudes toward different categories of stakeholders. Values' influence on staff is especially important in healthcare, given its many vulnerable stakeholders. A good example of a values statement aiming to instill expected behaviors is that of Dignity Health (formerly Catholic Healthcare West), a large hospital system in California, Arizona, and Nevada (Dignity Health 2017):

> Dignity Health is committed to providing high-quality, affordable health care to the communities we serve. Above all else we value:
>
> **Dignity:** Respecting the inherent value and worth of each person.
>
> **Collaboration:** Working together with people who support common values and vision to achieve shared goals.
>
> **Justice:** Advocating for social change and acting in ways that promote respect for all persons and demonstrate compassion for our sisters and brothers who are powerless.
>
> **Stewardship:** Cultivating the resources entrusted to us to promote healing and wholeness.
>
> **Excellence:** Exceeding expectations through teamwork and innovation.

Dignity Health (2008, 2) also has a document titled "Standards for Mission Integration" that addresses organizational identity, spirituality, ethics, and community health at both local and system levels. It states, "The Standards for Mission Integration reflect the future we, as a system, are aspiring to realize. The Standards provide us with a framework to identify, measure and improve the ways in which the mission of our health care ministry is carried out. They also are a tool that will help us assess how our values are being lived out in the day-to-day operations of our organization. Each facility is expected to establish and support an overall mission integration process, supported by an annual plan."

These standards expand on Dignity Health's written values and provide key metrics for evaluating how successfully the system is implanting its organizational identity, spirituality, and ethics. For example, local indicator ethics standard 9 states (Dignity Health 2008, 7):

> [Dignity Health] promotes ethical integrity in organization and business practices and in patient care.
>
> A. Each facility uses a structured process of ethical reflection for strategic, business and management decision-making and priority setting.
> B. Employee recruitment and evaluation integrates measures to gauge congruence with [Dignity Health] core values.
> C. Each facility has an Ethics Committee for clinical ethics policy development, education and case consultation, or has the resources of an Ethics Committee available to it. Each Ethics Committee:
>   - Is appropriately chartered within the organization;
>   - Maintains minutes for submission to the appropriate local hospital Board;
>   - Has interdisciplinary membership;
>   - Engages in regular education for itself, the organization and the medical staff;
>   - Has guidelines for policies and case consultation.
>
> D. Each facility integrates [Dignity Health]'s Philosophy of Mistake Management, Event Reporting Policy and Safe Harbor Provision into employee orientation and training programs, and promotes a non-punitive environment and culture that supports timely and appropriate reporting of mistakes.
> E. Each facility receives a rating of one (1) or two (2) in the Organization Ethics section of its JCAHO survey.

Dignity Health further reinforces its values by producing an annual corporate social responsibility report. In this report, Dignity Health outlines goal achievement that reflects its established values and relates anecdotes of ways its goals, mission, and values are being fulfilled. For instance, as shown in its "Sustaining Our Healing Ministry: Fiscal Year 2012 Social Responsibility Report," Dignity Health describes how its actions are affecting its key stakeholders and fulfilling its strategic priorities. The following excerpt explains how it has been addressing the needs of its vulnerable populations (Dignity Health 2013, 21):

> At the local level, each hospital assesses its community's health assets and needs on a triennial basis and then develops and annually updates a community benefit plan that addresses unmet health priorities identified in collaboration with community stakeholders.
>
> Community benefit programs take into consideration the socioeconomic barriers that often lead to poor health and offer programs that evidence supports can have a measurable effect. In Dignity Health communities, 100 percent of the community health needs assessments identified chronic disease as an unmet health need. A system-wide community benefit initiative focuses on improving health and avoiding hospitalizations. . . . In 2012, Dignity Health hospitals invested $2 million in evidence-based, chronic disease self-management programs that served more than 13,000 individuals, resulting in only 5 percent of the program participants using hospital or emergency room services in the six months following the intervention.

Dignity Health's approach is one example of how values can be instilled in an organization. Managers can accomplish this objective through a variety of means. Periodic and annual reviews such as those prepared by Dignity Health can be helpful. However, the actions of top executives exert a greater influence on organizational behaviors. Ultimately, executives are responsible for establishing values and ensuring ethical conduct. In general, employees gauge whether an organization's values have been incorporated into its culture by their perception of executives' behavior.

Line employees often perceive the organizational environment differently from executives. Therefore, to better assess the gap between existing, written values and actual behavior and culture, organizations should consider a structured values review process. This process might include the creation of a work group to examine the organization's beliefs and practices rigorously. The work group could host a series of focus groups that include clinical and nonclinical staff to learn which values reflect actual practice and identify behaviors that run counter to them. After a series of four to five focus groups, the work group would be able to identify common themes and gaps that need attention. From this information, the group could create an improvement plan and enact it with the direct support and participation of a top executive.

As mentioned earlier, annual employee evaluations should directly incorporate the values of the organization. For example, employees could be rated on each value. An evaluation based on Dignity Health's values might read as follows:

> In what ways does the employee exemplify Dignity Health's values? Review the following list of values and comment on where the employee excels and where the employee could improve. Please provide job-related examples.
>
> A. Dignity:
> B. Collaboration:
> C. Justice:
> D. Stewardship:
> E. Excellence:

Mission

An organization's mission is an enduring statement of core organizational purpose that distinguishes it from other organizations and identifies the scope of its operations in terms of products and markets. Scholars and management consultants popularized mission statements in the 1980s. By 2006, about 85 percent of large companies had written mission statements (Holland 2007). Yet some claim that companies do not use mission statements effectively, and about 80 percent of mission statements are boring and unmemorable:

> Cookie cutter statements are not going to inspire anyone. Worse, they fail to provide any strategic direction. What is missing in these statements is imagination. . . . I am talking about words, visions and missions that inspire and excite us. Adventures and goals that take us out of our mundane everyday lives and help make us part of something bigger than ourselves. We all want to be part of something great, something memorable. . . . We must believe that this "bigger" thing is going somewhere exciting or has the potential to be a winner. It has to be bigger than we are. It has to embody deep-seated hopes and dreams that are inherent in every human being. (Persico 2017)

To inspire an organization's mission should be the foundation of its strategic direction and reflect its values. The mission indicates which stakeholders are most important, and its fulfillment is the basis for judging an organization's success. As shown in exhibit 6.5, how a mission statement is constructed can make a big difference.

The statement should be written in the language of the organization's stakeholders, not jargon that might be popular in the business literature. Average people rarely find such jargon compelling—for example, comedy writers, such as "Weird Al" Yankovic (Kohli 2014) and Scott Adams of *Dilbert* have both mocked the business jargon often used in mission statements (Adams 2017).

EXHIBIT 6.5
Attributes of Good and Bad Mission Statements

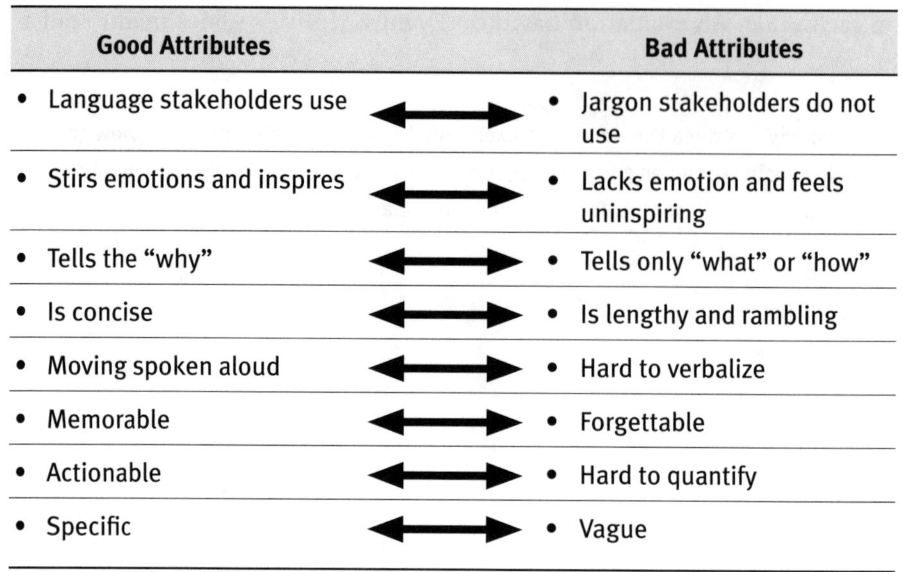

Good Attributes		Bad Attributes
• Language stakeholders use	⟷	• Jargon stakeholders do not use
• Stirs emotions and inspires	⟷	• Lacks emotion and feels uninspiring
• Tells the "why"	⟷	• Tells only "what" or "how"
• Is concise	⟷	• Is lengthy and rambling
• Moving spoken aloud	⟷	• Hard to verbalize
• Memorable	⟷	• Forgettable
• Actionable	⟷	• Hard to quantify
• Specific	⟷	• Vague

Source: Adapted from Koenig (2016).

Moreover, if an employee, a patient, or a community member cannot understand the language used, it should be revised. The primary purpose of mission statements is to communicate measurable, definable, and actionable objectives clearly to internal and external stakeholders (Sufi and Lyons 2003). To do so, statements must be concise and touch employees' hearts (George 2001). A mission becomes meaningful only when it begins to affect the behavior and actions of stakeholders (Darbi 2012).

For example, although most people worldwide have heard of Walt Disney, many may have difficulty understanding the company's mission statement and reconciling their perceptions of the company with it (Walt Disney Company 2013): "The Walt Disney Company's objective is to be one of the world's leading producers and providers of entertainment and information, using its portfolio of brands to differentiate its content, services and consumer products. The company's primary financial goals are to maximize earnings and cash flow, and to allocate capital toward growth initiatives that will drive long-term shareholder value."

A mission should keep management focused on meeting the needs of key stakeholders. The mission should be a guide to establishing actionable goals, performance measures, and structures aimed at creating value for stakeholders. The mission should address the organization's reason for being (what the organization does), why it does what it does, and for whom it does it, not just what it does. As a direct outgrowth of the organization's values, the mission guides leaders to make ethical choices and allocate resources appropriately. It is the foundation on which to base the answer to the question, are we doing the right things for the right reasons (Walston 2017)?

Key components of a mission statement include a definition of the organization's product or service, the organization's standards and values, and the population or key stakeholders the organization serves. The mission also sets boundaries beyond which the company does not venture. Some missions target a specific customer base. For example, an organization may state in its mission that it serves a special demographic segment (e.g., women, children) or a particular region.

The purpose of the mission statement is to describe the organization's competitive advantage: what the organization does differently or better than others (Walston and Chou 2012). The mission statements of organizations in an industry often are too similar, using similar common jargon and lacking elements that distinguish them from their competitors. Healthcare is not immune from these problems. Common mission statements include such wording as "providing world-class services" and "setting the community's quality standards." This lack of difference is frequently reflected in public relations materials that focus on the soft, caring aspect of healthcare employees. Most organizations over time tend to imitate their competitors and copy their structures, policies, and practices. This isomorphism suggests that, especially in fields such as healthcare, in which goals are ambiguous and great uncertainty exists, organizations may copy others as a result of external pressures from laws, accreditation rules, and professional associations (DiMaggio and Powell 1983).

Although the content of successful companies' missions varies, generally missions should contain (1) the services or products offered, (2) the values and standards that distinguish the organization, and (3) the market(s) in which the organization operates. Organizations express missions in many ways. Some are precise; others are lengthy. A mission statement should be long enough to be distinctive and guide an organization's strategies but concise enough that employees can remember and apply it. If a mission statement is too long, no one will recall and use it effectively to drive strategies and actions. For instance, Avon has a mission statement of 249 words "that cover everything from surpassing competitors to increasing shareholder value to fighting breast cancer" (Zetlin 2013). Clearly, few will remember or even read a statement this long. Short mission statements are easier to remember and communicate. For example, Nike's mission statement is very short: "To bring inspiration and innovation to every athlete in the world." As a rule of thumb, mission statements should contain no more than 35 words (Nike 2017).

Moreover, a mission should provide credible information about an organization. Again, while the mission statements of some successful companies do not appear to correspond to their line of business, a mission is more credible when employees and customers can relate the statement to the organization's actual actions and products or services. A mission statement that incorporates terms or content that is discordant with the organization's operations is unlikely to inspire stakeholders and motivate staff. For example, consider Coca-Cola's mission statement (Coca-Cola Company 2013):

> Our Roadmap starts with our mission, which is enduring. It declares our purpose as a company and serves as the standard against which we weigh our actions and decisions.
>
> - To refresh the world . . .
> - To inspire moments of optimism and happiness . . .
> - To create value and make a difference.

Although a highly successful company, Coca-Cola's mission statement does not accurately describe the products it offers. The phrase "to inspire moments of optimism and happiness" has little to do with beverages.

Like companies in other sectors, healthcare organizations should not use nondescript, generic statements—for example, "providing the highest quality of care for the lowest possible cost"—that in some derivation appear in many mission statements. Such declarations are virtually meaningless. In this example, the lowest possible cost is clearly zero. One might surmise from this mission that the organization aims to spend little or nothing and rely largely or exclusively on volunteer services.

The experience of King Faisal Specialist Hospital (KFS) of Saudi Arabia, related in exhibit 6.6, demonstrates the development of a meaningful, distinctive mission statement. KFS had to determine what its actual purpose was and what functions existed to support that purpose. Instead of embracing multiple purposes, the hospital determined that its primary reason for existence was the provision of specialized medical services. Education and research were important but only secondary to KFS's focus—patient services.

Too often, mission statements bear little relationship to a company's actual operational focus. To be more than a public relations device, the mission needs to reflect all key aspects and behaviors of an organization (Holland 2007). Many healthcare organizations' mission statements are fixated on quality and omit critical factors, diminishing the mission's impact on their performance (Clarke 2009).

This issue is pronounced for many for-profit healthcare organizations whose mission (and sometimes vision) statements do not address the financial returns required by their key stakeholders. Statements of for-profit companies that do not include expected returns—a primary purpose of for-profit companies—are less credible and often may fail to motivate employees, especially when their leaders focus intensely on profitability. In these situations, employees commonly feel that their leaders' actions contradict their organization's stated mission.

EXHIBIT 6.6
Determining the Real Mission That Drives an Organization

King Faisal Specialist Hospital (KFS), a 936-bed tertiary facility in Saudi Arabia focused primarily on highly sophisticated and complicated cases, was affiliated with a medical school and had many residents but did not provide education. The hospital had developed a semiautonomous research center that had studied a number of different topics. KFS's mission stated, "The KFS Hospital will provide medical services of highly specialized nature and promote medical research and education programs, including postgraduate education training, as well as contribute to the prevention of disease."

To facilitate its planning process, the hospital hired a consultant. Subsequently, KFS's top managers held a meeting to discuss the hospital's mission statement and determine whether it should be changed. The consultant identified four main purposes for the existence of the hospital in the mission statement:

1. Provision of highly specialized (tertiary and quaternary) services
2. Promotion of medical research
3. Promotion of educational programs, including postgraduate training
4. Prevention of disease

Discussion ensued regarding the actual importance of these four areas at KFS Hospital. The meeting attendees finally agreed that the real purpose of the hospital was to serve as the referral center for tertiary and quaternary services in Saudi Arabia and that the other three reasons were secondary to this focus. One person pointed out that the hospital provided few preventive services. Following extensive comments and wordsmithing, the group agreed on the following mission statement: "The KFS Hospital exists to provide the highest quality, specialized healthcare through an integrated education and research setting."

This statement clarified that the real purpose of the hospital was the provision of specialized healthcare and that the research and educational programs were engaged to help provide the specialized patient services and therefore should be directly tied to a process to increase the sophistication and competence of the provision of highly specialized healthcare.

Source: King Faisal Specialist Hospital (2017).

For example, a prominent for-profit healthcare system lists the following as its mission and values statement, which is silent on profitability and return on investment (HCA 2017):

> Mission and Values
> Above all else, we are committed to the care and improvement of human life. In recognition of this commitment, we strive to deliver high-quality, cost-effective healthcare in the communities we serve.
>
> In pursuit of our mission, we believe the following value statements are essential and timeless:

- We recognize and affirm the unique and intrinsic worth of each individual.
- We treat all those we serve with compassion and kindness.
- We trust our colleagues as valuable members of our healthcare team and pledge to treat one another with loyalty, respect, and dignity.
- We act with absolute honesty, integrity, and fairness in the way we conduct our business and the way we live our lives.

Yet in the author's experience, this system focuses extensively on profitability, with its pretax income almost $4 billion in 2015 (MarketWatch 2017).

Compare this mission statement to that of Novartis, a for-profit global pharmaceutical company (Novartis 2017):

> We want to discover, develop and successfully market innovative products to prevent and cure diseases, to ease suffering and to enhance the quality of life.
>
> We also want to provide a shareholder return that reflects **outstanding performance** and to adequately reward those who invest **ideas and work** in our company.

This statement balances quality and profits and more accurately captures the company's overall purpose.

Organizations should review their mission statements periodically to evaluate their effectiveness and relevance and ensure that organizations' actions are in line with their missions. The following questions can help organizations identify aspects that are missing or in need of modification. Does the mission (Sufi and Lyons 2003) do the following?

1. Define the organization's products or services and the markets in which it competes
2. Communicate where the company is and where it is going
3. Define and express concern for its key stakeholders
4. Motivate employees and reflect actual daily practice
5. Discuss the organization's commitment to economic objectives of prosperity, growth, and profitability
6. Incorporate the organization's basic beliefs, values, aspirations, and philosophical priorities
7. Indicate the competence or competitive advantage that distinguishes the organization from its competitors
8. Suggest the level and nature of the organization's social commitment

In summary, mission statements must inspire and call employees to action by being meaningful and free of jargon. One academic estimated that only 10 percent of mission statements say something meaningful (Holland

2007). Missions should direct organizations to focus their energies, help leaders develop action plans and allocate resources, and both constrain and guide strategies and tactical actions.

Vision

The third part of an organization's strategic intent is its vision. While some organizations combine their vision and mission, the two have different purposes. The vision is the organization's desired future state—what it wishes to become—while the mission describes the organization's existing purpose and practices. A clearly articulated, widely held vision can highly motivate employees (Walston 2017).

Leaders should understand and use the vision to build goals and strategic actions. It should be intrinsically tied to employees' work so that they feel proud and excited to be part of a design much bigger than themselves. The vision also should challenge and stretch the organization's capabilities and image of itself and set a time horizon of at least five to ten years. Organizations create visions through a visualization process in which leaders imagine what the organization should be. Good vision statements ground and direct an organization and give shape to its future and are especially helpful during turbulent times of change.

As described in exhibit 6.7, employees who understand the real purpose and vision of their organization and believe they are working toward a meaningful end will be more fully committed to their jobs. Stressing financial returns and profits alone will not inspire this level of motivation.

Vision statements can be even more important in not-for-profit organizations. Without a primary bottom-line focus, not-for-profits can use an effective vision as a guide to meeting the challenges of their environment (Kilpatrick and Silverman 2005). A concise vision written in clear language can provide specific, meaningful ideas to solidify an organization's goals and direction.

EXHIBIT 6.7
Who Has the Vision?

A man was passing by a work site where bricklayers were building a wall. It was still too early in the construction process to see what they were building. The man stopped and asked, "What are you doing?" One worker answered, "I am laying bricks." The man continued on his walk and then stopped to talk to a second worker further along the construction site. Again, the man asked, "What are you doing?" The second worker responded, "I am building a tall, strong wall." The man thanked the second worker and continued walking. Near the end of the work site, the man stopped a third time to ask another worker the same question. The third worker faced the man and stated, "I am building a cathedral for the glory of God."

Whose response captured the essence of a vision, and how do you think it influenced the quality of his work?

An organization can evaluate its vision statement by asking the following questions:

- Does the vision place the organization on the correct path to where it wants to go?
- Are the organization's current strategic actions consistent with the vision?
- What needs to happen this year, next year, and in three years to achieve the vision?
- Will achievement of the vision meet key stakeholders' needs? How?
- Does the vision depict a future that will be challenging to achieve, yet is attainable?

Like missions, visions should be relatively short and written in understandable language. Employees should be able to remember the statement's key components easily. Poor vision statements often include bland, generic phrases, interweave goals and objectives, and speculate on the unknown. For example, the author consulted with one hospital in the northwestern United States that embarked on a five-year project to change its culture and dramatically lower its costs. The vision, set by the CEO, was to say "welcome to a journey of change." Employees were confused and seemed cynical about the vision. It was unclear about the hospital's desired outcomes and did not motivate employees as the CEO had hoped.

Visions should be specific enough that someone not familiar with the organization would still be able to identify the industry to which it belongs. For example, one company's vision—"First for customers, first for employees, and first for shareholders"—is so nonspecific that it could be from any industry. As a result, it was of little benefit to the company. In contrast, the vision of LifePoint Hospitals, a national for-profit healthcare system, is clear and concise and identifies the healthcare sector (LifePoint Hospitals 2017):

> We want to create places where:
>
> - Patients choose to come for healthcare,
> - Physicians want to practice, and
> - Employees want to work.

In addition to customizing the vision for the field, LifePoint's vision specifies three key stakeholder groups and measurable outcomes.

On the other hand, some organizations create visions that are too specific, long, and complex to be useful. For example, the vision statement of Snohomish County Long Term Care & Aging is rather long and complicated (Snohomish County 2012):

Snohomish County Long Term Care & Aging is dedicated to creating and sustaining:

- a caring and compassionate community that fully understands the aging process and the issues involved in meeting the needs of older persons
- a community that endeavors to improve the quality of life for older persons, their families and caregivers in Snohomish County
- a community composed of older persons who maximize their independence and have freedom in life choices
- a community where older persons are respected, valued and accepted as individuals who both contribute to and are supported by the community
- a community that supports and reaches out to older persons who are disabled, isolated, low-income, persons of color, limited English speaking, or any who face barriers to full participation in programs and services.

This vision for a compassionate, elder-friendly community would ensure that all older persons, especially older adults who are vulnerable or disabled:

- have adequate income for retirement
- have their basic need for food, nutrition and shelter met,
- have access to affordable health care, including dental care, mental health services and prescription medications,
- have meaningful opportunities, both paid and volunteer, to remain active in the community,
- are supported in their efforts to plan and manage their own lives,
- are protected from abuse, neglect and exploitation,
- are linked to the community, regardless of their geographic location, income, cultural background or ability to speak English,
- are able to readily gain information and assistance in accessing services,
- have affordable housing options and a transportation system providing access to community activities and services
- benefit from a physical environment that encourages connection rather than isolation.

Although the second paragraph states the desired outcomes of this vision, there appear to be far too many potential metrics. The length of this vision statement and its multiple aims make it difficult to remember and to incorporate into strategic decisions.

In summary, a vision should

- be part of an organization's strategic intent,
- express what the organization wants to become,

- foster commitment and galvanize employees to action,
- be short enough to remember and be understandable, and
- show employees what they are striving for and give meaning to their work.

Chapter Summary

Organizations are created for the benefit of their stakeholders. At the same time, stakeholders support and invest in organizations. Many different groups of stakeholders exist, and some are more important to an organization than others. Key stakeholders should be highly involved in the creation and implementation of an organization's strategic intent. Strategic intent consists of values, missions, and visions. For organizations to enjoy sustainable prosperity, they must be driven by their mission and vision and be committed to practicing a set of values. Companies' strategic intents will vary, according to the purpose of an organization. In healthcare, a wide variance is found between not-for-profit and for-profit organizations, depending on the type of service. More than three-fourths of hospitals in the United States are not-for-profit; more than 80 percent of home health agencies, dialysis centers, and medical device and pharmaceutical companies are for-profit. Whatever the strategic intent, organizations' actions should be consistent with their mission and vision.

Values guide an organization's decisions and actions. They state what is and is not acceptable behavior; they are the foundation of the organization's culture. The aim to maximize profits will not motivate employees over time. Values can be essential principles guiding all of an organization's actions and forming the basis of its culture. Values should create the ethical environment in which all employees function, informing organizational decisions and helping to resolve conflicts.

An organization's mission is an enduring statement of core organizational purpose that distinguishes it from other organizations and identifies the scope of its operations in terms of products and markets. Missions describe what a company does, why, and for whom. Most companies possess written mission statements. Yet many are not well written or are not used effectively to motivate employees. To inspire an organization's mission should be the foundation of its strategic direction and reflect its values. The mission indicates which stakeholders are most important, and its fulfillment is the basis for judging an organization's success. A mission should use clear, understandable language, not jargon. It becomes meaningful only when it begins to affect the behavior and actions of stakeholders. It is the foundation for the answer to the question, are we doing the right things for the right reasons? At minimum, mission statements should contain (1) the services or products offered, (2) the values and standards that distinguish the organization, and (3) the market or markets in which the organization operates.

Vision statements point to a future state the organization seeks to emulate. While some organizations combine their vision and mission, the two have different purposes. The vision describes the organization's desired future state—what it wishes to become—while the mission describes the organization's existing purpose and practices. To be effective, mission and vision statements must be credible and clear. Leaders should understand and use the vision to compose goals and strategic actions. The vision also should challenge and stretch the organization's capabilities and image of itself and set a time horizon of at least five to ten years.

Chapter Questions

1. What is a stakeholder? What are some common groups of stakeholders in healthcare?
2. Why would groups' or individuals' interest in and power to influence an organization determine whether they are key stakeholders? What other factors might be considered?
3. Does an organization's strategic intent always need to specify a mission, a vision, and values separately? Why or why not?
4. How might an organization's culture reflect its established values?
5. What are the three essential components of a mission?
6. Why do many organizations fail to use their mission and vision effectively?
7. What is the purpose of a vision?

Chapter Cases

Case Studies

In the case studies section at the end of the book, read and discuss one of the following cases: "An Orthopedic Group Decides to Construct a Specialty Hospital," "The Struggle of a Safety Net Hospital," or "Build a New Service Because of a Large Donation?" Answer the questions at the end of the case.

The Unknown Mission and Vision

A consultant was asked to work with a large academic medical center's top leaders on their strategies and future plans. The leaders exhibited a great

(continued)

passion and desire to improve their organization and meet forthcoming challenges. However, they felt that the center's direction was inconsistent. Some indicated that it seemed to adopt each fad and then discard it almost as quickly. Others felt that the center had good strategic goals but did not seem to implement them.

To address these concerns, the consultant presented the principles of values, mission, and vision. As a learning exercise, he asked the leaders to comment on missions and visions he had gathered from several healthcare organizations, including the center's own mission and vision. Discussion ensued regarding the good and bad points of the different missions and visions. At the conclusion of this discussion, the consultant asked the group to identify the organizations to which the missions and visions belonged. Many guesses followed. When they came to the center's mission and vision, no one recognized the statements as the center's own.

Questions

1. Why do you think the leaders did not recognize their own mission and vision?
2. How does this lack of recognition tie in with their perception of inconsistency in the center's efforts?

Mission Matters Merger

In the 1980s, two healthcare organizations with distinct cultures attempted a merger that soon ran into trouble. How, and why, are mergers difficult? Consider the following history.

In 1975, Idaho Falls, Idaho, had two hospitals: Community Hospital of Idaho Falls and Idaho Falls Hospital. The first was managed by a community board and the latter was controlled by Intermountain Health Care (IHC), a regional healthcare system based in Salt Lake City, Utah, more than 200 miles away. To control costs of duplicate management and services, the two hospitals merged in 1978 to form the Idaho Falls Consolidated Hospitals, with two campuses: Parkview and Riverview.

However, the merger dissolved in 1984, and the board of the Community Hospital of Idaho Falls asked Hospital Corporation of America (HCA) to manage the Parkview facility and eventually replace it with a new healthcare facility. Local physicians wanted a single regional medical center, and eventually IHC and the Idaho Falls Community Hospital boards signed an agreement to build a joint venture hospital managed by HCA. In 1985, ground was broken for the HCA Eastern Idaho Regional Medical Center (EIRMC), which opened its doors to patients on December 22, 1986. The 1,074 employees of Parkview and Riverview Hospitals were terminated at midnight on December 21, 1986, and hired by EIRMC one minute later. The members of the medical staff no longer had to cross town to see their patients at two facilities. Significant savings to the community and reduced healthcare costs were predicted.

Although IHC controlled only 49 percent of the joint venture, it expected a collaborative relationship. Senior leaders of IHC trusted that HCA would work with them to maintain reasonable hospital charges and develop appropriate services for the Idaho Falls community. As one leader later reflected, he thought a handshake and promise would suffice.

However, almost immediately, the differences in missions arose and quickly became pronounced. What HCA and IHC thought was good for the community and for themselves appeared incompatible. As a for-profit, HCA's managers immediately focused on reducing costs and increasing prices. IHC, on the other hand, desired cost efficiencies, but nothing as austere as those pursued by the HCA. It also wanted prices to remain lower. But IHC did not manage the facility and only had influence at the board level.

Employees also struggled to work together. The cultures of the two previous hospitals had been very different. Turnover increased and conflicts erupted. These issues and differences became very clear when the board, which was made up of HCA and IHC leaders, was presented with the first EIRMC budget. The profit expectations were more than double what IHC would earn in one of its solely owned facilities. The CEO of IHC wanted this merger to work, but could it?

Questions

1. Why is the merger having difficulty? What factors cause mergers to fail?
2. How does having distinct missions affect how an organization structures its processes and outcomes?
3. What could be done to solve the problems? Is merging a for-profit with a not-for-profit doomed to failure?
4. Can organizations with such different missions merge? If so, how?

Chapter Assignments

1. Use class discussion and reading to infer the potential effect of various statements of strategic intent on organizations' strategic behavior.
   a. Choose two for-profit and two not-for profit hospitals, and identify their values, missions, and visions.

   b. Compare their values, mission, and vision statements. Are there any significant or subtle differences? If you feel they are the same, why?
   c. Does each statement contain the minimum content discussed in this chapter?
   d. Do you think these statements really guide the organizations' strategic actions? Why or why not?
2. Look at the following three mission statements, and evaluate them using the mission evaluation criteria given in this chapter. Which components does each of these statements contain? Lack? What would you recommend to improve these missions? Which could you as an employee understand and use best?

   a. "The American Red Cross prevents and alleviates human suffering in the face of emergencies by mobilizing the power of volunteers and the generosity of donors" (American Red Cross 2017).
   b. "Together with our customers and partners, we are creating a sustainable future for healthcare. Together we are charting a course to better health" (McKesson 2013).
   c. "Discover. Teach. Heal" (UC Irvine Health 2017).

3. Many healthcare organizations have been subject to state and federal fines and criminal investigation. Identify an organization that did not act in accordance with its values, mission, and vision and incurred criminal or civil fines as a result. In a one-page paper, describe how the organization's activities did not reflect its written strategic intent and propose lawful actions it could have taken to embrace its written values and achieve better outcomes.

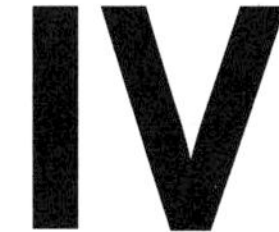

PART

IV

UNDERSTANDING ORGANIZATIONAL POSITION

Understanding one's position in a market is a critical aspect of strategy development. An organization must understand its competitors and recognize its competencies, capabilities, and weaknesses. Chapters 7, 8, and 9 explore organizations' dependence on their environment and offer means of analyzing and understanding it. Environmental factors such as the availability of key employees, new technology, laws, and competitors significantly affect an organization's strategies. Chapter 7 evaluates the external environment and its influence on organizations' actions, and chapter 8 examines the internal environment as a means of identifying organizations' capabilities and opportunities. An understanding of both environments is important to position oneself in a strategically appropriate manner. Chapter 9 provides valuable financial tools for evaluating organizations' financial performance.

Organizations can use environmental review to check the validity of their *assumptions*—propositions taken for granted and often based on limited evidence. To craft effective strategies, organizations must challenge past assumptions. In many cases, assumptions are incorrect and faulty. Faulty assumptions may arise from false traditions or new realities in an ever-changing world. As Dov Seidman (2011, 2) states, "We are in the grip of . . . false assumptions. In other words, our thinking and twentieth-century habits of thought and behavior are getting in the way of responding to the new realities that require attention in the twenty-first century."

Healthcare is no exception. Past assumptions about healthcare in the twenty-first century promoted by "experts" suggested that hospital inpatient care would be rare, health maintenance organizations (HMOs) would provide most health insurance, and only integrated healthcare delivery systems would be successful. Each of these assumptions proved to be unfounded (Burns and Pauly 2002). Organizations that based their strategies on these assumptions spent huge sums of money to form structures and design networks that came to be of little strategic benefit. Organizations that fail to correct faulty assumptions suffer.

By periodically scanning the environment, an organization can gather updated information and adjust its assumptions. Environmental assessment also enables an organization to better understand its and its competitors' strengths and weaknesses and evaluate the opportunities and threats it faces and may face in the future.

CHAPTER

7

THE EXTERNAL ENVIRONMENT AND STRATEGY

> "It's hard to plan a business with this many outstanding questions," said Ceci Connolly, CEO of the Alliance for Community Health Plans, which represents not-for-profit insurers.
>
> . . . observers acknowledge that congressional GOP leaders themselves don't know what they're going to put in the ACA's place—or precisely how they'll do it.
>
> —Harris Meyer, "Outlook for 2017: Healthcare Re-reform," 2016

Learning Objectives

After reading this chapter, you will

- comprehend Michael Porter's Five Forces model and its application to healthcare strategy,
- recognize market factors that increase competition,
- be aware of industry and market conditions that affect organizational strategies,
- be able to describe the concept and use of strategic groups,
- know how to use the concept of driving forces when developing strategy,
- be familiar with the techniques of PEST and force field analyses, and
- appreciate the concept of scenario analysis and how it can best be used.

What will be the future of healthcare? Many prognosticate, but the future is unknown. As stated at the opening of the chapter, the external environment, including governmental changes in policy, have tremendous impacts on healthcare. Major changes in the healthcare environment may dramatically affect how care is provided and managed. Advances in technology may allow more patient treatment in outpatient settings. For example, Deloitte predicts that "mobile health applications, telemedicine, mHealth, remote monitoring, and ingestible sensors" will permit physicians and patients to track symptoms in real time (Gov 2020 2017). The Institute for the Future concurs that healthcare information technology will generate abundant data that will allow physicians to better understand the health of their patients and enable patients to take more control of their care (Adler et al. 2009).

Some of these advances in technology may prove to be very disruptive to the field, including the following:

1. Artificial intelligence that can give providers access to clinically relevant, real-time data
2. Immunotherapies that may effectively treat various cancers
3. Liquid biopsies that can monitor tumors noninvasively
4. Gene editing that can make targeted modifications to DNA
5. Three-dimensional printing that can potentially customize human transplants and tissue repair (Das 2016)

The Healthcare Finance Management Association highlights the shift to value-based healthcare provision, the involvement of consumers as they take greater ownership of their care, and higher degrees of consolidation for healthcare insurers and providers as substantial changes on the horizon of healthcare (Healthcare Financial Management Association 2017).

Though the future is unknown, healthcare leaders need to understand the direction of the potential change and its impact on level and intensity of competition, and they must be prepared to shift their strategies and reallocate resources to achieve better mission advantage.

Any company must understand its relationship to the external environment and its strategies and products. This understanding is even more critical in the midst of change. Today the healthcare sector is faced with transformation. Johnson & Johnson recognizes this shift and states that it is "acutely aware of the need to evaluate our business against the changing health care environment." Globally, it observes the following changes:

- Populations of developed nations are rapidly aging
- Middle classes are expanding and demanding greater access to quality healthcare
- Patients are becoming more involved in their own healthcare decisions (Johnson & Johnson 2016)

These are only a fraction of the transforming dynamics in healthcare today. As shown in the introduction to this chapter, many predict significant changes that touch the entire healthcare ecosphere. The external environment comprises many interactive and complex factors important for effective strategic thinking. Various tools have been developed to assist with organizing environmental data to provide meaningful strategic information. This chapter discusses some of the more common methods of analyzing and examining the external environment.

Porter's Five Forces Model

In the early 1980s, Michael Porter (1985, 1980) developed the **Five Forces model**, a framework for identifying factors affecting the degree of market competition and the ability of established organizations to influence prices. As its name suggests, the Five Forces model (see exhibit 7.1) focuses on five forces that shape competition in an industry (Hitt, Ireland, and Hoskisson 2016):

Five Forces model A framework devised by Michael Porter that identifies five factors affecting the degree of competition in a market and the ability of established organizations to influence prices: (1) the potential for new entrants, (2) the threat of substitute products, (3) the power of suppliers, (4) the power of buyers, and (5) rivalry among competing sellers.

1. Possibility of new entrants: the risk and increased competition associated with the threat of new entrants
2. Threat of substitute products: increased competitiveness as a result of the availability or possible availability of substitutes for buyers' needs
3. Power of suppliers: the degree of suppliers' bargaining power and supplier–seller collaboration
4. Power of buyers: the degree of buyers' bargaining power and seller–buyer collaboration
5. Rivalry among competing sellers: the level of competitive pressures associated with market conditions and actions among rival sellers in an industry

Competitive forces vary from one industry (and often from one market) to another. Although Porter created the Five Forces model to examine the level of competition between industries and thus determine which industry might realize greater profits, the concept can also be used to understand the factors driving competitive forces within industries and markets. The forces exerting the greatest influence on competition vary among industries and markets. For example, the potential substitution of generic drugs for brand-name drugs is a significant influence in the pharmaceutical industry, while the threat of new entrants highly affects competition among healthcare recruitment companies.

The four outside elements in exhibit 7.1 strongly influence the rivalry among sellers of a product or service. The stronger the intensity of any of the five forces, the greater the level of competition. Likewise, the stronger the aggregate of the five forces, the greater the industry or market rivalry. As competition increases, competitors' ability to control prices and generate profits decreases.

EXHIBIT 7.1
Porter's Five Forces Model

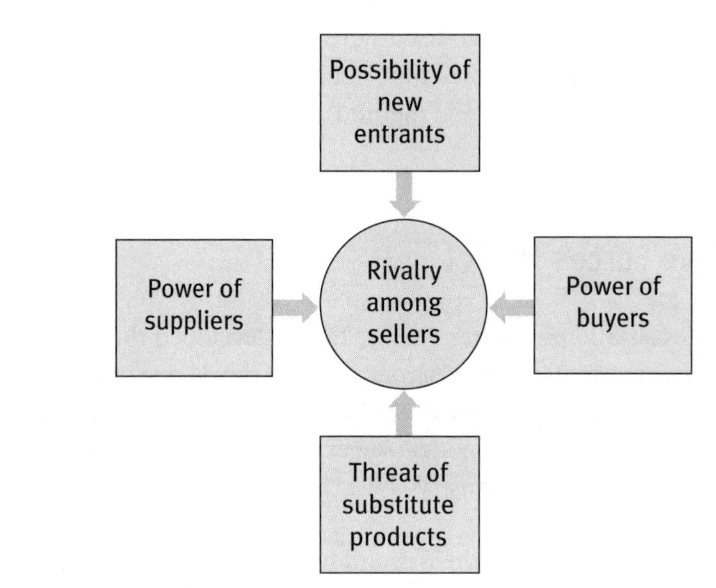

Pressures from the Threat of New Entrants

Porter (1980) stated that the threat of new entrants into an industry is a major factor affecting the intensity of rivalry and resultant profitability. New entrants bring new capacity and capabilities and change existing market relationships. Greater competition over price and quality may ensue, and incumbents may lose market share. As a result, they generate less revenue and their unit costs increase.

New entrants come not only from outside an industry but often also emerge from within when current industry members looking for growth opportunities expand into new geographic settings or introduce new products that compete with those of other incumbents (Hitt, Ireland, and Hoskisson 2016). For many existing hospitals, the greatest threat of entry is posed by for-profit systems seeking to expand into their markets or physician groups and to develop specialty facilities.

In the 1990s, the largest for-profit hospital company, Columbia/HCA, threatened to enter many markets, creating a great deal of tension and worry for incumbent hospitals. Many not-for-profit hospitals fought hard to keep Columbia/HCA out. In one year, more than 30 pending deals for expansion by Columbia/HCA were revoked or revised by regulatory, civic, and community opposition (Kuttner 1996; Watkins 1997). Just the threat of a for-profit entity entering a market significantly changed the behaviors of many market incumbents.

Barriers to entry
Obstacles that impede an organization as it seeks to enter a market.

Barriers to Entry

The degree of threat posed by new entrants depends on present barriers to entry. **Barriers to entry** are obstacles that impede a firm as it seeks to enter a market. They are outlined in the following section.

Economies of Scale

Economies of scale arise when the unit cost of a product or service declines as volume is added. Economies of scale exist primarily in organizations in which fixed costs—costs that do not vary with changes in volume—are a significant portion of the business's cost structure. As volume is added, fixed costs are spread across a larger base and the cost per unit decreases. The presence of economies of scale discourages organizations from entering markets because new entrants will not have the large volumes incumbents do and thus would risk having a cost-per-unit disadvantage. Companies may gain economies of scale through better use of plant and facilities, manufacturing, purchasing, research, marketing, and distribution (Porter 1980).

Economies of scale
Reductions in unit cost as a result of an increase in number of products or services produced.

For instance, contrast the difference in economies of scale between the opening of a hospital and the opening of a physician recruitment agency. The construction of a hospital requires a large capital expenditure to build nursing units, support space, ancillary equipment (e.g., radiology, laboratory), and a network of physicians who will refer patients to the facility. A large patient volume would be required to support these large, fixed expenses, and if the organization does not achieve this large number of patients, the cost per patient could be high. These factors reduce the prevalence of entry by new hospitals into markets in which incumbent hospitals have large economies of scale. In contrast, the economies of scale are minimal in a physician recruitment agency. The majority of costs are associated with recruitment activities (variable costs), and volumes do not significantly affect the cost per recruitment. Therefore, new agencies can enter the market with relative ease.

Some suggest that there are limited economies of scale available from merging hospital operations. Mergers save perhaps 15 percent, at most (Beckham 2016b).

Cost Disadvantages Not Related to Scale

Entrants often face cost disadvantages not related to scale. Existing organizations may enjoy benefits conferred by their experience or position on the learning curve, ownership of proprietary technology (e.g., patents), established partnerships with complementary organizations and networks (e.g., insurance plans, physician networks), favorable locations, governmental subsidies, and lower facility costs. These factors can become strong deterrents to new entries.

Customer Loyalty

Customers' loyalty to established products may be a significant barrier to entry because new organizations must spend heavily on promotion or substantially lower prices to change customers' perceptions and convince them to switch to new products. These up-front expenditures for marketing and promotion are not recoverable if the new organization is unsuccessful.

Sunk Costs

Large financial investments required to successfully enter a market deter entry, especially investments that cannot be recovered (i.e., *sunk costs*) or would be difficult to recover if the venture fails. The heavy financial investments required up front for building pharmaceutical manufacturing facilities and hospitals, for inventories and marketing, and for insurance are all difficult to recover in such cases. For example, FHP International, once a large HMO in the western United States, built a hospital in Salt Lake City in the 1990s, only to find that—after it opened—the hospital was not needed. The company retreated from owning a hospital in this market and sold the facility for a fraction of the price of its construction. The hospital was later mothballed and required tax subsidies to convert it to retail and commercial space (Jones 1999).

Switching Costs

Switching costs
The costs associated with changing a product, brand, marketplace, or supplier.

Switching costs are real or perceived costs associated with changing a product, brand, marketplace, or supplier. Costs can be monetary, psychological, or physical. The higher these costs are, the more difficult it can be for customers to change. Contract cancellation penalties and software incompatibilities with new hardware are common switching costs. An example in healthcare is the psychological cost of changing primary care physicians. Insurance companies that have restrictive physician networks may have difficulty attracting new customers if customers perceive that the change and new restrictions will cost them psychologically.

Access to Distribution Channels

Entrants may not have easy access to distribution channels. Products and services are exchanged within some type of distribution channel. Companies may have their own distribution channel or use another organization's channel. The best products will not sell unless consumers have access to them through a distribution channel. Pharmaceutical and healthcare equipment companies (e.g., Pfizer, Roche, GE, Toshiba) have extensive networks of salespeople. The more exclusive distribution channels are toward existing companies, the more difficult it is to enter a market. For example, many insurance companies (managed care firms) have established exclusive contracts for services. As Healthcare.gov explains, exclusive provider organizations are managed care plans in which services are covered only if one uses doctors, specialists, or hospitals in the plan's network (except in an emergency). Providers outside these contracts desiring to enter these markets often find it difficult to do so (Healthcare.gov 2017).

Governmental Policy

Governmental policy can complicate or even block entry into a market. Legislative barriers include licensure, permits, and regulatory rules. Healthcare is highly regulated by the government. Extensive professional licensure, construction permits, and regulatory review are required to ensure quality and moderate costs. In addition, many US states still sponsor **certificate of need (CON)** laws, which require organizations to obtain approval from a state planning agency before beginning a major capital project. The CON programs were created to restrain healthcare costs. As of December 2016, 37 states had active CON laws (National Conference of State Legislatures 2016). Likewise, many US states require unnecessary supervision and paperwork that restrict nurse practitioners' (NPs) scope of practice. In 2016, 29 states did not allow them full authority to practice, though most evidence does not support these restrictions (Pohl et al. 2016).

Certificate of need (CON)
State laws in the United States that require organizations to obtain approval from a state planning agency before beginning a major capital project.

The greater the number and strength of these barriers, the more difficult entry is for new organizations. Conversely, when these factors are not present or are weak, new organizations may easily enter markets and increase competition and rivalry.

The following questions can be used to assess the strength of barriers to entry. A greater number of positive answers suggests a favorable, less competitive market environment. Negative answers to the majority of the questions indicate that the market environment is likely to be competitive and difficult to enter.

- Do you have a unique process or product that is protected by patent?
- Are customers loyal to your brand and product?
- Does your type of business require high start-up costs?
- Are the assets needed to operate your type of business unique and hard to obtain?
- Are your business's processes and procedures difficult to learn?
- Would a new rival have difficulty purchasing key inputs?
- Would a new competitor have difficulty finding customers?
- Would it be difficult for a new entrant to attract enough customers and resources to operate efficiently?

The Threat of Substitute Products

The prevalence of substitute products can also meaningfully affect the level of market rivalry. Consumers select products and services on the basis of a mix of quality, cost, and features. Closely related industries almost always produce products that can be substituted for each other but differ with respect to quality, cost, and features. Substitute products can come from another industry or originate from existing competitors (Porter 1980). For example, contact lenses and glasses are a substitute for corrective laser surgery, a service provided by a different industry. Alternative medicine (e.g., acupuncture, naturopathy) in place of prescription drugs is another example of a cross industry substitute. Examples of substitutes in a common sector—healthcare—include physician specialists versus primary care providers and medical versus surgical treatments. Consumers substitute one product or service for another on the basis of their perception of the trade-offs between the quality, cost, and features of the products or services.

Organizations can blunt the threat of substitutes by understanding their existing customers' preferences, recognizing shifts, and differentiating their brands. However, the presence of substitutes pressures incumbent organizations to lower their prices and may stimulate innovation. The strength of substitutes' competitive pressure depends on whether the substitutes are readily available to customers. For instance, the competitive effect of a surgery center opening across the street from a hospital would be much greater than the effect of one opening ten miles away. Substitutes' price structure also influences the level of competition. Substitutes priced lower than an established product can exert intense competitive pressure. Lower prices may provoke competitive responses from incumbent organizations; companies may engage in price wars, increase their advertising, or introduce new product features or designs.

A substitute's key attributes also may affect the level of competition. Key attributes include the perceived quality of the product, including its performance. Newly introduced substitute products often are lower quality and lower priced than established products. Over time, however, product quality and pricing change to more directly compete with existing products.

Technological advances have introduced substitutions in healthcare. For example, in the 1990s laparoscopic surgery replaced traditional surgery for gallbladder removal, hernia repair, and appendectomies. Likewise, medications have almost completely replaced surgery for the treatment of peptic ulcer disease (Kotler, Shalowitz, and Stevens 2008).

Executives can evaluate the threat of substitutes by answering the following questions:

- Does your product offer more benefits than its substitutes do? If so, why are the benefits of your product valued by consumers? Are the benefits sustainable?
- Is the price for your product the same or less than the price for comparable substitutes?
- Is it difficult (monetarily or psychologically) for your customers to switch to another product?
- Are customers loyal to your existing products and brands?

Power of Suppliers

Suppliers exert competitive pressure when they have sufficient bargaining power to influence prices and the terms of their sales. Powerful suppliers can extract concessions from their buyers. Suppliers are powerful if they are few in number and more concentrated than buyers. Likewise, if an industry purchases a small proportion of sellers' product volume and the rest is sold to buyers in a different industry, and the product is important to buyers' business, suppliers' power is enhanced (Porter 1980). Suppliers consist of a wide array of organizations, ranging from unions (suppliers of workers), intermediaries such as HMOs and insurance companies, and retail outlets to wholesalers and manufacturers of raw materials.

Sellers in healthcare have become more concentrated in the recent past. Consolidation has occurred in hospitals, pharmaceutical drug companies, insurance companies, medical supply companies, and physician groups and has generally increased suppliers' power. The bargaining power of sellers has become strong in some of these markets. For example, certain medications necessary for the treatment of cancer and bacterial infections are sold by only a few pharmaceutical companies. In 2011, these firms produced an inadequate supply of approximately 180 drugs, which caused prices to rise as much as twentyfold (Harris 2011). Likewise, exclusive suppliers of specialized drugs can charge high prices. The three highest priced drugs in 2016 for a 30-day supply were Sovaldi (hepatitis C, $81,000), Harvoni (hepatitis C, $79,200), and Cinryze (hereditary angioedema, $72,100) (Ramsey 2016).

Insurance companies, which supply patients to physicians and hospitals, have completed significant mergers since the 1980s. This consolidation has substantially increased the market share and supplier power of a few large plans. By 2014, one of the largest US healthcare insurance companies controlled more than 80 percent of the large group market in seven states (Alabama, Alaska, Arkansas, Mississippi, North Dakota, South Carolina, Vermont). This dominance has enabled insurance companies to aggressively increase their premiums and enjoy higher profits (Trish and Herring 2015).

The following questions can be used to ascertain suppliers' relative bargaining power in a market. The greater the number of positive responses, the lesser the suppliers' power; the greater the number of negative responses, the greater the suppliers' power and, potentially, the greater the competition.

- Is there a large number of potential suppliers for your critical inputs?
- Are there potential substitutes for your critical inputs?
- Do your purchases from certain suppliers represent a small portion of your business?
- Would it be difficult for your supplier to enter your business and sell directly to your customers?
- Are you well informed about your supplier's product and market?

Power of Buyers

The power of buyers is almost the mirror image of the power of suppliers. Buyers can have little or extensive market power, depending on their size, their number, and the nature of the market. Transactions between buyers and sellers create value, but when buyers have greater power, the sellers may lose a large portion of that value, along with profits. Buyers enjoy more power when they are large relative to sellers and purchase a large part of a business's output. Individuals can pay the displayed price, wait for a sale, or take their business elsewhere, but overall their power is much weaker than that of organizations and groups that collectively purchase (Hitt, Ireland, and Hoskisson 2016).

In contrast to supplier power, buyer power increases if switching costs are low, the number of buyers is small relative to the number of sellers, the demand for the product is marginal, buyers have a good understanding of the purchase, buyers can acquire sellers (backward integration) fairly easily, and the products sellers offer are not critical to the buyers' business. Tension is always present between buyers and sellers, and their relative power depends on these market factors.

As mentioned, larger buying groups have greater negotiating power and receive concessions on price and delivery times, special features, and other factors. Healthcare buyers include group purchasing organizations; pharmaceutical wholesalers; medical-surgical distributors; independent contracted distributors; and providers, such as healthcare systems, integrated delivery networks, ambulatory surgery centers, and physician offices (Burns and Wharton School colleagues 2002).

Group purchasing organizations (GPOs)
Alliances formed to give member organizations greater negotiating power and concessions on price, delivery times, and quality when purchasing products or services.

Initially formed by clusters of hospitals and later expanded to include other providers, **group purchasing organizations (GPOs)** increase their bargaining power over suppliers by bringing organizations together to make group purchases from product and nonlabor vendors. Most hospitals and a growing number of non-acute care facilities use the services of GPOs today. Although there are more than 50 GPOs in the United States that serve the healthcare field, seven large GPOs accounted for 90 percent of hospitals' purchases in 2015, excluding Veterans Administration and Department of Defense hospitals (Definitive Healthcare 2016). These seven are listed in exhibit 7.2. These very large GPOs control billions of dollars of purchases annually. Their immense size and importance exert power over sellers; as a result, GPOs secure lower prices and better service for member hospitals and their respective systems. Purchasing managers believe that GPOs negotiate prices that are 10 to 16 percent lower than the prices any one organization in the group could negotiate on its own; GPOs saved more than $55 billion for hospitals in 2013 (Burns and Wharton School colleagues 2002; Healthcare Supply Chain Association 2014).

As mentioned, the importance of the buyer's size is relative to the seller's size. A buyer does not have to purchase billions of dollars of products to have an influential impact. For example, in many markets, health management organizations—small when compared to a national market—may exercise power in their local markets to obtain significant price concessions.

EXHIBIT 7.2
Top Seven GPOs

GPO Name	Location
AmerisourceBergen	Charlotte, NC
Cardinal Health	Alpharetta, GA
HealthTrust	Irving, TX
Intalere	St. Louis, MO
McKesson Pharmaceutical	Dublin, OH
Premier Inc.	San Francisco, CA
Vizient Inc.	Chesterbrook, PA

Source: Definitive Healthcare provider analytics database, accessed May 2017. Used by permission.

The following questions can help organizations ascertain the strength of buyers' power in a market. If the majority of the answers are positive, buyers have limited power; if the majority are negative, buyers have strong market power.

- Do you have enough customers that the loss of one will not significantly damage your business?
- Does your product account for a relatively small expense for your buyers?
- Is it difficult to understand your market, and are buyers poorly informed?
- Is your product unique and differentiated in the minds of your buyers?
- Would it be difficult for your buyers to purchase one of your competitors and then produce the products you offer?
- Would it be difficult for customers to switch from your products to those of your competitors?

Rivalry Among Competing Organizations

The intensity of rivalry may vary in different markets. Companies generally seek to gain better market positions, greater sales and market share, and other competitive advantages. To achieve gains in these areas, organizations may lower their prices, add new or different features to their products (e.g., higher quality, better product performance), emphasize their brand image, offer a wider selection of products and services, expand their distribution network, offer low-interest financing, increase their advertising, provide longer warranties, or improve customer service, among other strategies (Hitt, Ireland, and Hoskisson 2016; Porter 1980).

Rivals react to each other's strategies. Many factors moderate the extent of such competition, including the anticipated actions of rivals. Responsive actions vary by organizations' mission, culture, and management processes and often are difficult to predict. In most industries, actions by one organization commonly are copied or countered by its rivals. The pattern of action and response may escalate into a cycle of move and countermove, weakening all businesses involved. Price wars can be especially detrimental because initial price cuts are easily matched, potentially reducing the overall profitability of the industry and weakening individual organizations.

As discussed previously, the extent of rivalry relates to the number of organizations in a market. Rivalry is intense in perfect competition and much less so in oligopolies. However, other factors also influence the degree of competition. As shown in exhibit 7.3, these factors include the equality of organizations' strengths, the degree of product differentiation, the height of exit barriers, different ownership types, and the rate of demand growth.

Equality of Organizations' Strengths

Various organizational factors affect the nature of rivalry in a market. For instance, the more similar organizations are in terms of size, market share, and competitive capability, the greater the market rivalry. Distribution of market share also affects the level of competition. The level of rivalry can vary dramatically depending on whether market share is concentrated among a few organizations or more evenly distributed, regardless of the number of organizations in the market. For example, oligopolies exist in many configurations. In some markets, one organization is dominant, while in others, two or more organizations may dominate the market. Markets dominated by one organization tend to be less competitive, while more evenly distributed market share encourages rivalry.

The level and nature of competition affect organizations differently, depending on the organization's market position and the market's structure. The competitive pressures that large organizations experience tend to be much different from those experienced by their smaller competitors. Smaller organizations' actions often have little effect on their large rivals and elicit little or no reaction. On the other hand, similarly sized organizations often compete intensely. Therefore, within markets, smaller, equally sized organizations may experience greater competitive pressures than a large, dominant firm might.

Exhibits 7.4, 7.5, 7.6, and 7.7 provide market share data on three oligopolies experiencing different competitive interactions. In Indianapolis, Indiana, a few healthcare systems control a substantial portion of the market. The systems of Indiana University Health (formerly Clarian Health), Ascension

EXHIBIT 7.3
Organizational and Product-Related Factors Affecting Rivalry

- Equality of organizations' strengths
- Degree of product differentiation
- Height of exit barriers
- Different ownership types
- Rate of demand growth

EXHIBIT 7.4 Market Distribution by Inpatient Beds in Indianapolis, Oklahoma City, and Utah Wasatch Front Acute Care Hospital Markets, 2013

Indianapolis[1]			Utah Wasatch Front[2]			Oklahoma City[3]		
Health System or Hospital	**Beds**	**% of Market**	**Health System or Hospital**	**Beds**	**% of Market**	**Health System or Hospital**	**Beds**	**% of Market**
Indiana University Health	1,778	42.0	Intermountain Healthcare	2,025	51.0	INTEGRIS Health	924	27.0
Ascension Health (St. Vincent)	988	23.0	HCA	868	22.0	HCA	728	21.2
Community Health Network	775	18.0	IASIS Healthcare	580	14.0	SSM Health Care (St. Anthony)	551	16.1
Franciscan Alliance	299	7.0	University of Utah Health Care	504	13.0	Mercy	344	10.0
Wishard Memorial Hospital	293	7.0				Community Health Systems	283	8.2
Westview Hospital	67	2.0				Health Management Associates	255	7.4
Indiana Orthopaedic Hospital	38	1.0				Oklahoma Heart Hospital	145	4.2
						McBride Orthopedic Hospital	78	2.2
						Community Hospital of Oklahoma	49	1.4
						Lakeside Women's Hospital	23	0.7
						Oklahoma Spine Hospital	23	0.7
						Surgical Hospital of Oklahoma	12	0.4
						Northwest Surgery Hospital	9	0.3
						Orthopedic Hospital	8	0.2

[1]Indianapolis market includes hospitals in Indianapolis, Mooresville, Carmel, and Avon.

[2]Utah Wasatch Front market includes hospitals in Sandy, American Fork, Tremonton, Brigham City, Layton, Heber City, Murray, West Jordan, Bountiful, Salt Lake City, Ogden, Payson, Orem, Park City, Riverton, and Provo.

[3]Oklahoma City market includes hospitals in Oklahoma City, Edmond, and Midwest City.

Note: Some of the hospitals included in this table are joint ventures with some of the systems.

Source: Data from American Hospital Directory (2017).

EXHIBIT 7.5
Indianapolis Market Share by Bed, 2013

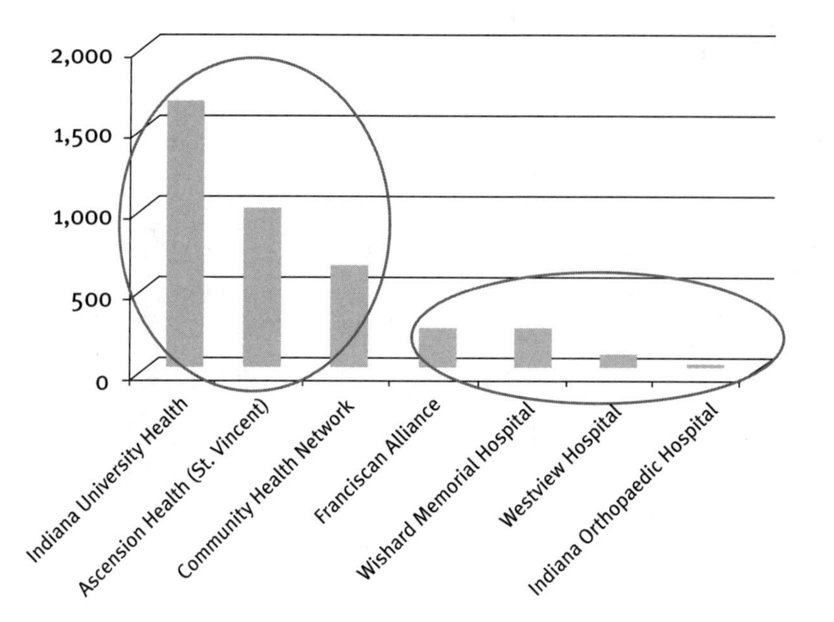

Source: Data from American Hospital Directory (2017).

EXHIBIT 7.6
Utah Wasatch Front Market Share by Bed, 2013

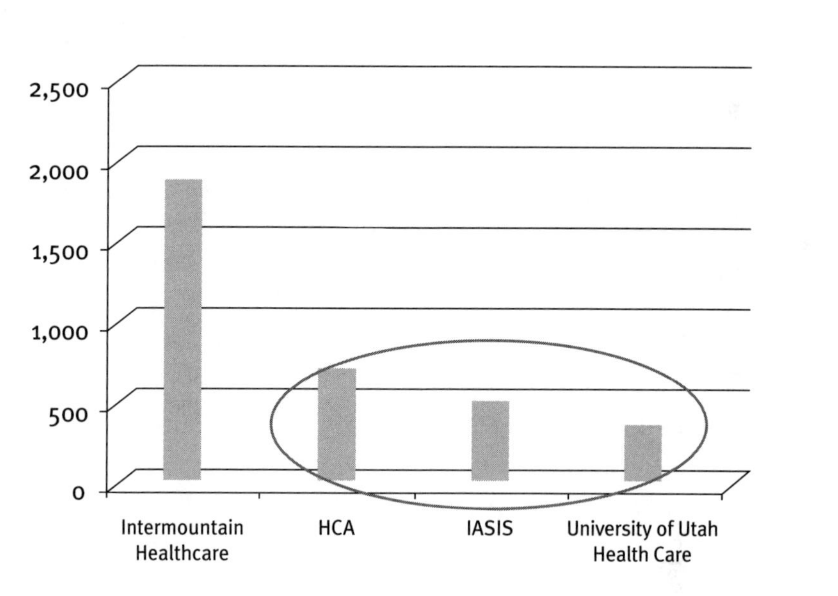

Source: Data from American Hospital Directory (2017).

EXHIBIT 7.7
Oklahoma City Market Share by Bed, 2013

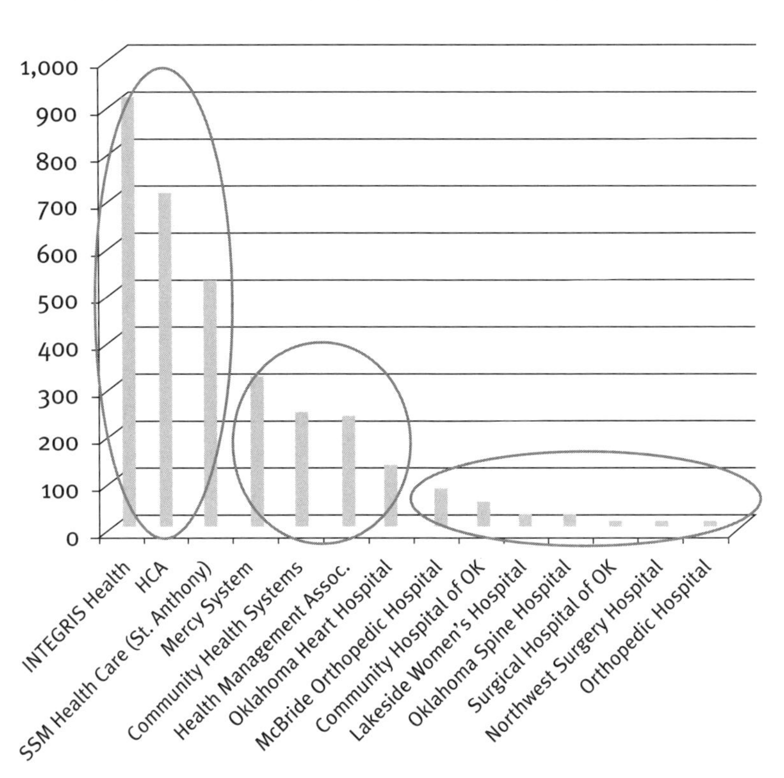

Source: Data from American Hospital Directory (2017).

Health (St. Vincent), and Community Health Network each have approximately 20 percent or more of the market share of hospital beds, while the rest of the market combined (one system and three hospitals) controls about 17 percent. As discussed earlier, the three dominant systems tend to compete primarily among themselves and mostly ignore the strategic activities of the smaller hospitals and system. In Oklahoma City, Oklahoma, three groupings suggest intragroup competition. In the first grouping, INTEGRIS Health System, Hospital Corporation of America (HCA), and SSM Health Care (St. Anthony) compete primarily with each other. In the second grouping, four hospitals compete primarily among themselves, and a third cluster is made up of small, mostly proprietary hospitals that compete directly with each other. The Utah Wasatch Front market is distinct in that Intermountain Healthcare (IHC) is the dominant organization, controlling more than 50 percent of the inpatient bed market. Three firms—HCA, University of Utah Health Care, and IASIS Healthcare—each control 13 to 22 percent of the market. IHC, as the dominant firm, likely leads the market with minimal rivalry, and the other firms mostly react to IHC's strategic moves. The three other systems compete more fiercely with each other.

Degree of Product Differentiation

The ability to differentiate a product can also affect the degree of market rivalry. Products that are not significantly different from those of competitors or are weakly differentiated create little or no brand value. Lack of brand loyalty increases competition and enables rivals to convince buyers to switch products more easily. When buyers perceive little difference among products' attributes and features, they can negotiate with ease, mostly on the basis of price.

In contrast, products that are strongly differentiated have distinct attributes that can generate strong brand loyalty and deter customers from switching to another product, thereby dampening rivalry. For example, insurance companies often perceive little difference in the quality of care offered at different hospitals; quality is generally assumed equal among facilities. Therefore, negotiations for managed care contracts between insurance companies and hospitals often are centered on pricing, enabling insurance companies to extract cost concessions (in a market with multiple hospitals of equal size). On the other hand, many perceive brand-name prescription drugs to be different from their generic equivalents. As a result, there is little direct competition between manufacturers of brand-name and generic drugs. Instead, the pharmaceutical companies spend their energies and budgets primarily on advertising and other activities to maintain this perceived difference.

Height of Exit Barriers

Exit barriers
The costs an organization will incur if it exits a market.

The height of **exit barriers**—the costs an organization incurs from exiting a business—also moderates the level of rivalry in a market. Exit barriers are economic, strategic, or emotional factors that keep organizations from leaving an industry, even when they have failed to achieve their mission outcomes. Competition may arise between organizations that have heavily invested in their facilities and would be unable to recover those costs if they left the market. Exit barriers are higher when an organization has specialized assets that they cannot easily move or reuse for another purpose. Hospitals and pharmaceutical manufacturing facilities have high exit costs because their buildings and equipment are difficult and expensive to convert for other purposes.

Exit barriers also include the prevalence of high fixed costs (i.e., high investments that often are difficult to use for other purposes) in an organization; strategic interrelationships that would be lost; emotional aspects, such as loyalty to customers and employees; and governmental and social restrictions (Porter 1980). High exit barriers in an industry may generate excess capacity, limit requisite productivity, and raise competitive pressures.

Different Ownership Types

Organizations' ownership is yet another factor that can affect the degree of rivalry in a market. Market competition is greater among rivals of different ownership types. Ownership differences often breed distrust and uncertainty about rivals' potential actions because cultures and norms regarding acceptable decisions and business practices vary with ownership type. Corporate-owned and freestanding organizations in the same industry often engage in greater competition than do organizations of the same ownership type (Porter 1980).

Many healthcare markets are composed of organizations of different ownership types. In the United States, for-profit healthcare providers, insurance companies, and not-for-profit organizations compete in the same markets. As mentioned in chapter 6, about 21 percent of hospitals and 80 percent of home health agencies operate as for-profit companies. Intense rivalry can arise between for-profit and not-for-profit organizations in the same market.

Rivalry and Demand

Rivalry is greater in industries in which consumer demand is low or decelerating. When consumer demand is high, producers have growth opportunities and strategies often focus on attracting new customers. When demand slows or declines, organizations grow primarily by drawing existing customers away from rivals. Organizations commonly predict future demand on the basis of past increases in demand. When the rate of demand slows unexpectedly, organizations may be left with unneeded facilities and capacity. Those in this situation may seek to undercut their competitors through price competition and fierce sales tactics.

For instance, in the mid-1980s Medicare and Blue Cross Blue Shield began paying hospitals on a prospective payment system (PPS) basis, which incentivized providers to reduce the frequency and intensity of patient services. As a result, the number of hospital admissions and inpatient stays declined significantly (Scheffler et al. 1994). Having anticipated continued demand for inpatient services prior to the implementation of PPS, many hospitals had large construction projects under way that were no longer needed after implementation. The reduced demand created high excess capacity for inpatient services. At some facilities, entire floors were left unused. Hospitals became much more willing to negotiate contracts with insurance companies at highly discounted rates, in some cases as much as 40 to 60 percent lower than published rates.

Organizations often seek to lessen the intensity of their rivalries by locating their facilities in more favorable markets. Some industry and market structures are much more conducive to favorable business conditions. As discussed in chapter 2, organizations that have monopolistic power have little competition. However, even in competitive markets, organizations can reduce price competition by differentiating their products from those of their competitors (e.g., offering innovative or novel features), strengthening personal relationships to build customer loyalty, distributing their product through novel channels, and focusing on a unique market segment.

The following questions can be used to ascertain the favorability of market conditions. The more positive the answers to these questions, the more positive (less competitive) the market environment:

- Is the number of competitors small?
- Does one organization clearly lead the market?
- Is the market growing?
- Does your organization have low fixed costs?
- Can your product be stored and sold at a later time?
- Are competitors pursuing a low-growth strategy and making few investments to develop their products?
- Is your product unique and different from other available products?
- Would it be easy for your competitors to exit the industry?
- Is it difficult for your customers to switch from your product to another?

Strategic Groups

Strategic groups Clusters of organizations that use the same or similar strategies in an industry. By classifying organizations into strategic groups, leaders can better analyze the structure of an industry.

Strategic groups are clusters of organizations that use the same or similar strategies in an industry. Although differences matter, competition tends to arise most often among organizations that have similar strategies. Although various groups of businesses may be part of an industry, only organizations that employ similar strategies may be direct competitors. Strategists see identifying strategic groups as the first step in analyzing the structure of an industry (Porter 1980). The concept of strategic groups has been referred to as "one of the most valuable analytic concepts in the armory of the strategist, practitioner, or researcher" (Hatten and Hatten 1987, 340). By segmenting industry competitors, analysts refine their view of organizations' market positions and gain a better understanding of how the organizations interact and compete.

Strategic groups are distinguished on the basis of factors such as price or quality, geographic coverage, degree of vertical integration, product breadth, and choice of distribution channels. The factor or factors used to form strategic groups depend on which best capture essential strategic differences among the organizations in an industry. Members of a strategic group tend to have a similar strategic focus and comparable market share and are similarly influenced by or respond similarly to environmental conditions and competitive actions and changes (Hitt, Ireland, and Hoskisson 2016; Leask and Parker 2007; Porter 1980).

Hospitals, physicians, health insurers, distributors of health products, drug companies, and organizations in other healthcare sectors can be segmented into strategic groups on the basis of a variety of factors. For example, physicians might be segregated by size of practice and whether the practice is a single or multispecialty organization. Segmentation of drug companies might be based on global presence and breadth of products. Hospitals may be grouped by national or regional chain. The organizations in a strategic group employ somewhat similar strategies, offering similar products and seeking to attract similar customers. The strategic actions of one organization in a group affect the other members of the group. Thus, a certain level of interdependency exists among the members of a strategic group.

However they are segmented, strategic groups tend to be reasonably stable because of **mobility barriers**—intraindustry obstacles that impede organizations in a strategic group from joining and competing in another group. Mobility barriers include advertising, research and development expenditures, distribution channels, breadth of product line, patents, and objectives that might be difficult to achieve without large expenditures of time and money (Hitt, Ireland, and Hoskisson 2016).

Mobility barriers
Intraindustry obstacles that impede organizations in a strategic group from joining and competing in another group. Examples of mobility barriers include advertising, expenditures on research and development, distribution channels, breadth of product lines, and patents.

Strong mobility barriers enable organizations in industry segments or strategic groups to enjoy greater profitability than they would if they were outside their strategic group. For example, strong mobility barriers—patents, distribution channels or sales forces, and other factors—separate large, brand-name drug companies (e.g., Pfizer, Roche, GlaxoSmithKline, AstroZeneca, Merck) from generic drug companies (e.g., Teva Pharmaceutical, Mylan, Novartis-Sandoz, Allergan, Sun Pharmaceutical). A generic drug company would struggle to find the necessary resources (i.e., finances, staff, research) to produce brand-name products and compete with established brand-name companies. These mobility barriers keep generic drug manufacturers in competition with similar firms (i.e., each other) and distinct from the major brand companies.

Strategic groups can be mapped to gain a graphic perspective on rivals' geographic position. Generally, the closer the members of a cluster are located to one another, the greater the competition among them. For instance, exhibit 7.8 provides a strategic group analysis of the pharmaceutical industry. The dimensions examined in the exhibit are the size (revenues) and the focus on generic versus brand products. As shown, there is a very large revenue distance between the generic and brand-name companies. Given their focus and revenues, the two groups compete minimally against each other.

Driving Forces of the Industry

Part of an environmental analysis prior to developing and implementing strategies includes identifying key industry driving forces. **Driving forces** are the major factors causing change in an industry. All industries are affected in some way by changes in technology, demographics, politics, culture, and economics. However, different forces affect industries unevenly and may have differential impacts on organizations in an industry. By identifying driving forces,

Driving forces
The major factors causing change in an industry.

EXHIBIT 7.8
Pharmaceutical Strategic Groups

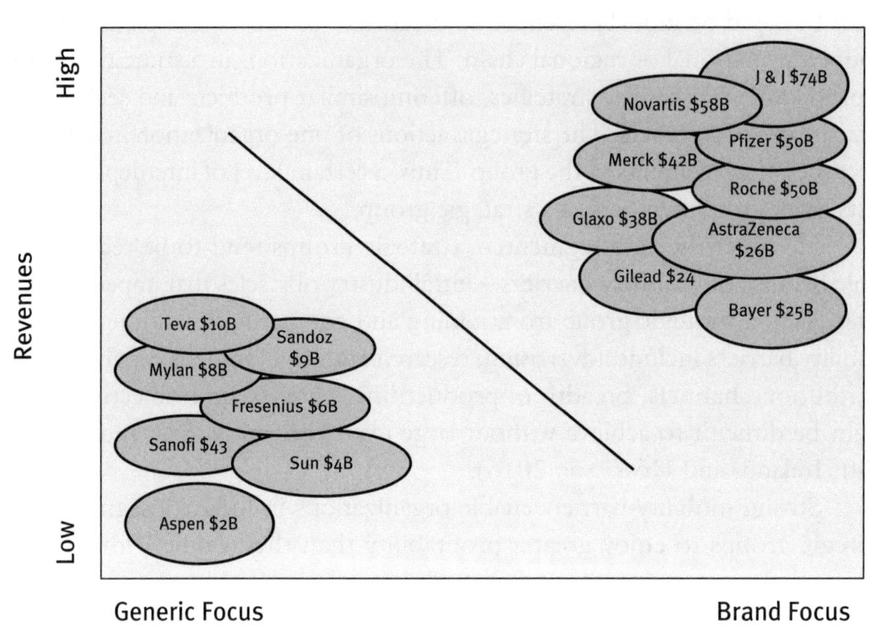

Sources: Hogg (2015), Pharmaceutical-technology.com (2016).

organizations can develop strategy to prepare for their possible effects. The following forces are some of the most common in healthcare:

- *Changes in consumer demand.* Consumers expect to become much more involved in decision making about the healthcare they receive. Demand is also anticipated to increase as populations age and more chronic diseases prevail.
- *Technological changes.* The use of the Internet and information technology is changing the way people interact, share information, and create business processes.
- *Workforce availability.* Shortages of healthcare personnel in nursing, ancillary services, and certain physician specialties are predicted to worsen. Shortages have become a global problem.
- *Political changes.* New state and national laws on healthcare access and reimbursement requirements have been and may be passed.

PEST analysis
An analytical method of deriving forces that are driving change in an industry. Categories of forces explored include political, economic, social, and technological.

PEST Analysis

One analytical method for deriving driving forces is political, economic, social, technological analysis, or **PEST analysis**. Political factors include laws, regulations, and governmental policies that support or hinder an organization's plans. Economic factors include macrolevel data, such as national purchasing power, wealth distribution, workforce availability, financial growth, and inflation. Social factors include population demographics, attitudes, and lifestyles, among others. Technological factors encompass research and development, innovation potential, the rate at which technology is advancing, and the breadth of consumer use of emerging and existing technologies.

Force Field Analysis

Force field analysis elaborates on PEST analysis by determining whether the identified forces support or undermine an organization's plans. Forces that promote achievement can foster the organization's goals, while those that hinder it should be mitigated (Schwering 2003). Force field analysis has long been used to analyze problems and develop effective action plans that are multidimensionally focused on key driving forces (Bailey 1994; Lewin 1951). It graphically displays the forces that encourage and those that hinder the action or goal under consideration. Exhibit 7.9 illustrates the forces affecting the closing of a service. The forces on the right promote the change, while those on the left hinder it.

Force field analysis
A technique used to evaluate whether environmental influences support or undermine an organization's decisions or plans.

EXHIBIT 7.9
Force Field Hindering or Promoting Analysis

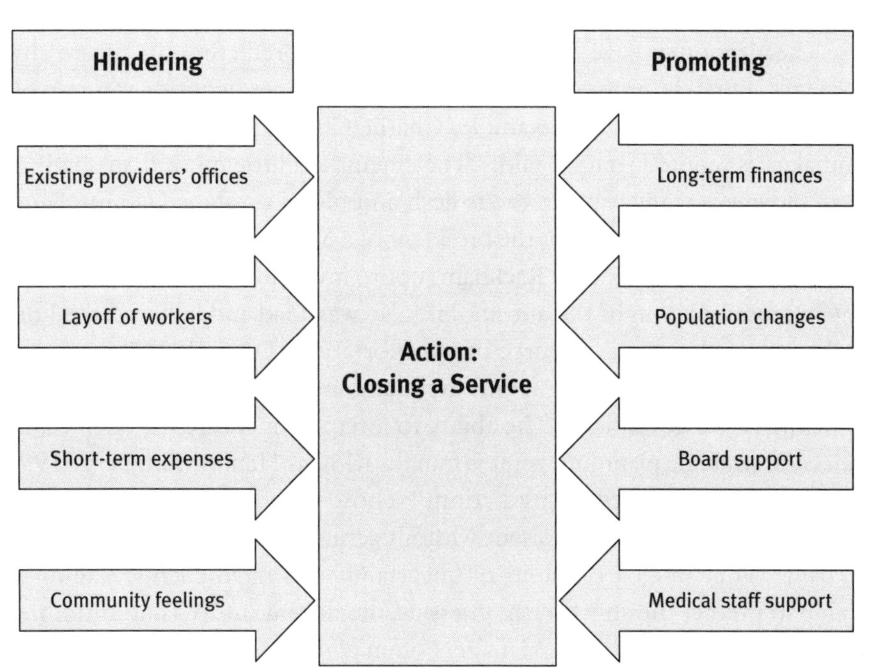

Driving forces can be identified through brainstorming, surveys, and the input of key stakeholders. Questions such as the following can be used to facilitate discussion:

- What factors account for our present situation?
- What factors are keeping us from accomplishing our goals?
- What factors are helping us achieve our goals?

Scenario Analysis

Scenario analysis A technique of proposing alternative futures that could come to pass if a specified environmental change occurs. This type of analysis is used by leaders to better understand and plan for future contingencies.

Scenarios are stories that describe the effect environmental changes could have on an organization. They are "plausible, not probable or preferable, portraits of alternative futures" (Leufkens et al. 1994, 1137). **Scenario analysis** sensitizes leaders to different possible environments in ways that traditional graphs and written plans do not. It helps organizations prepare the knowledge and means they will need to deal with different futures and "Scenario planning typically includes both qualitative and quantitative analyses to illustrate the trade-offs between different futures and their relative impacts on different community goals. This robust discussion of trade-offs and identification of a preferred set of strategies based on that trade-off discussion can lead to more thoughtful, effective, and resilient plans" (Federal Highway Administration 2016). It has been suggested as a good tool for healthcare planning and strategic decision making (Vollmar, Ostermann, and Redaelli 2015).

Leaders often have difficulty evaluating and predicting the future environment accurately, especially major shifts in consumer behavior triggered by technological advances. For example, Charlie Chaplin, a silent film actor and filmmaker, is reputed to have said, "The cinema is a little more than a fad. . . . What audiences really want to see is flesh and blood on stage" (QuoteFancy.com 2017). Likewise, in 1903, the president of a Michigan savings bank advised Henry Ford's lawyer, Horace Rackham, not to invest in the Ford Motor Company because he thought the automobile also was a fad and believed the horse would remain the primary source of transportation (Dunn 2016).

Managers still tend to spend great amounts of time and resources on predicting future conditions. The ability to forecast the future has been central to classical strategic planning, yet it is fraught with, as Henry Mintzberg (1994, 109) stated, "the fallacy of prediction." Those who attempt to predict the future generally extend the present without actually knowing what conditions will exist. While in environments of uncertainty and rapid change one might be able to predict the short term, guessing the distant future is no more than gambling (Beckham 2016a). Managers often compensate for this uncertainty by creating high, middle, and low projections. Classification by potential can refine predictions but in many cases does not consider major contingencies that could radically change the organization's environment.

Scenario generation helps organizations examine the assumptions on which its strategies are based; opens discussion about potential eventualities; and reveals new environmental patterns, trends, and changes that could enable a company to shift the way it operates significantly (Luke, Walston, and Plummer 2004). An early user of scenario analysis was the Royal Dutch/Shell Group. Use of this technique positioned the group for the major changes that occurred in the oil markets in the 1970s (Wack 1985).

The use of scenario planning is appropriate when significant future uncertainties exist as a result of

- rapidly advancing technologies;
- potential shifts in customers' preferences;
- major market power shifts by consolidation (or diversification) of distribution channels, suppliers, or buyers; or
- changes in government regulations.

Scenarios can help most when the environment is complex and characterized by many key unquantifiable factors and few sources of reliable data are available (Schnaars 1987).

One can break scenario analysis into four steps:

1. Examination of key factors in the external environment
2. Identification of key uncertainties and driving forces
3. Creation of scenarios
4. Integration of scenarios into strategic planning

Analyzing and determining key external environmental factors involves scanning, monitoring, and assessing key environmental forces to identify the uncertainties the organization is facing. These uncertainties should be separated into two categories: those that are predetermined and those that really are uncertainties. For instance, the increasing number of elderly is a predetermined factor, while the potential for biotechnology is an uncertainty.

In the second phase of scenario analysis, the two most critical uncertainties are selected, often on the basis of the highest perceived probability of occurrence and highest potential impact on the organization (Schwenker and Wulf 2013). This selection could be accomplished through a survey of key stakeholders, during a retreat, or by some other decision-making process. As shown in exhibit 7.10, many critical market forces were narrowed to two: consumer activism and rate of inflation. These two uncertainties form the axes of a four-quadrant scenario matrix. The four scenarios describe how the market would be under different environmental conditions. Each scenario has different strategic implications that may require different competencies and resource allocations.

EXHIBIT 7.10
Using Scenario Analysis to Determine Managed Care Strategy

Providers' strategies for contracting with managed care organizations have changed significantly since the 1990s, although what they should be in the future is unclear. To help healthcare managers prepare for the implementation of managed care strategies, Krentz and Gish (2000) constructed a scenario analysis. In their analysis of the external environment, they identified these critical market forces:

- Collective bargaining for physicians
- Consolidation of health plans
- Employee benefit structures
- Federal healthcare reform and universal access
- Medicare managed care
- Healthcare inflation
- Health plan models
- Impact of consumerism
- Provider payment structure
- Physician practice structure

From among these critical market forces, they selected healthcare inflation and the role of the healthcare consumer as the critical forces anticipated to have the greatest potential impact overall. These two factors were used to create the following chart:

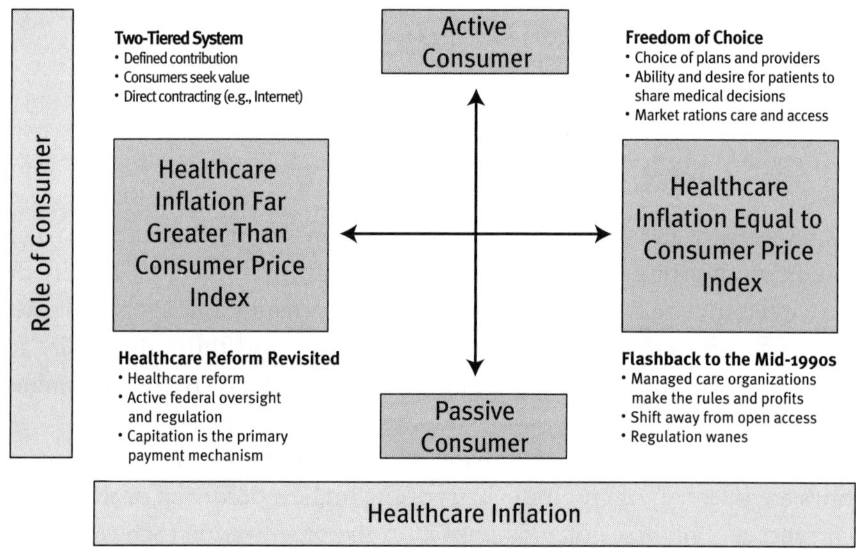

The four scenarios in the chart describe providers' potential futures:

- *Two-tiered system*. Medical costs greatly exceed general inflation, and consumers take an active role in their healthcare decision making. Employers use a defined contribution model for healthcare coverage;

EXHIBIT 7.10 Using Scenario Analysis to Determine Managed Care Strategy *(continued)*

employees receive a fixed amount per month to spend on healthcare. New purchasing channels emerge, facilitated by the Internet and health insurance exchanges. Branding and product differentiation through consumer report cards are crucial. Consumers are price sensitive.

- *Freedom of choice*. Consumers are active, and medical inflation is reasonable. Companies offer their employees a choice of plans under a defined benefit arrangement. Market forces of supply and demand ration care and access.
- *Flashback to the mid-1990s*. Increases in medical costs are relatively modest, and consumers are passive. Managed care payers dominate the market and have the power to set the terms of contracts. Open-access products change to closed-panel models controlled by gatekeepers. Federal legislation diminishes. Hospitals and physicians seek to merge.
- *Healthcare reform revisited*. High medical cost inflation and passive consumers prompt federal intervention. The federal government actively oversees and regulates both providers and payers. Providers focus on corporate compliance. As a result of capitation, risk shifts from payers to hospitals and physicians, who consider integrated delivery models. Information technology is essential to managing risk.

After evaluating these scenarios, Krentz and Gish (2000) identified the following strategic implications:

Strategic Implication	Two-Tiered System	Freedom of Choice	Flashback to the Mid-1990s	Healthcare Reform Revisited
Contracting through new distribution channels	X			
Traditional consumer goods strategies	X			
Branding and differentiation	X	X		
Measurement of quality	X	X	X	X
Selective panel participation		X		
Corporate compliance resources				X
Consolidation to gain leverage			X	X
Shared contracting vehicles			X	X
Physician–hospital integration			X	
Risk management skills			X	

Source: Adapted from Krentz and Gish (2000). Reprinted with permission from *hfm* magazine, September 2000; copyright Healthcare Financial Management Association.

In addition, managers should identify and monitor events that signal a shift toward a scenario. These events, or *trigger points*, could be technology breakthroughs, changes in laws and regulations, market shifts, or world events (Luke, Walston, and Plummer 2004).

Understanding External Market Data

Leaders must understand the implications of external market data not just for their organizations but also for their competitors. Along with the information discussed in this chapter, competitors' market shares by key services should be collected, and market dominance and influence by service should be quantified. Managers should note and understand competitors who have reputational and special service advantages. Customer surveys may be required to obtain data on market providers' quality and reputation. Underserved areas and markets also should be identified. Gaps in services that consumers need should be recognized and noted. Likewise, managers should identify and track the presence and growth of alternative and innovative services. A thorough and systematic approach to evaluating the external environment is critical to developing successful strategies.

Chapter Summary

Porter's Five Forces model is commonly used to examine competition in markets. The forces include the risk of entry, the threat of substitute products, the power of suppliers and buyers, and rivalry among competitors.

Organizations also use the concept of strategic groups to understand market rivalry more thoroughly. Organizations in a market that have similar characteristics are grouped to examine strategic differences among the resulting clusters. Strategic groups tend to remain relatively stable because of mobility barriers that impede organizations from shifting to compete in a different group.

The idea of driving forces helps analysts define and understand the critical influences affecting organizations. Common influences include shifts in consumer demand, technological changes, workforce issues, and political fluctuation. Political, economic, social, and technological (PEST) analysis is one analytical method of deriving driving forces. Force field analysis is another excellent tool used for this purpose. This type of analysis produces a graphical display of forces that are encouraging and restricting an organization's actions or achievement of a goal.

Last, scenario analysis can help organizations prepare for the events of tomorrow. This type of analysis identifies critical environmental uncertainties and projects alternative future scenarios. Understanding how the future may be different if critical environmental factors change enables leaders to question their assumptions and determine potential resource and competency needs.

Chapter Questions

1. Which of Porter's Five Forces are more dominant in healthcare than in other fields? How does the strength of these forces vary among healthcare sectors?
2. Identify some switching costs in healthcare. What could a healthcare organization do to minimize the impact of switching costs?
3. What are the major substitutes for hospital care? How do these substitutes vary by hospital service?
4. Are insurance companies buyers or suppliers for hospitals? What about physicians? Why is this designation more difficult to make in healthcare?
5. How does product differentiation affect the level of rivalry in a market?
6. How are products and services in healthcare different from one another?
7. How is quality determined in healthcare? How is clinical quality different from service quality?
8. How can strategic groups be used to determine market competitors?
9. Can mobility barriers be created by industry incumbents? If so, why would they desire to create them?
10. How can driving forces be used to envision the future?

Chapter Cases

Case Studies

Read and discuss one of the following cases: "The Virulent Virus," "The Battle in Boise," "Dissolving a Long-Standing Affiliation and Moving On," or "Value in Capitation for Hospitalists?" in the case studies section at the end of the book. Answer the questions at the end of the case.

Power of a Healthcare Insurance Supplier

Heightened supplier power often induces responses from buyers. As described in the following case, the consolidation and market power of the insurance company Anthem created situations that required responses from

(continued)

Anthem's buyers. This case is a compilation of actual events. When you have finished reading the case, answer the questions that immediately follow.

It is the summer of 2003. The Physicians' Group Clinic (PGC) in Indianapolis has a dilemma. The largest insurance company in the state, Anthem, had been doing business in Indiana for 50 years as Blue Cross and Blue Shield of Indiana. However, in the early 1990s, the company merged with Blue Cross plans in Kentucky, Ohio, Connecticut, New Hampshire, Colorado, Nevada, Maine, and Virginia and changed its name to Anthem, Inc. These acquisitions occurred at the same time the insurance company was pushing to gain more market share in Indiana. As of 2003, Anthem controls 20 percent of the nongovernmental health insurance in the state. Although PGC always has had a friendly relationship with Anthem's representatives, the insurance company is offering different incentives that could profoundly affect the clinic's business.

Anthem is proposing to increase the number of PGC patients covered by its insurance substantially. Currently, Anthem's patients account for 13 percent of PGC's business. The proposal offers a larger group of Anthem HMO patients and reimbursement at a per member per month rate. The physicians analyze the suggested rate and feel that the amount is adequate to cover all costs, including overhead, and generate some profit. The proposed contract also offers monetary incentives for providing efficient care. If PGC accepts this contract and the promised volumes materialize, the number of PGC patients covered by Anthem would increase to 22 percent.

The physicians discuss the positives and negatives of the contract. They are unhappy with their Medicaid reimbursement, which is about 15 percent lower than their direct costs. If they accept Anthem's proposal, they could decrease the number of Medicaid patients they agree to in order to accommodate the new patient load. On the other hand, they are worried about becoming so dependent on Anthem's business. What would prevent Anthem from cutting their reimbursement in the future and imposing other requirements? The physicians need to decide whether to accept or reject the Anthem proposal.

Questions

1. How would Anthem's relationship and negotiating power with the physician group change if the physicians accepted the proposal?
2. Why might this physician group want to build a strong relationship with a small number of insurance companies (i.e., suppliers)?
3. What should the physicians do?
4. What might PGC do to reduce the supplier power Anthem could have over PGC in the future?

5. What other recommendations can you make?

Decisions Under Uncertainty for 2017

It is December of 2016. The NHL Health System has many decisions to make. Its capital budgeting process requires that the largest capital investments, those more than $5 million, be approved by the corporate office. This year, as normal, there are more than 30 requests, and the requests total more than $250 million. However, 2016 is also a year of heightened uncertainty surrounding the US healthcare sector. NHL has hired a prominent consulting group to advise it on the risks and contingencies it should consider. Key areas of uncertainty that the consulting group identified include the following:

1. *The fate of the Affordable Care Act (ACA)*. Republicans have promised to repeal the ACA, but its replacement remains far from clear. Bad debts and charity care across the system have dropped by $6 to $10 million per year as a result of more having insurance or Medicaid coverage.
2. *A move to value-based purchasing*. More of Medicare payments are now tied to the demonstration of value and satisfaction. Many predict that the fee-for-service system cannot last and that healthcare organizations must move to a population-based system founded on value indicators.
3. *Drug prices*. One of the largest increases in hospital costs has been the escalating cost of drugs. Many suggest that these increases will continue.
4. *Consolidation*. Many healthcare systems have merged in the recent past and many continue to seek partners. NHL has absorbed a few smaller systems but has been hesitant to combine with a large system.

Top management will be making decisions on the capital budget items next week.

Questions

1. How might these uncertainties affect Porter's Five Forces (the power of buyers, suppliers, substitutes, entry, rivalry)?
2. Do a PEST analysis. What additional factors would you include as key uncertainties?
3. Create a scenario analysis for this situation. What would be the two key critical uncertainties? Scenarios?

Chapter Assignments

1. Select a healthcare company with which you either are reasonably familiar or on which significant public information is available, and perform a PEST analysis.
2. Develop a list of ten barriers to entry for the following healthcare organizations: (a) hospitals, (b) physician practices, (c) nursing homes, (d) health insurance companies, and (e) pharmaceutical companies. How and why do the barriers to entry vary among these different healthcare groups?

CHAPTER

8

THE INTERNAL ENVIRONMENT AND STRATEGY

> Hospital and health system CEOs today must be equipped with certain core competencies to effectively navigate the constantly and rapidly changing healthcare environment. Andrew Ziskind, MD, managing director of Huron Healthcare, outlined seven core competencies for leaders. . . .
>
> 1. Increase your organization's capacity for innovation. Keeping up with the pace of change and discovering ways to stay ahead of the curve are crucial. . . . Innovation should be incorporated as a strategic priority. . . .
> 2. Become agile. . . . Having the ability to change direction, make decisions and execute quickly is imperative for success for healthcare providers of all sizes.
> 3. Get the most from your data. . . . To get the most from data, analytics that produce meaningful insights must be embedded into daily workflows to guide clinical care and operations. . . .
> 4. Keep an open mind to unconventional partnerships. . . . Organizations will need to be open to new partnerships, evaluate potential suitors carefully and have the flexibility to act on them.
> 5. Consider new business and care delivery models to manage financial risk. . . . Organizations should seek models that enable them to provide "the right services in the right locations" while simultaneously improving outcomes and diminishing risk. . . .
> 6. Cultivate asset agility. Organizations that have less capital will still be able to respond to market changes more comprehensively.
> 7. Foster a stronger culture of management. To effectively shepherd their organizations through change, healthcare leaders must support a culture rooted in discipline and accountability, using real-time performance management to produce results.
>
> —Tamara Rosin, "Hospital CEOs: 7 Core Competencies for Future Organizational Success," 2016

Learning Objectives

After reading this chapter, you will

- understand how to evaluate a company's internal environment and capabilities,
- recognize the value of benchmarking against other organizations,
- comprehend the use of trended data,
- be familiar with methods of evaluating key organizational strengths and weaknesses,
- know how to perform a stakeholder analysis,
- be able to conduct a SWOT analysis,
- discern the proper uses and misuses of SWOT analysis,
- grasp the use of TOWS analysis,
- appreciate how internal analysis helps an organization develop strategic direction to meet its mission and vision,
- be informed about the concept of value chains and their uses, and
- be capable of performing a portfolio analysis.

For strategic planning to be effective, leaders must comprehend the strengths, weaknesses, competencies, and challenges presented by their organization's internal environment. The internal environment comprises personnel, intellectual property, and tangible assets, among other elements. This chapter discusses methods of analyzing organizations' composition and components.

Organizational capabilities
Internal resources, such as physical assets, human resources, reputation, culture, and processes and routines that enable an organization to accomplish its mission.

A common phrase in the 1980s among not-for-profit healthcare providers was "no money, no mission." Organizations cannot accomplish their missions unless adequate resources are available. Money is a critical resource, but organizational capabilities and competencies are just as critical. Nonfinancial internal resources include physical assets, human resources, reputation, culture, and organizational processes and routines, among others. Exhibit 8.1 identifies key internal resources, both financial and nonfinancial.

Core competencies
Activities "that a company performs proficiently that [are] also central to its strategy and competitive success." (Thompson et al. 2016, 93)

An organization's capacity to integrate its resources to achieve a desired objective depends on its **organizational capabilities**—the proficiency with which it performs internal activities. Capabilities develop from organizational learning and experience. When combined in unique combinations, capabilities form **core competencies** that have important strategic value. As shown in the discussion at the opening of the chapter, core competencies are central to fulfilling a company's mission and can place an organization in a position of competitive advantage. They are created by superior resources and put to use in a way that other organizations may find difficult to replicate—the essence of

EXHIBIT 8.1
Key Internal Resources

Marketing
- Products and services
- Pricing
- Promotion
- Reputation
- Distribution
- Location
- Brands

People
- Management
- Technical specialists
- Innovation specialists
- Sales force

Operation and Facilities
- Processes
- Facilities and equipment
- Cost management and efficiency

Finances
- Profitability
- Capital structure
- Inventory management
- Billing and receivables management

what makes an organization unique in providing value to its customers. Exhibit 8.2 illustrates the development of internal resources into strategic results.

Resources are inputs into an organization's production process. They are either tangible or intangible. **Tangible resources** include land, buildings, plant, equipment, cash, and personnel. **Intangible resources** consist of reputation, brand names, employees' skills, and industry knowledge. Tangible resources are more easily acquired than intangible resources. Organizations can purchase land and equipment and construct buildings, whereas reputation, brand image, and knowledge develop over time through experience and interactions with other organizations.

Tangible resources
An organization's physical assets, including land, buildings and plant, equipment, cash, and personnel.

Intangible resources
Nonphysical resources, including reputation, brand name, skills, and knowledge.

The intangible components of core competencies—not the tangible ones—are what make core competencies difficult to copy. Core competencies underlie the value customers derive from an organization; they are the functions an organization fulfills better than anyone else. Generally, organizations should identify and concentrate on only three to four core competencies (Hitt, Ireland, and Hoskisson 2016).

To be valuable, resources must be rare, difficult to imitate, and lack substitutes. For example, reputation is a critical resource for many healthcare companies because it can take many years to establish, making it hard to duplicate. As stated in exhibit 8.3, reputation may be a healthcare organization's most important attribute. Likewise, exhibit 8.4 describes how name recognition and reputation can be valuable tools. Organizations often are willing to pay significant amounts of money to use a name with a positive reputation.

Similarly, clinical knowledge and specialized facilities, even if rare and expensive, may not sustain an organization's strategic advantage if competitors can easily create substitutes. For instance, INTEGRIS Health, the largest healthcare system in Oklahoma, partnered with a for-profit firm in 2006 to offer the sixth proton therapy center in the United States. Although the

EXHIBIT 8.2
Development of Internal Resources into Strategic Results

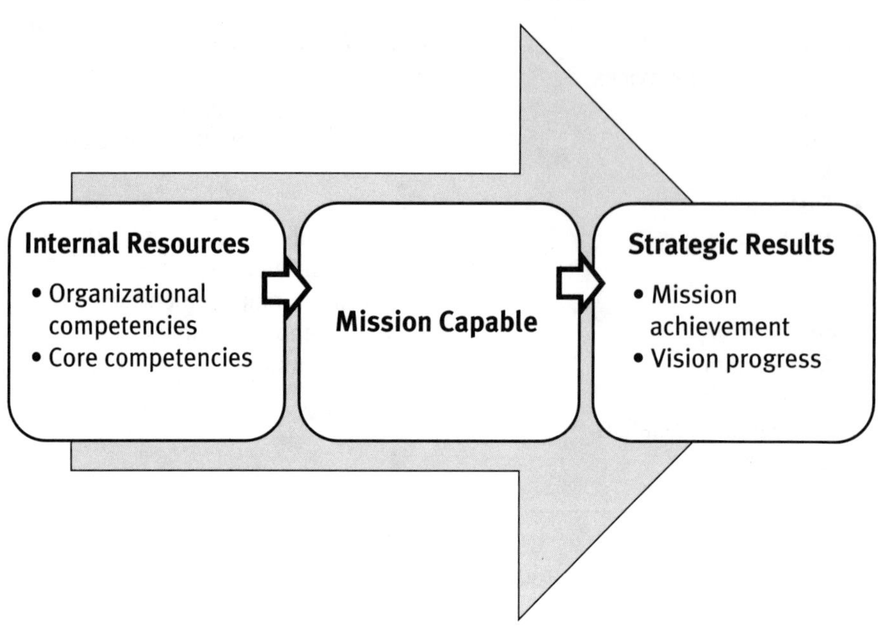

cost-effectiveness of this expensive treatment has been questioned (each center costs up to $200 million) and the need for two facilities in the small state of Oklahoma was suspect, shortly after INTEGRIS Health made its announcement, the University of Oklahoma declared that it also would purchase proton therapy equipment and offer a competing service (Simpson 2007). This decision would make Oklahoma one of the few states to have two proton therapy

EXHIBIT 8.3
The Importance of Reputation

"A hospital's reputation may be its most important attribute. A report by the National Research Corporation found 60 percent of consumers said a hospital's reputation is 'very important' when considering it for future needs."

Source: Quoted from Flanagan (2016).

EXHIBIT 8.4
The Value of Name Recognition and Reputation

When HCA merged University, Presbyterian, and Children's hospitals in Oklahoma City in 1990, it initially named the cluster "University Health Partners." A decade later, it found that patients and the community had little awareness of this nondescript name. After conducting focus groups, HCA realized that the name of the University of Oklahoma medical school was much more recognized. Seeing an opportunity to leverage the power of reputation, in 2001 HCA paid the University of Oklahoma $1.5 million for the use of its name over the next decade and rebranded the complex as "OU Medical Center."

Sources: *Journal Record* (2001), Lackmeyer (2001).

units. By 2016, only 25 centers were in operation across the United States with 11 others planned (National Association for Proton Therapy 2017). The duplication of INTEGRIS Health's investment diluted the system's strategic advantage and diminished the value of its resources.

Academics have long taught that organizations must accumulate the proper mix of tangible and intangible resources to ensure successful implementation of their strategies and sustain their strategic value (Barney 1991; Mintzberg, Ahlstrand, and Lampel 1998; Wernerfelt 1984). As mentioned earlier, physical assets are more easily duplicated, so competitive advantage must be achieved through the integration of physical, human, and organizational resources. Culture has been suggested as an effective and durable barrier to imitation because it is difficult to replicate (Barney and Hesterly 2014). Of course, an effective culture is also difficult to create in the first place.

Leaders should periodically examine their organization's capabilities and core competencies to understand more thoroughly the linkages and synergies among the organization's resources and the sustainability of its capabilities and competencies. The following questions are useful in this type of analysis (Hitt, Ireland, and Hoskisson 2016):

1. How does the organization bundle resources to build capabilities and core competencies that create value for customers?
2. Could the organization align its resources in a better way to improve its capabilities and core competencies?
3. Is it likely that environmental changes will make the organization's core competencies obsolete?
4. Are substitutes for the organization's core competencies available or soon to be available?
5. Could the organization's core competencies be easily imitated?
6. If the answer to questions 3, 4, or 5 is yes, what should the organization do to protect or improve its core competencies?

Internal Environmental Analysis

Internal environmental analysis
Evaluation of an organization's products, assets, operations, and other factors to determine whether the organization is carrying out its mission effectively and efficiently.

Internal environmental analysis involves obtaining, analyzing, and understanding data on the internal environment. Although the information that is collected and examined varies by the type of healthcare organization, data about the organization's capabilities, core competencies, and key stakeholders are essential to all organizations' internal environmental analyses. A wide variety of data should be organized and evaluated to determine whether an organization is carrying out its mission effectively and efficiently. Data relevant to internal environmental analysis include the following measures:

- Financial information (see chapter 9)
  - Operational cost and revenue data
  - Cash flow
  - Capital costs and projections
- Data on human resources
  - Staffing shortages and projected needs
  - Turnover reports
  - Training and development issues
  - Employee satisfaction scores
- Customer (patient) information
  - Demographics by service line
  - Volumes by major insurance type (e.g., Medicare, Medicaid, indemnity, health maintenance organizations [HMOs])
  - Quality measures
  - Consumer satisfaction scores
- Physician information
  - Unique competencies and specialties
  - Key performance data by specialty, physician age, and geographic location
  - Productivity measures
  - Specialty deficits
- Value-based performance data (For more information, see www.cms.gov/Outreach-and-Education/Medicare-Learning-Network-MLN/MLNProducts/Downloads/Hospital_VBPurchasing_Fact_Sheet_ICN907664.pdf)
  - Clinical care
  - Safety
  - Patient and caregiver-centered experience of care or care coordination
  - Efficiency and cost reduction

However, data alone can be relatively meaningless. For example, if a hospice reports 201 visits in the town of Bakerville this year, is this measure good or bad? Does it indicate that the hospice has progressed toward fulfilling its vision? Data are meaningful when they are compared to other data. In many cases, this comparison is expressed as a ratio. For instance, the managers of the hospice would be much more enlightened if the report showed that the 201 visits represented 80 percent of total patient visits among all hospices in Bakerville this year, up from 150 visits, or 60 percent of total visits, last year.

Organizations can compare their data to their past performance and to other organizations' data. There are advantages to using each method, but each is also problematic. For example, **benchmarking** data against data of similar organizations can catalyze change. If an organization is trailing its competitors on certain measures, leaders can set performance targets and goals aimed at closing that gap. Organizations should strive to be the best in their core competency areas; comparing organizational data to outside benchmarks helps an organization determine whether its core competencies truly lead the market. If it does not, this comparison tells the organization the level of effort it will have to make to attain excellence.

Benchmarking
Comparison of internal data to those of outside organizations for purposes of evaluating an organization's performance.

Illustrating this concept, exhibit 8.5 benchmarks data from three Illinois hospitals against survey data from the state and national levels. The comparison suggests that the hospitals are underperforming in a few areas. To address this situation, the hospitals could set target measures aimed at improving their communications, response times, and room quietness.

EXHIBIT 8.5
CMS Hospital Compare Data, 2016

	Adventist Bolingbrook Hospital (%)	Advocate Good Shepherd Hospital (%)	Franciscan St. James Health (%)	Illinois Average (%)	National Average (%)
Patients who reported that their nurses "always" communicated well	77	81	75	81	80
Patients who reported that their doctors "always" communicated well	79	78	74	82	82
Patients who reported that they "always" received help as soon as they wanted it	60	62	56	69	69
Patients who reported that their pain was "always" well controlled	68	72	63	72	71
Patients who reported that staff "always" explained their medications before administering them	61	62	57	65	65
Patients who reported that their room and bathroom "always" were clean	76	72	68	75	74
Patients who reported that the area around their room was "always" quiet at night	61	50	63	62	63
Patients who reported YES, they would definitely recommend the hospital	65	73	62	71	72

Source: Data from Medicare.gov (2017).

As mentioned earlier, benchmarking against other organizations can be problematic. In many cases, organizations use different methods to calculate data and find themselves comparing apples to oranges. In addition, benchmark data are almost always a few years old; the data in exhibit 8.5—the most current data available as this book goes to press—are generally from 2015. Along with the possibility of being outdated, a benchmark is just an assessment of something at a given point of time and does not account for continuing improvements or trends. The hospitals' data or the state and national data may have changed over time. At the time the data were collected, the displayed hospitals may have been making consistent progress in the area of patient satisfaction or the situation may have been stagnant or worsening.

Trend data
Data that portray changes over time (generally from one year to the next).

Trend data portray changes from one year to the next. Year-to-year information enables an organization to determine the direction in which it is moving. Exhibit 8.6 provides data for Alta Bates Medical Center, a large hospital in the San Francisco Bay area. Data for five years are given. One can see that the number of the hospital's inpatient surgeries consistently dropped until 2015, while outpatient surgeries increased until 2013 and then dropped to 2015. Comparison of year-to-year data from the same organization should be based on consistently defined data, not divergent information. By examining data over time, leaders also can predict organizational statistics for future years. If not compared to data from outside organizations, however, trend data do not indicate how well the organization is performing, only how its performance is changing. Even if the trend shows improvement, the statistics still may be much worse than the statistics of market competitors.

Therefore, organizations should use both benchmarking and trending to evaluate internal data effectively. Benchmarking enables external comparisons and goal setting, while trending tracks an organization's progress over time.

Organizations generate hundreds, perhaps thousands, of statistics. For purposes of strategic management, they should only use a few for analysis. Selection of statistics is an important decision and can be instrumental to the

EXHIBIT 8.6
Inpatient Utilization Trend Report, Alta Bates Medical Center

Statistic	FY 2011	FY 2012	FY 2013	FY 2014	FY 2015
Inpatient surgeries	3,317	3,286	2,812	2,574	3,022
Inpatient surgery operating room minutes	555,872	550,091	357,750	337,549	507,525
Outpatient surgeries	2,401	2,682	4,197	3,987	2,752
Outpatient surgery operating room minutes	248,410	268,773	325,41	321,834	273,234

Source: Data from Office of Statewide Health Planning and Development (2017b).

success and failure of strategic efforts. Three simple guidelines will help leaders choose appropriate statistics. The data should

1. help measure achievement of the organization's mission and progress toward its vision,
2. reflect important stakeholder needs, and
3. be accurate and timely.

Consider the mission and vision of Texas Health Resources, one of the largest faith-based, nonprofit systems in the United States:

> Mission statement: To improve the health of the people in the communities we serve.
>
> Vision: Texas Health Resources, a faith-based organization joining with physicians, will be the health care system of choice.

To determine whether the mission and vision are being achieved, Texas Health Resources should examine internal statistics that reflect these statements. Is the health of people in its service area improving? How can it track, document, and trend this information? Do most residents living in the market area choose Texas Health Resources' providers for medical care? What is the population's impression of Texas Health Resources relative to other providers in the same service area?

Exhibit 8.7 explains how Texas Health Resources breaks down its strategy into initiatives aligned with its mission, vision, and values. A senior system

EXHIBIT 8.7
Texas Health Resources' Use of Mission-, Vision-, and Value-Based Objectives

Utilizing the metaphor of a journey up a transformational mountain, Texas Health Resources has embraced a 15-year plan that defines five strategic/transformational themes: (1) strengthening culture, (2) engaging physicians, (3) adopting a comprehensive view of quality, (4) ensuring a cost-effective system, and (5) becoming an integrated provider and coordinator of care.

Each theme is driven by specific strategic initiatives (a total of 16 among them) that cascade down the organization and into the fabric of this regional healthcare system, whose 25 acute care, transitional, rehabilitation, and short-stay hospitals serve a population of more than 6 million. Texas Health Resources also includes a network of more than 250 ambulatory facilities and offices with net revenues in excess of $4 billion.

The 16 strategic initiatives are listed on a single sheet of paper that has become known as the "strategy on a page" or the "value equation"—efforts taken to fulfill the system's mission and vision and live its values. A

(continued)

EXHIBIT 8.7
Texas Health Resources' Use of Mission-, Vision-, and Value-Based Objectives *(continued)*

senior system champion and specific action plans are assigned to each initiative. The senior system champion chairs a steering team; identifies assumptions, constraints, and dependencies; and selects performance indicators. Texas Health Resources' senior executive council, under the direction of the chief strategy officer, monitors the progress of the 16 strategic initiatives and reviews the value equation in detail biannually.

In addition to systemwide strategies, action plans and tactics that align with systemwide efforts are developed for each individual hospital/facility. The importance of aligning the system's hospitals and other facilities cannot be overstated. For example, Texas Health Presbyterian Hospital Dallas has an entity-specific steering team chaired by a hospital executive who sits on the systemwide steering team. As a result, the hospital has line of sight on systemwide efforts and at the same time is nimble enough to respond to issues specific to its geographic area. The Dallas steering committee identified an emerging Burmese population that is not present throughout the region. By so doing, the systemwide steering team instituted an initiative to address the needs of this emerging population, set goals and measures, determined the membership of the initiative's steering team, defined major deliverables and timing, and confirmed key issues/risks involved in the initiative.

For an example of Texas Health Resources' approach to strategy, one of the initiatives driving the "strengthening our culture" theme—"Getting Serious About Service"—is to advance the system's mission, vision, values, and promise and adopt service standards. Getting Serious About Service speaks to the creation of educational programs on patients' healthcare experience, room service, bilingual translation services, diversity training, and other efforts. Another example is an initiative under the "engaging physicians" theme. The acquisition of a large primary care physician group with more than 250 locations throughout the Dallas/Fort Worth metro area aligns with the strategy-on-a-page initiative to provide clear reasons and ways for Texas Health Resources to engage independent and employed physicians.

Source: Berrett (2012). Used with permission.

champion and explicit performance indicators are assigned to each initiative, and data are tracked and monitored biannually.

Following the example set by Texas Health Resources, executives should recognize and analyze appropriate data to ascertain how well the organization is meeting the needs of its key stakeholders. Stakeholders have different needs, so leaders should identify and use different indicators to ensure these needs are met. For instance, a for-profit hospital's key stakeholders might be (1) owners and shareholders, (2) physicians on its medical staff, (3) employees, (4) patients, and (5) the community. To examine how well the hospital is meeting the needs of each of these stakeholder groups, it could gather the following statistics:

- Owners and shareholders: profitability, return on investment, asset turnover, earnings per share, and rate of net revenue growth

- Physicians: admission trends and physicians' satisfaction with the hospital's technology, facilities, staffing, and management
- Employees: employee productivity and the results of employee satisfaction surveys
- Patients: market share trends; patients' satisfaction with the hospitals' facilities, nursing staff, physician staff, and quality of care; and patients' willingness to return to the hospital for care in the future
- Community: the community's perception of the hospital's reputation and image

Exhibit 8.8 is a sample matrix that could be used for gathering and organizing stakeholder data. Stakeholders can be asked to rate their level of satisfaction with the statistics listed in the chart on the basis of a Likert scale (e.g., 1 = very low, 2 = low, 3 = neutral, 4 = high, 5 = very high). If the survey is repeated over time, trends can be identified. Managers should compare survey results to desired results to determine whether gaps exist, and areas needing improvement can be addressed.

Effective healthcare leaders obtain and use internal data from many sources to guide their decisions. Internal statistics and information can be obtained from budget reports, ad hoc studies, external reports, and periodic surveys. Informative data are timely and address the identified question or need. They also are defined consistently. As discussed earlier in this chapter, definition consistency is especially important when one compares internal data to other organizations' data. For instance, the author found that one large international hospital had seven different definitions for patient length of stay. This statistic was meaningless until the hospital agreed on a standardized definition.

National associations and government entities provide definitions for many measures. For example, in 2002, the US government's Interdepartmental Committee on Employment-based Health Insurance Surveys approved a list of definitions of health insurance terms that the Bureau of Labor Statistics subsequently published (see the list at www.bls.gov/ncs/ebs/sp/healthterms.pdf). Likewise, Blue Cross Blue Shield Association (www.bcbstx.com/insurance-basics/understanding-health-insurance/glossary) and the American Hospital Association (www.ahadataviewer.com/glossary/) have published definitions of common healthcare terms.

Despite their best efforts to meet the needs of their stakeholders, organizations frequently find it impossible to meet the needs of all stakeholder groups. Employees may want higher wages, investors may demand greater returns, and customers may request lower prices. To meet these multiple demands, organizations have to balance their efforts and prioritize stakeholders' benefits and support. As organizations develop their mission and vision, it is important to consider which stakeholders are most crucial, what benefits they require, and what support they provide to the organization.

EXHIBIT 8.8
Key Stakeholder Satisfaction Matrix

Key Stakeholder	Statistic	2018 Statistic	Trend	Desired Result	Gap: Actual to Desired
Owners/ shareholders	Profitability				
	Earnings per share				
	Revenue growth				
Physicians	Technology*				
	Facilities*				
	Staffing*				
	Management*				
Employees	Benefits*				
	Culture*				
	Management*				
Patients	Market share trends				
	Facilities*				
	Food*				
	Nursing staff*				
	Physician staff*				
Community	Perceived reputation				
	Perceived image				

*This statistic reflects stakeholders' satisfaction with the item listed.

Managers can use different analytical methods to identify and prioritize key stakeholders and decide how and when they should be involved in strategic planning and management (Bryson 2004). Basic stakeholder analysis includes the following steps:

1. *Identify key stakeholders.* All stakeholders are identified through brainstorming, surveys, or some other means, and then key stakeholders are selected from among them. Exhibit 8.9 suggests that key stakeholders have both a high interest in the organization and high power to influence the organization. Core organizational strategies should address this key group.
2. *Determine key stakeholders' expectations.* Stakeholders judge the organization's performance on the basis of their expectations. In a

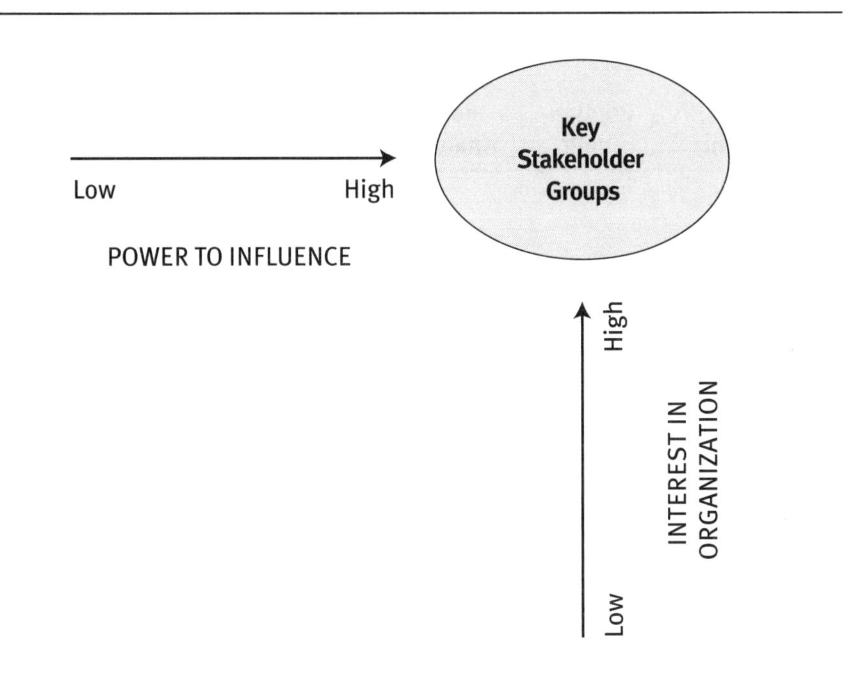

EXHIBIT 8.9
Key Stakeholder Groups

hospital, for example, patients—clearly a key stakeholder group—might judge the hospital by its cleanliness, its food, the friendliness of its staff, and access to care. Clinical networks—key stakeholders of HMOs—might judge an HMO by its reimbursement level and the helpfulness of network personnel.

3. *Judge key stakeholders' perception of the organization's performance.* Key stakeholders' perception of how well the organization is meeting their expectations could be evaluated on a numerical scale (e.g., from 100 [excellent] to 0 [terrible]), by colors (e.g., green = good, yellow = fair, and red = poor), or on a Likert scale (e.g., 7 = excellent, 6 = very good, 5 = good, 4 = adequate, 3 = poor, 2 = very poor, 1 = extremely poor).
4. *Identify changes needed to satisfy key stakeholders.* Changes required to improve key stakeholders' satisfaction can be identified from their perceptions of the organization's performance. Changes might entail increasing their level of involvement in strategic planning, adding programs and facilities, or improving service.
5. *Determine the proper level of involvement of key stakeholders.* Key stakeholders' involvement in strategic planning and management depends on the value their abilities, interest, and availability could add to these functions. Likewise, their degree of involvement might vary by planning stage. Their degree of empowerment can also vary by organizational function or activity. As shown in the sample chart in exhibit 8.10, ways of involving key stakeholders include (Bryson

EXHIBIT 8.10 Sample Chart for Determining the Level and Type of Key Stakeholders' Involvement

Levels of Involvement	Preplanning	Environmental Analyses	Goal Setting	Implementation	Outcome Monitoring and Evaluation
Inform					
Consult					
Participate					
Direct					

2004) (a) informing (keeping them updated on activities and actions), (b) consulting (seeking their opinions and providing them feedback on their input), (c) participating (inviting key stakeholders to serve on committees and task forces), and (d) directing (having key stakeholders take ownership of selected planning stages, functions, and activities).

For example, a hospital could inform a key governmental agency of milestones during strategy implementation, have its physician group collaborate on the implementation of key goals, and empower its union to oversee aspects of strategy monitoring and evaluation.

6. *Incorporate needed changes into strategic plans.* Organizations maintain key stakeholders' support by including any changes required to meet their needs in strategic plans.

SWOT analysis An analytical tool used to develop an overview of an organization's strategic situation and better understand its environment. This type of analysis examines four important aspects of an organization: its strengths and weaknesses (i.e., the internal environment) and its opportunities and threats (i.e., the external environment).

Use and Misuse of SWOT Analysis

SWOT analysis is an easy-to-use tool for developing an overview of a company's strategic situation and a better understanding of its internal and external environment. It is probably the most commonly used strategic planning mechanism. SWOT analysis works best when an organization has already gathered internal and external data. It has been called "the doorway to strategic planning" because it can synthesize large quantities of data into specific issues that need to be addressed in the strategic planning process (Nauert 2005). As illustrated in exhibit 8.11, SWOT analysis examines four important aspects of an organization: (1) its *s*trengths, (2) its *w*eaknesses, (3) its *o*pportunities, and (4) its *t*hreats. Strengths and weaknesses are components of an organization's internal environment, while opportunities and threats are forces that fit under its external environment.

Strengths are important capabilities, characteristics, and competencies that enable an organization to compete successfully or that set it apart from its

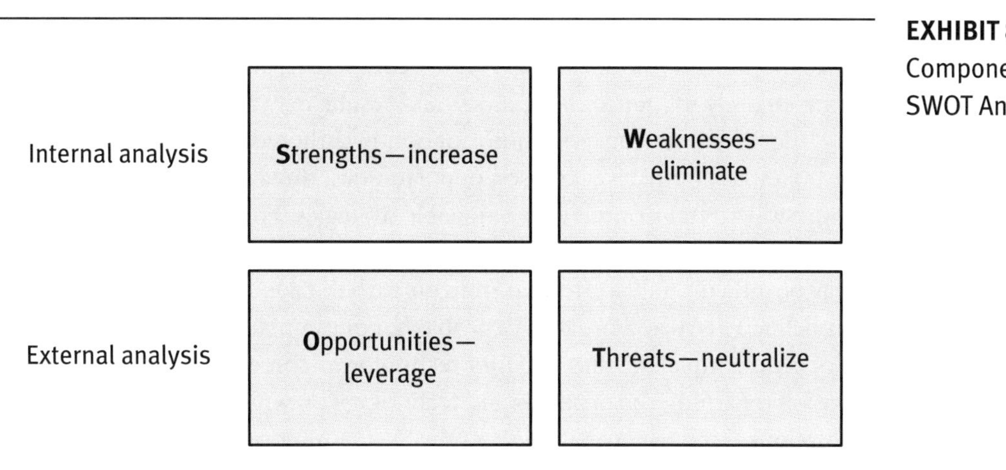

EXHIBIT 8.11
Components of SWOT Analysis

competitors. Examples of strengths include name recognition, patents on key technology, cost advantages, skilled employees, and loyal customers.

Weaknesses are characteristics that place an organization at a disadvantage in the marketplace. It may perform certain tasks poorly in comparison to its competitors or just fail to fulfill certain functions. Weaknesses might include a poor reputation and market image, old facilities, poor customer relations, and inefficient operations.

SWOT analysis is popular because it can be conducted with little preparation and used in a variety of situations and contexts, from small departmental meetings to large corporate gatherings. It can be used to examine an organization's market position, a product or a brand, a business idea, a potential acquisition, and outsourcing opportunities, among other purposes. All that needs to be done to conduct a SWOT analysis is to gather a group of people who have knowledge about the organization or a segment of the organization, although participants generally are chosen because of their stakeholder position. Participant groups typically consist of 5 to 25 individuals led by a facilitator, who identify strengths, weaknesses, opportunities, and threats through brainstorming. The facilitator needs as little as a piece of chalk and a blackboard, sticky notes, or a flip chart and markers to fashion a two-by-two SWOT chart. Because of the flexibility of SWOT analysis and its ease of administration, it is used across all industries.

However, because of its ease of use, SWOT analysis tends to be misused. The author has seen complete strategic planning efforts erroneously driven almost exclusively by SWOT analysis, but given its many inherent weaknesses, relying too much on SWOT analysis can be problematic. Too often, SWOT analysis is initiated without giving thought to background and trend information. A typical SWOT analysis ignores trend and other data and almost never considers organizational charts and graphs. Participants arrive with only their existing ideas and perspectives, which may reflect their biases and misperceptions. Also, unless the facilitator is highly competent, powerful individuals may inappropriately influence the analysis, and results may be inaccurate or biased.

Furthermore, once the information is gathered and classified into the four boxes (strengths, weaknesses, opportunities, threats), there may not be an obvious way to transform it into actionable strategies. For example, if the SWOT analysis identifies strengths and opportunities that all other competitors also have, it may be difficult to discern what strategic path to take. In many cases, long lists of ill-defined items accentuate this problem. For example, if participants identify "poor product quality" and "inferior technology," there is no depth of detail or precision regarding the products and technology on which they are basing their perceptions. Likewise, participants in the SWOT almost never present evidence justifying their perceptions . As a result, feelings and anecdotes—neither of which may be factually accurate—often dominate SWOT analysis.

Another problem is participants' failure to rank and prioritize their results, which makes it difficult to identify critical areas. Few organizations can focus on 20 to 30 opportunities; narrowing priorities to 7 to 10 items makes implementation of resulting strategies more likely. Some have suggested that a more structured analysis is needed to distill the lists from SWOT analysis into core competencies and core problems that can more easily be linked to plans of action to preserve and leverage strengths and eliminate weaknesses (Coman and Ronen 2009).

Suggestions for the Effective Use of SWOT Analysis

Properly performed SWOT analyses can meaningfully inform strategic planning. The following suggestions can mitigate the aforementioned problems and improve the results of SWOT analysis:

- Use a trained facilitator.
- Review the organization's mission and vision to remind participants that the SWOT analysis is directly related to these statements.
- Gather helpful data and provide them to participants prior to the meeting.
  - Consider conducting surveys or focus groups to obtain key data.
  - Prepare and distribute white papers, if needed. (**White papers** are documents written by experts that examine business problems and potential solutions. They are used to educate readers and help people make decisions.)
- Consider using other process methods to arrive at better information, such as nominal or Delphi groups (see the glossary at the end of the book) that can rank data more efficiently.

White paper
An authoritative paper or analysis of an issue or a problem.

- Weight or rank SWOT items to establish strategic priorities. Select no more than seven to ten critical factors to address strategically.
- Use more than one word to explain comments. For example, "technology" listed as an opportunity provides no details.
- Use SWOT analysis as a basis for a gap analysis to determine where the organization is now and where it wants to be.

Exhibit 8.12 provides a template that can be used to guide a SWOT analysis. The questions in each quadrant can facilitate identification of an organization's strengths, weaknesses, opportunities, and threats.

Implementation Suggestions

SWOT analyses often end with nicely made lists that are not translated into strategic action. Before conducting a SWOT analysis, an organization should determine how the resultant information will be used. It might be used in the strategic planning processes, in the budgeting cycle, or for other decision making. Whatever the purpose, the following questions can help participants turn the results of the SWOT analysis into strategy (Thompson et al. 2016):

- Which weaknesses need to be eliminated immediately?
- Do new strengths need to be developed to meet existing or future challenges?
- Can any current strengths be given less emphasis or downgraded?
- What actions need to be taken to reduce the organization's weaknesses?
- Which market opportunities should be top priority?
- Which opportunities can be ignored for now?
- Which threats are significant and need to be addressed immediately?

Another way to better use and focus the results of a SWOT analysis is to categorize items by degree of certainty and impact. The degree of certainty projects the likelihood of occurrence from "unlikely" to "almost certain." Likewise, the impact of key items can be classified from "insignificant" to "catastrophic." For example, as shown in exhibit 8.13, the strengths, weaknesses, opportunities, and threats generated in a brainstorming session can be placed in one of four quadrants based on combinations of degree of certainty and impact. This arrangement enables participants to understand visually which items rank higher in priority. Clearly, items placed in quadrant 2 (high impact and very probable) must be addressed, while issues in quadrant 3 (low impact and improbable) generally can be discarded.

Items can be further refined and prioritized by assigning each a numeric value ranging from 1 (low) to 5 (high) for both degree of uncertainty and

EXHIBIT 8.12
SWOT Analysis Template

Organization's mission and vision ______________________________

____

Strengths
- What are your best capabilities?
- Which assets are most important to your mission and vision?
- What are your core competencies?
- What differentiates you from your competitors?
- Who are the most important people on your staff?
- How strong are your finances?
- How loyal are your customers?
- What unique resources do you have?
- How advantageous is your location?
- How do you compare to your competitors in terms of price, value, and quality?
- What proprietary knowledge, superior technological skills, or important patents do you possess?
- Do you have important alliances or joint ventures?

Weaknesses
- In what critical areas do you need to improve?
- What necessary expertise or staff do you currently lack?
- In what areas do your competitors have an advantage?
- Do you rely on one set of customers too much?
- Do you lack adequate cash flow and capital reserves to meet current and future needs?
- Do you have adequate profit (income) levels?
- Do you lack needed capabilities?
- Do you have too much debt?
- Does the organization's culture align with its strategic direction?
- Are administrative or structural issues impeding you from achieving your mission and vision?
- Are your costs higher than those of your competitors?

Opportunities
- What external changes present possible opportunities?
- Are these changes technological? Customer related? Legislative?
- What trends are likely to affect your industry?
- Might you be able to attract and acquire important capabilities you do not have?
- Is any of your competitors failing to meet its customers' needs?
- What areas of growth might you be able to expand into?
- Are there niche markets you are not serving?
- Could you package your products or services differently to better meet customers' needs?
- Would any partnerships or alliances help you meet your mission and vision?

Threats
- Is any of your competitors better positioned than you?
- Are there organizations that might enter the market and become new competitors?
- Could key staff be hired away?
- What effect will new laws have on your organization?
- Could new technology destroy your core competencies?
- Do you have any insurmountable weaknesses?
- How will demographic changes substantially affect your existing products and services?
- Are your partners happy with the current arrangement?
- What are the major threats in the next five years to achieving your mission and vision?

Note: Questions should be selected on the basis of the topic and context of the analysis.

EXHIBIT 8.13
Ranking SWOT Items by Degree of Certainty and Impact

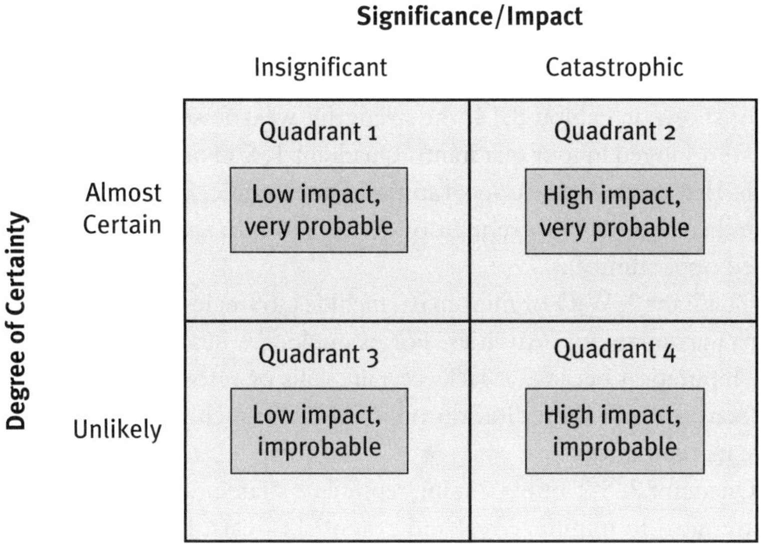

impact and then multiplying these values to obtain a total score (Nauert 2005). For example, if participants identified an increasing elderly population, market entry by a for-profit organization, and genomic therapy for cancer as opportunities and threats, they might be scored accordingly:

SWOT Issue	Degree of Uncertainty	Impact	Total Score
Increasing elderly population	5 (high certainty)	3 (moderate impact)	15
Market entry by for-profit organization	4 (reasonable certainty)	5 (high impact)	20
Genomic therapy for cancer	1 (low certainty)	5 (high impact)	5

Given these rankings, the organization should give the highest priority to the threat of market entry and secondary priority to the opportunity presented by an increasing elderly population.

TOWS Analysis

TOWS analysis
A variant of SWOT analysis that helps leaders make better strategic decisions. Leaders compare external opportunities and threats to internal strengths and weaknesses to determine whether their organization's strengths can leverage its opportunities, minimize its threats, and so forth.

TOWS analysis expands on the concepts of SWOT analysis to help leaders make better strategic decisions. Similar to SWOT analysis, TOWS analysis examines the same categories of external and internal environmental factors but focuses more on the external environment. It explores strengths, weaknesses, opportunities, and threats and then links the four categories to facilitate strategy development (Oxford College of Marketing 2017).

As shown in exhibit 8.14, the strengths, weaknesses, opportunities, and threats are arranged in four quadrants. Quadrant 1, S-O or maxi-maxi, examines strengths that can leverage opportunities. For example, an organization could leverage the strength of its reputation to expand into a secondary market (an identified opportunity).

Quadrant 2, W-O or mini-maxi, includes strategies that minimize weaknesses to maximize opportunities. For example, if a healthcare system has an average reputation because it lacks certain skills or resources (a weakness), it could focus on new accreditation opportunities, such as Magnet status, to improve its reputation.

Quadrant 3, S-T or maxi-mini, represents strategies that use an organization's strengths to minimize real and potential threats. For example, a dominant, well-funded healthcare organization could use its financial resources (a strength) to purchase smaller rivals that have novel business models (threats).

The strategies in quadrant 4, W-T or mini-mini, aim to minimize weaknesses and threats simultaneously. Organizations that have significant external threats and severe internal weaknesses may be poorly positioned and have few development opportunities. Strategies generated from this quadrant often are aimed at survival and implementation of major changes to improve weaknesses before the threats can overwhelm the organization. Examples include divestiture to another organization and merger.

EXHIBIT 8.14
TOWS Analysis

	List of internal strengths 1. 2. 3.	List of internal weaknesses 1. 2. 3.
List of external opportunities 1. 2. 3.	Quadrant 1: S-O (Maxi-Maxi)	Quadrant 2: W-O (Mini-Maxi)
List of external threats 1. 2. 3.	Quadrant 3: S-T (Maxi-Mini)	Quadrant 4: W-T (Mini-Mini)

Value Chain

Another tool widely used to analyze internal organizational competencies is the value chain. Introduced by Michael Porter (1985), a **value chain** is a graphical representation of key internal activities an organization performs to create stakeholder value. Usually presented in a graphic format as shown in exhibit 8.15, the value chain provides a framework for analyzing an organization's strengths and weaknesses across the flow of product or service development.

Value chain
The key internal processes or activities that an organization performs to create value for its stakeholders. The value chain provides a framework for analyzing an organization's strengths and weaknesses across the flow of product or service development and delivery.

As shown in exhibit 8.15, the ultimate stakeholder value is mission achievement. In most value chains, profitability or margin is the mission and a proxy for organizational success. Profitability is an appropriate outcome for many healthcare organizations, especially for-profits whose mission is to provide economic returns to stakeholders. However, for others with greater community responsibilities, the desired value chain outcome may be mission based. For example, a public health department might define success as improved community health outcomes, and a community hospice might base its success on serving a greater number of terminally ill patients.

Value chains consist of two broad categories of activities: (1) primary activities, which principally create value for customers, and (2) support activities, which sustain and enrich the primary activities. For example, the primary value-creating activities of a physician's office include managing supplies, drugs, and equipment; performing examinations, treatments, and surgeries; referring patients to other services; contracting with insurance companies; and providing follow-up service to patients (e.g., home visits, Internet contact).

Support activities, on the other hand, include maintaining an organization's infrastructure (i.e., culture, leadership, and processes), human resources management (i.e., recruitment, hiring, firing, training, labor relations), product

EXHIBIT 8.15
Value Chain for Support and Primary Activities

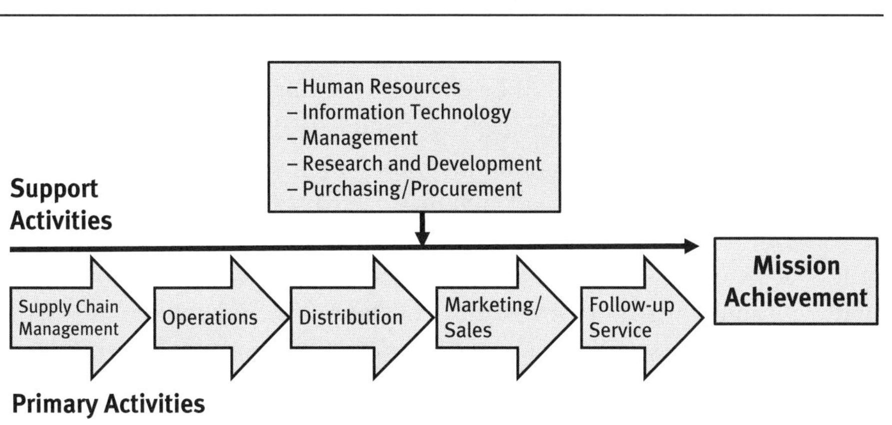

research and development, and development of technology. Different healthcare organizations have different components, and certain components are more important in some types of organizations than in others. For instance, pharmaceutical companies emphasize inventory and research and development, while a medical device company might be more concerned about service.

Value chains can help leaders recognize critical activities that produce value. For example, many organizations today are under pressure to reduce costs and maintain or improve quality. By mapping a value chain and identifying the relative value found in each activity, organizations can improve their efficiencies. Each activity should further the achievement of the organization's mission. The following questions are useful in value chain analysis:

- Are any activities not producing value?
- Does the sequence of activities produce the best value?
- Is coordination across activities appropriate? Do handoffs between activities present any problems?
- Do the teams involved in each activity have the proper mix of skills? Would the addition of any skills significantly improve the value produced by each activity?
- Is the right information collected, integrated, and used across segments? Does a lack of information thwart the creation of value?
- Is the organization's structure aligned with the value the organization intends to create?
- Which support and primary activities do you perform better than your competitors, and which do you not perform so well?
- Could any of the organization's current services or products be outsourced to increase value?
- Could any currently outsourced services or products be better produced internally?

Multiple value chains can be combined to analyze the supply chain of producers, purchasers, and providers in an industry. Leaders can examine the value created by the exchanges that occur among suppliers, distributors, and customers (see exhibit 8.16). Functions performed at each point of transfer can be analyzed to ensure that they contribute value (Burns 2002). This type of analysis helps leaders more accurately understand the value sought and obtained by the consumer. As stated by Arthur A. Thompson and colleagues (2016, 102), "Accurately assessing a company's competitiveness entails scrutinizing the nature and costs of value chain activities through the entire value chain system for delivering its products or services to end-use customers."

EXHIBIT 8.16
Industry Value Chain

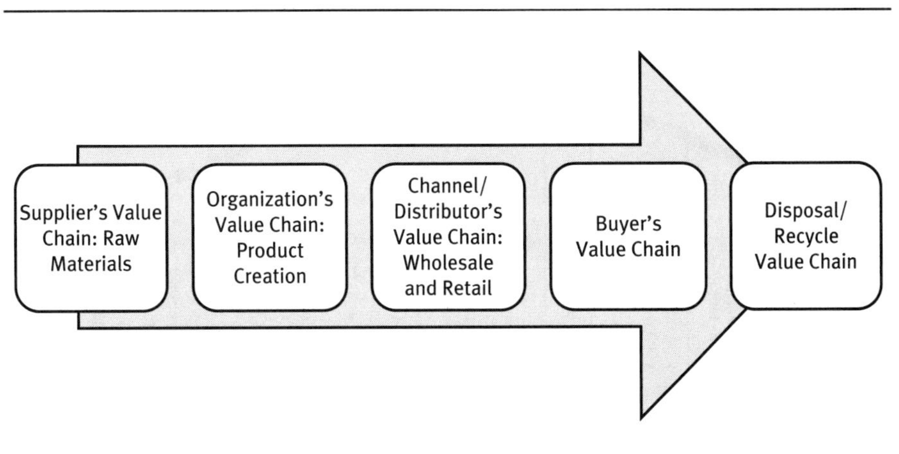

Sources: Adapted from Gimbert (2011), Rajagopalan (2015).

By looking at multiple value chains, as well as their interconnections and points of exchange, an organization can (Burns and Wharton School colleagues 2002)

- optimize the overall activities of organizations working together to create goods and services,
- manage and coordinate product processing from raw materials to end customers,
- develop efficient exchanges and processes that benefit all participating organizations, and
- build positive relationships between suppliers and customers to establish beneficial exchanges.

Kaplan and Porter (2011) suggest that the value chain framework also can be used to lower the costs and improve the quality of medical care. Care is delivered through a process of discrete activities that can be configured and integrated to produce greater value and optimal results. Exhibit 8.17 is a value chain for a neuro-oncological surgery unit. Note the division of support and primary activities and the different components that make up the delivery of care. Primary activities include prevention, diagnosis, preparation, intervention, recuperation or rehabilitation, and monitoring and long-term management. Support activities, including management of patient information, measurement of results, and patient admission, extend across the primary activities. By breaking down the delivery of care in this manner, an organization can evaluate the sequence of activities and value of each component.

In summary, a value chain breaks down the functions of an organization, a process, or a supply chain into its component activities. Porter's original value

EXHIBIT 8.17
The Care Delivery Value Chain

Who Is Who in a Hospital
Primary and support activities in the care environment, adapted from Porter.
Value chain in providing services in a neuro-oncological surgery unit.

Support Activities (that help primary activities by maintaining the right activity environment)

Knowledge Management							
Patient Information	Education and reminders for periodic visits. Advice on lifestyle	Advice to the patient on the diagnostic process	Explanation to the patient about options and support for his or her choice		Information to the patient on treatment and prognosis	Advice to the patient about the rehabilitation process and his or her different options	Advice to the patient and his or her family about long term risks
Result Measurement		CT, MRI, Angiographies, Biopsy, Stereotaxis			Measurements relevant to the type of surgery performed	Measurement of side effects and postoperative complications	Periodical CT, MRI scans (trimester, annual for a few years)
Patient Admission/ Entry	Visits to the neurologist	Consultation visits Visits to diagnostic unit, laboratory, etc. Visits to the emergency room	Visits to the hospital		Stay in the hospital	Consultation visits	Consultation visits
	Visits to primary care		Visits to external consultation		Visits to radiotherapy, or chemotherapy	Rehabilitation visits	Visits to laboratory department Visits to neuroimaging department
Primary Activities (directly related to providing healthcare)	**Monitoring/ Prevention** Medical history Neurological monitoring of seizures Checking risk factors, family history, etc. Clinical exams Genetic screening	**Diagnosis** Medical history Determination of specific nature of the illness Genetic evaluation Choice of treatment plan	**Preparation** Medical advice (risk evaluation) Preoperative informed consent Psychological counseling Evaluation by other specialists (plastic surgeons, etc.)		**Intervention** Surgery (craniotomy, stereotactic surgery, etc.) Adjuvant therapies (hormonal therapies, chemotherapies, radiotherapies)	**Recuperation/ Rehabilitation** Hospital and home care Psychological counseling Treatment of side effects or complications (flap infections, hair loss, nausea, deficiencies)	**Monitoring/ Long term management** Periodical neuroimaging tests Periodical clinical checkup Treatment of side effects or complications that persist for some time

Source: Pareras (2008). Used with permission.

chain was broken into primary activities that included inbound logistics (the way in which an organization receives and stores its inputs), an organization's operations (the basic activities involved in producing its product or service), outbound logistics (the activities involved in storing and distributing the final product or providing the service), marketing and sales (all activities involved in attracting and retaining customers), and service (the activities involved in providing support to customers, including developing user manuals, staffing help lines, and fulfilling warranties). Subsequent modifications to the original value chain enabled examination of more macro and micro processes, such as specific intracompany activities (micro) and the exchange of goods and services across multiple industries (macro).

Portfolio Analysis

Almost all businesses offer an array or portfolio of products and services. Large corporations often segregate products into strategic business units (SBUs), while smaller businesses may incorporate all of their products in one main unit. However the organization is structured, a fundamental strategic role of leaders is to determine the composition and mix of its products and services. To achieve an optimal mix, leaders need a means of systematically analyzing and evaluating their organization's portfolio to decide what resources to allocate to each product and service. A portfolio analysis

- comparatively evaluates the viability and future of the main components of an organization's business (SBUs or key products and services);
- graphically depicts the performance of an organization's products and services;
- examines the balance between cash flows and growth among key business components; and
- guides strategic allocation of resources—which products or services or SBUs should be funded, which should be trimmed, and which could be divested.

Beginning in the 1970s, various consulting firms developed methods of analyzing organizations' portfolios. These methods use objective criteria to categorize an organization's products and services statistically and visually. The Boston Consulting Group (BCG) decades ago used market growth and market share as primary measures in its growth-share matrix, shown in exhibit 8.18 (Hambrick, MacMilan, and Day 1982). Products and services (or SBUs) are categorized by the rate of their market growth and their relative market share. Suggestive names are given to represent the quadrants of the matrix.

EXHIBIT 8.18
BCG's Growth-Share Matrix

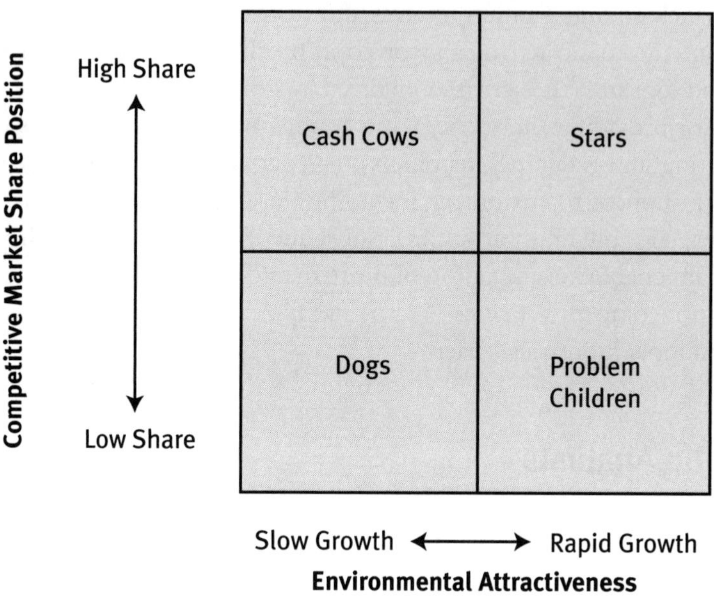

Stars grow quickly and have high market share. *Problem children* grow quickly but have low market share. *Cash cows* grow slowly but have high market share. *Dogs* grow slowly and have low market share. Implicit in this analysis is that low market share corresponds to low current profits and slow market growth correlates to potentially poor future profits.

Later, the General Electric (GE)/McKinsey nine-block matrix (also known as the *GE business screen*) substituted industry attractiveness for market growth and competitive advantage for market share. The matrix categorized each business unit or product according to an aggregate scoring in each of these two dimensions. Industry attractiveness is computed on the basis of the following factors:

- Market size and growth
- Market profitability
- Capital requirements
- Competitive intensity

Likewise, the competitive advantage of an organization or SBU is a composite of multiple factors:

- Market share
- Technological ability
- Product quality

- Service quality
- Price competitiveness
- Manufacturing, marketing, and distribution

Weighted factors for market attractiveness and competitive advantage can be computed for each SBU or product and arrayed in a 3 × 3 table as shown in exhibit 8.19. A product's or an SBU's location on the matrix helps leaders determine the level of investment it should receive. Products or SBUs that rank high on both dimensions should receive continued investment and be grown (built) because they have high profit potential. Conversely, those ranking low on both dimensions should receive little further capital allocation and be closely managed to maximize cash flow (harvest). Finally, those in the middle spaces should be improved to achieve a higher ranking (Luke, Walston, and Plummer 2004).

A modified method of portfolio analysis called the *mission-based matrix* is useful in sectors composed of many not-for-profit organizations (e.g., healthcare). The mission-based matrix adds a third dimension, mission contribution, to the GE/McKinsey matrix (see exhibit 8.20). This additional dimension quantifies the relevance of the SBU or product to an organization's mission. For instance, a healthcare system may own retail clinics, an HMO, a durable medical equipment company, indigent clinics, and outpatient surgical units. The importance of each may vary according to the system's mission. If a religious order concentrated on serving the poor sponsors the healthcare system, the indigent clinics may have the greatest importance. The mission-based matrix enables an organization to identify mission-essential units and products that could have been targeted for divestiture had it used the GE/McKinsey or BCG matrix (Luke, Walston, and Plummer 2004).

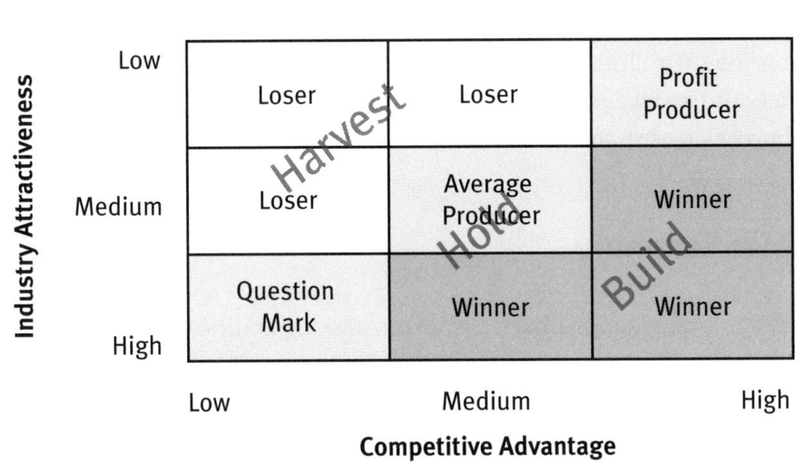

EXHIBIT 8.19
GE/McKinsey Nine-Block Matrix

EXHIBIT 8.20 Mission-Based Matrix

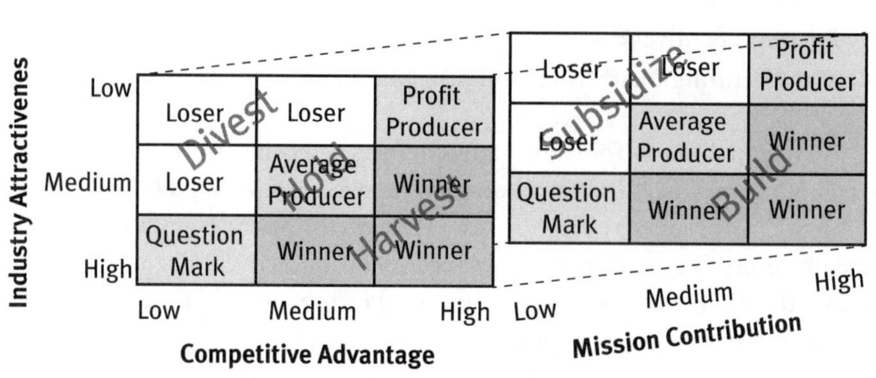

This further segmentation provides greater clarity on potential strategic actions. Products that have little mission value but are well positioned otherwise should be harvested. Excess cash flows from these products could subsidize products that are poorly positioned but critical to the mission. The firm might consider divesting the well-positioned, profitable products because well-positioned products have the best sales price.

Portfolio analyses can be problematic, however. As does any screening mechanism, it simplifies a complicated world. Even the more complicated models may ignore important factors. The dimensions, such as industry attractiveness, are difficult to define quantitatively and thus qualitatively emphasize certain aspects and ignore others, depending on the perspective of the leader performing the analysis. Even products and SBUs may be difficult to define, given the interdependence of products and processes. Furthermore, the dimensions used in portfolio analysis may not reflect profitability. A product may rank high on the dimensions yet because of other factors may generate little or no profit. To address this problem, some analysts add a profitability dimension. Even with its problems, however, portfolio analysis is a commonly known means of balancing cash allocations among units. This analysis can help leaders identify products and services that require cash infusions for future growth and established products that can provide the necessary cash flows (M. Martin 2015).

Chapter Summary

Valuable resources Resources that lack substitutes and are critical, rare, and difficult to imitate.

Healthcare organizations have resources and capabilities that managers can convert to products and services. To sustain its mission, an organization must have **valuable resources** from which to develop capabilities and core competencies. Resources that develop over time, such as a reputation, are rare and difficult to imitate and substitute.

Internal analyses evaluate internal resources by comparing meaningful data to those of other organizations and trending the data over time. Both benchmark and trend data are important to evaluating an organization's effectiveness and direction. Data chosen for analysis should reflect stakeholders' needs and can be gathered periodically from surveys, public sources, and operations.

Two methods often used for internal analysis are SWOT analysis and value chain analysis. SWOT analysis examines the internal and external environments by identifying strengths and weaknesses (internal) and opportunities and threats (external). To use SWOT analysis effectively, leaders must consider objective data in addition to subjective perceptions, rank and prioritize the results of the analysis, and be able to translate the results into strategy. TOWS analysis extends SWOT analysis by linking an organization's strengths, weaknesses, opportunities, and threats to clarify strategic direction. Value chain analysis is used to identify internal strengths and weaknesses and improve organizational processes and outcomes. Value chains are segmented into primary and support activities to evaluate the flow, processes, and interchange of information, services, and products. They can be used to examine an organization, a process, or an industry supply chain.

Portfolio analysis is a graphical method of assessing the value of an organization's products and services or SBUs. Products and services or strategic business units (SBUs) are categorized according to industry attractiveness and competitive advantage or market growth and share. This categorization helps leaders allocate resources appropriately. Mission-based matrixes expand on basic portfolio analysis by considering products' or SBUs' contribution to fulfilling and sustaining the organization's mission.

Chapter Questions

1. What are the differences between resources, capabilities, and core competencies?
2. To sustain a competitive advantage, an organization must have resources with what characteristics?
3. Can an organization gain and sustain competitive advantage by having cutting-edge technology? What problems are inherent in this approach?
4. Which of the following approaches is most likely to sustain an organization's strategic advantage? Why?
   a. Buying new equipment
   b. Being the first to add a new service
   c. Having a unique culture

5. What are the benefits and challenges of having culture as a core competency?
6. Why do data need to be translated into useful information?
7. How do benchmarking and trend data differ?
8. Why is it important to consistently evaluate data that reflect how well key stakeholders' needs are being met?
9. What is the value of gathering data over time and trending them?
10. What can be done to use SWOT analysis more effectively?
11. What is a value chain?
12. How can a value chain be used to improve different levels of an organization and an industry?
13. What are the pros and cons of using portfolio analysis? In your opinion, which dimensions contribute more information?

Chapter Cases

Case Studies

Read and discuss "The Virulent Virus" or "Dissolving a Long-Standing Affiliation and Moving On" in the case studies section at the end of the book. Answer the questions at the end of the case.

The Necessity of SWOT

A large, not-for-profit healthcare organization spent one year developing its first strategic plan. It involved both internal and external stakeholders, created a mission and a vision, gathered trend data, made projections, and identified strategic priorities and subsequent projects. After completing the first draft, it gave the document to various stakeholders for review and comment. Generally, the feedback was positive. However, one high-ranking governmental official remarked that the strategic plan was incomplete and not of high quality because it made no reference to SWOT analysis.

Questions

1. Is the governmental official correct? Should all strategic plans be informed by SWOT analysis?
2. What does a SWOT analysis provide? Could this information be generated in another way?
3. What is the value of using SWOT analysis? Are there disadvantages to using SWOT analysis?
4. Could a strategic plan be created solely on the basis of SWOT analysis? Why?

Determining How to Involve Stakeholders

Sue was just hired as the director of the Springfield Public Health Department. She had been an assistant director in a public health agency located in another state. She was excited to take her first director position. The previous director had been a very private person and rather reclusive. He had not involved many employees or community members in his decision making, and this tendency contributed to his resignation.

Sue understood that, to do well, she would have to involve the key stakeholders. However, she was not certain with whom to spend her time. Her first day she had what seemed like hundreds of people wanting to schedule an appointment with her. At the end of the day, she spoke with her administrative assistant to talk about her schedule. She noted that people wanting to see her included physicians, nurses, the director of a regional laboratory, three community members, two health promotion specialists, a past donor, the mayor, a housekeeper, a union representative, and a Medicaid agency manager, among others. The demand made her feel overwhelmed. She left for the day wondering with whom she should spend her time.

During the evening, she read guidelines regarding stakeholder management that the US Centers for Disease Control and Prevention (CDC) had published that suggested giving priority to stakeholders who can do the following:

- Increase the credibility of your efforts
- Be responsible for day-to-day implementation of the activities that are part of the program
- Advocate for or authorize changes to the program
- Fund or authorize the continuation or expansion of the program (CDC 2017a).

She also learned that she should classify her stakeholders according to level and type of involvement. She saw the following matrix and wanted to use it.

Levels of Involvement	Preplanning	Environmental Analyses	Goal Setting	Implementation	Outcome Monitoring and Evaluation
Inform					
Consult					
Participate					
Direct					

(continued)

She decided to identify her department's key stakeholders and classify them to their appropriate level of involvement.

Questions

1. Who are the key stakeholders? Working in a group, identify them based on the perceived power of influence in the organization according to the CDC guidelines.
2. What is each key stakeholder's appropriate level of involvement?

Chapter Assignments

1. In groups of three, pick a local healthcare organization with which you are familiar. Conduct a SWOT analysis on the organization. After completing the SWOT analysis, use the template in exhibit 8.12 to prioritize the strengths, weaknesses, opportunities, and threats you identified.
2. A large pharmaceutical company wants to ascertain how well it is meeting the needs of its stakeholders. The business development team determines that the key stakeholders it wishes to survey include physicians, retail pharmacists, and patients with chronic diseases who take multiple medications. Critical factors of interest include the company's reputation and the value of its medications relative to their cost. You are asked to develop the survey. Create a survey based on a five-point Likert scale that will provide your team with the information it needs on each stakeholder group.

CHAPTER

9

STRATEGIC FINANCIAL ANALYSIS

> To provide high-value care, an organization must (1) establish parameters of financial performance, (2) balance sources and uses of capital, (3) estimate a future financial trajectory, and (4) assess how changes to key assumptions will affect its financial position.
>
> Sound projections are integral to developing a realistic financial outlook, including setting goals and performance targets to keep the organization within its "corridor of control"—that is, balancing its strategic requirements and capital capabilities, while protecting its long-term financial integrity. This balance drives financial support for the organization's strategic direction.
>
> . . . Working from a realistic baseline plan, leaders must incrementally test the impact of major strategies or changes on the organization's ability to bridge the gap between projected results and targeted performance goals. . . . [As] leaders move beyond strategic cost-management toward strategic cost-transformation, trustees and senior executives should ask: Are we doing the right things? Providing the right services? Are we using the right venues and the right providers? Can we sustain these over the long haul?
>
> . . . Robust and disciplined financial planning is critical to providing high-quality, high-value care to patients. Traditional financial and capital planning still make sense in a changing business model, but hospitals and care systems today must be more focused on strategy. . . . Leaders . . . [should] be far more aware of the external environment and its changes, and then translate that knowledge internally, applying the analytics and planning, to create a portfolio of initiatives that define the organization's road map for success.
>
> —Cynthia Hedges Greising, "How Hospitals Should Approach Financial Planning in Changing Times," 2014

Learning Objectives

After reading this chapter, you will

- comprehend balance sheets and operating statements,
- know key financial ratios,
- see the importance of liquidity to an organization,

- recognize the relationship between assets and activity ratios,
- perceive the significance of debt ratios and their impact on organizations,
- be able to identify the major profitability ratios and the differences between for-profit and not-for-profit organizations,
- understand the time value of money and its use in financial analyses,
- be able to compute a net present value for a proposed project,
- be familiar with internal rate of return and the advantages and disadvantages of using this financial tool,
- understand payback and its use,
- be able to perform breakeven analysis, and
- grasp the use of sensitivity analysis.

Financial skills are important tools for the strategist. They cannot be separated from strategic thinking and strategic decision making but are increasingly important as an integral part of an organization's road map for success. Strategy revolves around making better decisions for the organization, which ultimately requires allocation of finite resources. One could say that actual, realized strategy (see chapter 1) is the placement of capital resources and not necessarily statements written in a strategic plan.

Managers use financial skills to ascertain the viability of acquisitions and the strength of competitors and to establish appropriate metrics for monitoring budgets and progress toward goals. Understanding an organization's financial position, as well as that of its competitors, can be a crucial skill for healthcare leaders. When formulating strategy, leaders must consider business cost structures, payment and reimbursement, cash flows, return on investments, operating budgets, pro forma financial statements, and capital budgeting.

Leaders without a solid knowledge of finance are at a severe disadvantage. Many of the major bankruptcies involving healthcare companies resulted from a combination of poor strategic and financial management. For example, as mentioned in chapter 4, the Allegheny Health Education and Research Foundation (AHERF), at one time Pennsylvania's largest statewide, integrated delivery system with 14 hospitals and more than 300 physician practices, imploded in 1998 because of a misguided strategic direction that incurred massive debt. AHERF's bond debt grew from $67 million in 1986 to $1.2 billion in 1998, while payment rates to its hospitals declined and annual losses from its owned physician practices exceeded $60 million. AHERF's inattention to finances while pursuing a rapid growth strategy invoked its collapse (Burns et al. 2000). Other health systems continue to struggle financially. In the first six months of 2016, seven hospitals and health systems filed for bankruptcy protection (Ellison 2016).

This chapter examines basic financial tools that support strategic thinking, including ratio analysis, net present value, return on assets, internal rate of return, and breakeven analysis. Readers are encouraged to read texts on healthcare finance to gain a greater depth of financial knowledge.

A leader uses financial skills in many aspects of strategy formulation. She can determine if a project is a good investment, ascertain what the existing and future sources and amounts of organizational capital are and will need to be, compare strategic alternatives, and monitor strategic initiatives. When strategic planning involves identifying targets for acquisition or potential partners, financial analyses clarify an organization's market position and options. Leaders do not need to be accountants or finance majors but do need to have the basic knowledge required to integrate finance with their strategic thinking, be able to ask the tough questions during strategic decision making, and understand the implications of their strategies for their organization's finances. Excellent strategic thinkers almost always have good financial skills.

Exploring a Company's Financial Strengths and Weaknesses

Ratio analysis
A quantitative analysis that uses financial data from an organization's financial statements to highlight its financial strengths and weaknesses.

An organization's financial strengths and weaknesses and capital capacity can be examined using **ratio analysis**. As discussed in chapters 7 and 8, knowledge of one's own and competitors' strengths and weaknesses informs the development and implementation of strategy. Ratios make data more interpretable and comparable and are used for many purposes. For example, a batting average of .350 is much more understandable than a statistic of 70 hits in 200 turns at bat. Likewise, a report indicating that a politician has garnered 52 percent of the vote in an election is more meaningful than a report indicating that the politician has received 2,562,124 votes.

Operating statement
A financial statement containing operating results for a specific period; includes revenues (monies taken in), expenses (monies paid out), and the difference between the two (profit or loss). Also referred to as a *profit and loss (P&L) statement*, *revenue statement*, *statement of financial performance*, *earning statement*, and *statement of operations*.

Most commonly, the data for ratio analysis come from organizations' operating statements and balance sheets. Most companies hire external auditors to examine their financial data periodically (typically annually) and issue an audited financial report. Although nonaudited statements and data may be adequate, if significant or important evaluations are being conducted, organizations should use audited reports.

Operating statements, also referred to as *profit and loss (P&L) statements*, *revenue statements*, *statements of financial performance*, *earning statements*, and *statements of operations*, contain financial activity for a specific period (generally a month, a quarter, or a year). Figures include revenues (monies taken in), expenses (monies paid out), and the difference between the two, which profit-seeking firms acknowledge as the *bottom line* or *net profit (loss)*. Not-for-profit organizations commonly refer to this difference as *change in net assets* or *excess of revenues over expenses* (Finkler and Ward 2006; Gapenski and Reiter 2015).

As discussed previously, ratios allow better comparisons. Organizations can compare themselves to competitors, peers, and state and national averages (medians). Averages will change over time based on industry conditions. For example, the median number of days of cash on hand has steadily increased over the past few decades; in 2008, the median was around 110 but increased to 200 days by 2015. In addition, days in accounts receivable were 45 days in 2009 but increased to 51 by 2015 (Associated Press 2016; Merritt Research Services 2017). Likewise, a healthcare organization's ratios will change depending on its use of capital and profitability.

Exhibit 9.1 shows the 2015 and 2016 statements of operations for Stanford Health Care (SHC), one of the largest academic medical systems

EXHIBIT 9.1 Stanford Health Care Consolidated Statements of Operations, Years Ended August 31, 2016, and August 31, 2015 (in thousands of dollars)

	2016	2015
Operating revenues		
Net patient service revenue	$4,019,285	$3,525,014
Provision for doubtful accounts	(126,280)	(131,601)
Premium revenue	72,292	62,893
Other revenue	122,996	98,718
Net assets released used for operations	9,372	15,663
Total operating revenue	$4,097,665	$3,570,687
Operating expenses		
Salaries, wages, benefits	$1,850,124	$1,428,100
Professional services	49,846	47,801
Supplies (purchases)	531,130	484,036
Purchased services	1,058,182	912,886
Depreciation and amortization	136,442	109,735
Interest expense	39,661	40,485
Other	389,199	359,368
Expense recoveries from related parties	(104,965)	(93,640)
Total operating expenses	$3,949,619	$3,288,771
Net operating income	$ 148,046	$ 281,916
Other revenues and gains	$ (78,142)	$ 107,320
Net income (excess of revenues over expenses)	$ 69,904	$ 389,236

Source: Data from Stanford Health Care (2016).

in California. The presentation of such statements varies by organization but generally is based on a common structure. SHC's statement is structured in the typical way: The first section includes the different forms of revenues or monies brought in, the next section lists expenses or monies paid out, and the last line is the difference between the two.

From the data in exhibit 9.1, one can see that SHC is a very big organization. In 2016, its businesses brought in revenues of more than $4 billion and spent almost $4 billion, producing a small net income of only $70 million, a decrease over the net income of $389 million in 2015. However, as discussed earlier, ratios would tell us more about SHC's financial situation.

Exhibit 9.2 shows SHC's balance sheets for 2015 and 2016. The **balance sheet** is a snapshot of an organization's financial condition at some point in time. In exhibit 9.2, these points in time were the last day of its fiscal years 2015 and 2016. The data are divided into assets, liabilities, and net assets. As shown in the exhibit, total assets equal total liabilities plus net assets (also called *equity* or *net worth*).

Balance sheet
A financial statement of an organization's assets, liabilities, and capital at a given point in time.

Again, one can see that SHC is a very large organization, having $690 million in cash, more than $800 million in current assets, $5.7 billion in total assets, and $1.5 billion in liabilities in 2016. However, like the figures in the operations statements in exhibit 9.1, the raw numbers on the balance sheet do not provide a lot of information about the efficiency and effectiveness of the company. Ratio analysis provides this information.

Financial Ratio Analysis

Leaders use data from both operating statements and balance sheets extensively in financial ratio analysis. Financial ratios enable an organization to determine its ability to pay its immediate debts (liquidity ratios), the efficacy of its use of assets (activity ratios), its capacity to cover long-term borrowing (debt ratios), and the reasonableness of its financial return (profitability ratios). This chapter does not discuss the many other ratios in these and other categories (e.g., market ratios). A few of the most commonly used ratios in each category are explored.

Liquidity Ratios

Liquidity refers to the ability to turn some asset into cash or a cash equivalent. All businesses have financial obligations. Employees must receive paychecks. Equipment and supplies must be purchased. Interest and principal on loans must be repaid.

Liquidity
An organization's ability to convert assets into cash.

Organizations should retain an adequate amount of cash or resources that can be easily converted to cash. This amount of working capital should not be too small or too large. Organizations often go out of business when they lack adequate working capital, even when they have significant assets. On the other hand, too much working capital may tie up resources in lower-producing assets that might be better put to use in another investment.

EXHIBIT 9.2 Stanford Health Care Balance Sheet Summary, Years Ended August 31, 2016, and August 31, 2015 (in thousands of dollars)

	2016	2015
Current assets		
Cash and cash equivalents	$ 690,460	$ 475,677
Short-term investments	103,627	101,677
Receivables, less doubtful accounts	559,993	550,721
Other receivables	92,961	75,427
Inventories	50,016	42,935
Prepaid expenses	36,273	35,486
Total current assets	$1,533,270	$ 1,281,923
Investments	132,273	127,860
Investments in university-managed pools	1,316,489	1,440,352
Assets limited as to use, held by trustee	235,788	580,701
Property and equipment, net	2,401,880	1,923,465
Other assets	137,637	163,578
Total assets	$5,757,337	$ 5,517,879
Liabilities		
Current liabilities		
Accounts payable and accrued liabilities	$ 335,995	$ 282,134
Accrued salaries and related benefits	236,819	202,859
Due to related parties	61,308	43,324
Third-party payer settlements	22,948	9,018
Current portion of long-term debt	13,756	13,932
Debt subject to short-term remarketing	228,200	228,200
Self-insurance reserves and other	43,232	34,918
Total current liabilities	$ 942,258	$ 814,385
Self-insurance reserves, net of current portion	118,994	120,364
Other long-term liabilities	355,683	234,855
Pension liability	65,463	51,220
Long-term debt, net of current portion	1,220,789	1,237,347
Total liabilities	$2,703,187	$ 2,458,171
Net assets		
Unrestricted	$2,469,170	$2,490,372
Temporarily restricted	577,086	561,642
Permanently restricted	7,894	7,694
Total net assets	$3,054,150	$3,059,708
Total liabilities and net assets	$5,757,337	$ 5,517,879

Source: Stanford Health Care (2016).

Two primary questions underlie the evaluation of liquidity:

1. Does the organization have enough liquid assets to meet its short-term obligations?
2. Does the organization have sufficient liquid assets to carry out planned financial transactions?

Four ratios are commonly calculated to examine the adequacy of an organization's liquidity. The first is the **current ratio**:

Current ratio
An organization's current assets divided by its current liabilities. This calculation determines the degree to which an organization can pay its current liabilities with liquid assets.

Current ratio = Total current assets ÷ Total current liabilities.

This liquidity ratio provides the number of times short-term obligations can be met by short-term assets. As it provides an indication of the ability to pay liabilities, a high ratio is better. The current ratio is a metric for determining how well a firm can pay its current liabilities (i.e., those due within 12 months) with its liquid assets. For example, based on the data in exhibit 9.2, SHC's current ratios for 2015 and 2016 are as follows:

	2016	2015
Total current assets ÷ Total current liabilities =	$1,533,270 ÷ $942,258 =	$1,281,923 ÷ $814,385 =
Current ratio	1.67	1.57

The results signify that SHC has about 1.67 more current assets than current liabilities in 2016. The generally acceptable range for this measure is about 2.0. Therefore, SHC's current ratio is on the low side of the acceptable range.

The second ratio is the **acid** or **quick ratio**:

Acid (or quick) ratio
The combined amount of an organization's cash and marketable securities divided by its current liabilities. This ratio examines an organization's ability to pay its current liabilities from cash and cash equivalents.

Acid (quick) ratio =
Cash + Accounts receivable + Short-term investments ÷
Total current liabilities.

The acid or quick ratio is a more short-run indicator of liquidity, as it removes the less liquid assets (i.e., inventory) from the current assets used in the current ratio calculation and examines the organization's ability to pay current liabilities with cash and cash equivalents. Inventory generally is not a liquid asset because it often cannot be sold for its purchased value, may be difficult to resell, and takes time to liquidate. Prepaid expenses are also not included in the ratio, as they are not assets available, but assets previously spent. Based on the data in exhibit 9.2, SHC's acid (quick) ratios for 2015 and 2016 are as follows:

	2016	2015
(Cash + Accounts receivable + Short-term investments) ÷ Total current liabilities =	$1,447,041 ÷ $942,258 =	$1,203,502 ÷ $814,385 =
Acid (quick) ratio	1.54	1.48

The generally acceptable rate is around 1.0. Therefore, SHC's liquidity appears sound; it would be able to pay all of its current short-term liabilities with its cash and marketable securities.

Days cash on hand
The combined amount of an organization's cash and marketable securities divided by its operating expenses less depreciation, all divided by 365. This liquidity indicator evaluates how many days an organization could pay its daily operating expenses without additional cash inflows.

The third ratio is **days cash on hand**:

Days cash on hand = (Cash + Cash equivalents) ÷ ([Total operating expenses – Depreciation and amortization] ÷ 365).

Days cash on hand is an important liquidity indicator. It evaluates how many days a company could pay its daily operating expenses without collecting additional cash inflows. Data from SHC's balance sheets and operating statements are used jointly to calculate this ratio:

	2016	2015
(Cash + Cash equivalents) ÷	$690,460 ÷	$475,677 ÷
([Total operating expenses – Depreciation and amortization] ÷ 365) =	([$2,747,405 – $152,686] ÷ 366*) =	([$2,495,052 – $143,521] ÷ 365) =
Days cash on hand	97	74

*Leap year

Days in accounts receivable
An organization's accounts receivable divided by its average daily revenue. This ratio shows how many days of billings are owed to the organization and the average time it takes a bill to be paid.

As is true of all financial ratios, the appropriate number of days cash on hand changes according to industry type and market conditions. The recommended range for not-for-profit healthcare organizations is now about 200 days, suggesting that SHC had less days cash on hand with 97 (2016) and 74 (2015).

The fourth ratio is **days in accounts receivable:**

Days in accounts receivable = Accounts receivable ÷ Average daily revenue.

Accounts receivable
The monies customers owe to a business for goods and services they have received.

This ratio is a measure of the efficiency of an organization's collections function. **Accounts receivable** are monies customers owe to a business for goods and services they have received. Outstanding bills for patient care and products that have been shipped to the customer but are not yet paid for are examples of accounts receivable. Because many healthcare transactions are paid for by third-party companies (e.g., insurance companies, Medicare, Medicaid), only a small percentage of the total bill is collected at the time of service and the third party is billed for the remaining amount. Healthcare companies tie up substantial amounts of cash by providing services and then waiting many days to be paid for services rendered. Not surprisingly, accounts receivable are usually the second largest asset of healthcare organizations, representing up to one-half of their total assets and about three-fourths of their current assets (Herbert 2012).

Days in accounts receivable shows both how many days of billings are owed and the average time it takes a bill to be paid. A small number is better because it indicates quick turnover from billings to cash:

	2016	2015
Operating revenue ÷ 365 days = Average daily revenue	$4,019,285 ÷ 366* = $10,981	$3,525,014 ÷ 365 = $9,658
Receivables, less doubtful accounts ÷ Average daily revenue =	$559,993 ÷ $10,981 =	$550,721 ÷ $9,658 =
Days in accounts receivable	51.0	57.0

*Leap year

SHC's days in accounts receivable decreased from 57.0 to 51.0. This ratio is comparable to the national median, as the average days in accounts receivable for US hospitals was 51 in 2015.

Activity Ratios

Leaders construct **activity ratios** to measure how efficiently an organization uses its resources. Generally, these ratios are determined by dividing the amount of generated revenues by the cost of the assets used to produce the revenues. Activity ratios are also known as **efficiency** ratios (Zelman et al. 2014). Activity ratios are particularly important to companies that sell products and generate inventories but also are meaningful to providers of services. Some of the common activity ratios include the amount of revenues generated per asset unit (asset turnover), the frequency of inventory change (inventory turnover), and average time to pay the organization's bills (average payment period). Because these ratios affect the availability and use of cash in an organization, sometimes they are also considered liquidity ratios.

Activity (or efficiency) ratios
Measures of how efficiently an organization uses its resources.

Take, for example, **asset turnover**:

Asset turnover = Operating revenue ÷ Total assets.

Asset turnover demonstrates the amount of money each dollar of asset creates in a defined period. The greater the amount, the more the organization benefits financially. SHC produces about $0.71 to $0.65 yearly for each $1.00 invested as assets:

Asset turnover
An organization's operating revenues divided by its total assets. This ratio identifies the amount of money each dollar of assets creates over a defined period.

	2016	2015
Operating revenue ÷ Total assets =	\$4,097,665 ÷ \$5,757,337 =	\$3,570,687 ÷ \$5,517,879 =
Asset turnover	0.71	0.65

Inventory turnover
The cost of supplies (cost of goods sold) divided by an organization's average inventory. This ratio measures the number of times inventory is used or sold during a specific period.

The ratio of **inventory turnover** is also important:

Inventory turnover = Total revenue ÷ Average inventory.

Inventory turnover measures the number of times an organization uses or sells inventory during a specific period, which is generally either a calendar year or a fiscal year. A low ratio suggests inefficient use of assets; inventory sits a long time on shelves and could become obsolete. By keeping a modest inventory, organizations free up cash for other purposes. However, excessively high turnover is not necessarily optimal because it may indicate inadequate stocking; stock outs could occur, and critical supplies may be unavailable.

In the following calculation, the year-end inventory on the balance sheet is assumed to be listed as "other current assets (inventory)" and represents the average inventory for the year:

	2016	2015
Total revenue ÷ Average inventory =	\$4,097,665 ÷ \$50,016 =	\$3,570,687 ÷ \$42,935 =
Inventory turnover	81.9	83.2

SHC's inventory turnover was 81.9 to 83.2 for the two years, suggesting that the average inventory item is replaced more than 80 times per year.

Average payment period
An organization's accounts payable divided by its annual purchases divided by 365. This ratio presents the number of days an organization takes to pay its credit purchases.

Organizations also use the **average payment period** ratio:

Average payment period = (Current liabilities × 365) ÷ (Total expenses less depreciation) ÷ 365).

This ratio represents how promptly an organization pays its bills. The average payment period is the number of days an organization takes to pay its credit purchases. Few customers today immediately pay for purchases with cash. Longer payment periods may indicate organizational cash problems, which may prevent the organization from taking advantage of trade discounts for prompt payments. On the other hand, too short a payment period may not be the best use of an organization's cash and may require it to have a large amount of working capital.

	2016	2015
Current liabilities ÷ (Total expenses less depreciation ÷ 365) =	(\$942,258 × 366*) ÷ (\$3,949,619 − 136,442) =	(\$814,385 × 365) ÷ (\$3,288,771 − 109,735) =
Average payment period	90.4	93.5

*Leap year

SHC's average payment period is consistently running over 90 days for the two years, which signifies that vendors are waiting for payment, on average, about three months.

Debt Ratios

Debt ratios (also known as **capital structure** ratios) show how an organization's assets are financed and assess its capacity to take on additional debt. Almost all organizations fund a portion of their assets through debt. This approach to funding, referred to as *financial leverage*, makes sense if an organization can borrow money at a rate that is significantly lower than the rate of return on the assets purchased through debt. Debt leverages an organization's equity by using others' monies to multiply its overall returns.

Debt (or capital structure) ratios Measures indicating how an organization's assets are financed and its capacity for additional debt.

Experts have not established a definitive standard for the optimal use of debt. Organizations too highly leveraged (having too much debt) may find it difficult to pay interest and principal and have little capacity for additional debt. This situation can create organizational stress and potentially foreclose opportunities. On the other hand, people may argue over what constitutes too little debt, depending on their attitude toward risk. Some organizations prefer to have little or no debt, while others attempt to maximize their income through the use of debt.

Some of the most common capitalization ratios include debt to total assets, net assets to total assets, and times interest earned. Calculation of the **total debt to total assets ratio** is straightforward:

Total debt to total assets ratio An organization's long-term debt divided by its net assets. This ratio measures the proportion of an organization's assets that is funded by debt.

Total debt to total assets = Total debt ÷ Total assets.

Total debt to total assets measures the proportion of assets funded by debt in a company's capital structure. In for-profit organizations, net assets are represented as equity, so this relationship is called the *debt-to-equity ratio*. The higher this ratio is, the greater the amount of debt financing.

Net assets to total assets
An organization's net assets divided by its total assets. In the case of a not-for-profit organization, this ratio indicates the proportion of assets that is financed by retained earnings and donations; in the case of a for-profit organization, this ratio indicates the proportion of assets that is financed by equity from profits and private contributions (the sale of stock and private investments). The higher the ratio, the lesser the debt and the greater an organization's capacity to borrow and to pay back existing debt.

	2016	2015
Total debt ÷ Total assets =	(\$13,756 + \$228,200 + \$1,220,789) ÷ \$5,757,337 =	(\$13,932 + \$228,200 + \$1,237,347) ÷ \$5,517,879 =
Total debt to Total assets	0.25	0.27

Relative to similar organizations, SHC has a modest total debt to total assets ratio, which suggests it has a reasonable capacity for additional debt and may not be heavily burdened by debt service. As a comparison, the 2017 healthcare national median is .06, and LifePoint Hospital, a for-profit hospital system, had a debt-to-equity ratio of 1.25 in 2017 (CSIMarket.com 2017). Although deriving meaning from a single ratio is always difficult, one might conclude that SHC is much better positioned than LifePoint, which has higher debt load.

The **net assets to total assets ratio** formula is equally straightforward:

Net assets to total assets = Net assets ÷ Total assets.

Net assets to total assets shows the proportion of assets financed by retained earnings and donations to not-for-profit companies or, in the case of for-profit organizations, equity from profits and private contributions (selling stock and private investments). The higher the ratio, the lesser the debt and the greater the organization's capacity to borrow and pay back existing debt.

	2016	2015
Net assets ÷ Total assets =	\$3,054,150 ÷ \$5,757,337 =	\$3,059,708 ÷ \$5,517,879 =
Net assets to total assets	0.53	0.55

It appears that slightly more of SHC has been financed by equity.

Organizations perform the calculation of the **times interest earned ratio** for for-profit organizations according to the following equation:

Times interest earned =
(Earnings before interest and taxes) ÷
Interest expense.

The times interest earned ratio demonstrates an organization's ability to produce the earnings or profit necessary to pay the interest on its loans. For-profit organizations use EBIT (earnings before interest and taxes) or EBITDA (earnings before interest, taxes, depreciation, and amortization) as the numerator. Not-for-profit organizations' EBIT may be called *retained earnings* or *net income*. These figures are divided by the interest expense for the relevant period. The higher the ratio, the greater an organization's ability to cover its interest payments.

	2016	2015
(Revenues – Expenses) + Interest expense = *x*	($4,097,665 – $3,949,619) + $39,661 = $187,707	($3,570,687 – $3,288,771) + $40,485 = $322,401
x ÷ Interest expense =	$187,707 ÷ $39,661 =	$322,401 ÷ $40,485 =
Times interest earned	4.73	7.96

SHC's times interest earned ratio decreased significantly between 2015 and 2016 as a result of a decrease in earnings. Compared to a sector average of 3.89, SHC appears well positioned to cover the interest expense (Zelman et al. 2014).

Times interest earned ratio
A ratio that shows an organization's ability to produce the earnings or profit necessary to pay the interest costs on its loans. For-profit organizations calculate it by dividing an organization's profits (EBIT or EBITDA) by its interest expense. For not-for-profit organizations, it is calculated by dividing an organization's net revenues less expenses plus interest expense by its interest expense.

Profitability Ratios

All organizations must produce more revenues than expenses to remain in business. **Profitability ratios** examine an organization's ability to produce this excess. These ratios are some of the most visible and common indicators of whether an organization is generating enough monies to fund its mission. They also can be used to compare the relative profitability of business lines, markets, and industries. A few of the most common ratios include operating margin, net margin, and return on assets.

Profitability ratios
Measures that examine an organization's ability to produce earnings or profits.

Organizations calculate **operating margin** as follows:

Operating margin = Total operating revenue –
Total operating expenses) ÷ Total operating revenue

This profitability ratio gives the income derived from patient care operations. Profitability ratios measure the degree to which the organization uses its financial and physical assets to generate a profit. The operating margin measures the percentage of revenues from operations—the organization's primary business(es)—that accumulate as profits or exceed expenses. In other words, the operating margin indicates how sustainable the business activity of an organization is. Many healthcare organizations have very low or even negative operating margins and are sustained by other, nonoperating-related revenues from governmental contributions, donations, and investments.

Operating margin
An organization's net operating income divided by its net operating revenues. This ratio measures the percentage of revenues from operations (the organization's primary businesses) that accumulates as profits and exceeds expenses.

	2016	2015
Net operating income ÷ Net operating revenue =	$148,046 ÷ $4,097,665 =	$281,916 ÷ $3,570,687 =
Operating margin	3.6%	7.9%

SHC's operating margin stood at almost 7.9 percent in 2015, which is considerably higher than the sector benchmark of 3 percent, but it dropped closer to the sector average to 3.6 percent in 2016 (Zelman et al. 2014).

Net margin
An organization's net income divided by its total revenues. This ratio demonstrates the actual flow of all revenues, including nonoperating revenues, into an organization.

Organizations calculate **net (or excess) margin** as follows:

Net margin = (Total operating revenue – Total operating expenses + Nonoperating revenue) ÷ (Total operating revenue + Nonoperating revenue).

This ratio builds on the operating margin to include all sources of income and expenses. Other sources of income aside from patient care operations have become increasingly important to hospitals. Net margin includes all sources of revenue, such as charges for products and services, donations, investments, and so forth. This ratio provides a clear picture of the actual flow of revenue into a healthcare organization. As mentioned earlier, many not-for-profit hospitals and other healthcare organizations tend to rely heavily on nonoperating revenue to sustain their products and services.

	2016	2015
Net income ÷ Total operating revenue =	$69,904 ÷ $4,097,665 =	$389,236 ÷ $3,570,687 =
Net margin	1.7%	10.9%

As shown, other revenue can both increase and decrease operating income. In 2016, SHC saw a significant decline in its net margin. However, in 2015, SHC's net income was high, yielding a 10.9 percent net margin.

Return on assets
A ratio calculated by dividing net profits by total assets showing the amount of earnings or profits gained for each dollar of invested assets.

Another profitability ratio is **return on assets (ROA)**:

Return on assets = Net income ÷ Net assets.

ROA measures the earnings or profits gained for each dollar of invested assets. The greater the earnings per each dollar of assets, the better the organization's financial performance and returns.

	2016	2015
Net income ÷ Net assets =	$69,904 ÷ $3,054,150 =	$389,236 ÷ $3,059,708 =
Return on assets	2.3%	12.7%

Again, as a result of the large shift in net income, SHC's ROA changed dramatically between 2015 and 2016. However, its average for the two years, about 7.5 percent, is significantly above the national benchmark of 4 percent (Zelman et al. 2014).

Comparative Use of Ratio Analysis

As previously discussed, ratio analysis informs strategic decisions. Comparison of various ratios to those of similar organizations is an excellent source of information. Exhibit 9.3 summarizes SHC's ratios discussed in this chapter and compares them to the national ratios for 2015, as well as the ratios for the state of California.

An organization can be better evaluated on the basis of aggregated ratios. The data in exhibit 9.3 suggest that SHC performs well except on its cash on hand and accounts payable. SHC's payment period is almost 4 times the national median and may be causing trouble with its vendors. Similarly, its current ratio is significantly lower.

Ratios, however, rarely provide definitive answers; rather, they often raise questions and highlight areas that organizations must evaluate further. Unexpected results can be examined by asking the following questions:

- Are there extraordinary reasons that explain the outcomes?
- What have past trends been?
- How do the ratios position the organization relative to other firms in the industry?
- Has a change in the type of product and consumer produced the results?
- What other major market shifts may have influenced the results?
- What are future expectations?
- What are the areas of most concern? Why?

For further financial ratios, see examples at the Healthcare Financial Management Association website at www.hfma.org/Content.aspx?id=1113.

EXHIBIT 9.3 Comparison of Stanford Health Care's Financial Ratios

Ratio	SHC		US Median Ratio	California Median Ratio
	2016	2015	2015	2015
Current ratio	1.67	1.57	2.05	2.36
Acid (quick) ratio	1.54	1.48	0.90	
Days cash on hand	97	74	200	
Days in accounts receivable	51	57	51	48.2
Asset turnover	0.71	0.65		
Inventory turnover	81.9	83.2		
Average payment period	90.4	93.5	64	58
Debt to asset ratio	0.25	0.27	0.36	0.372
Net assets to total assets	0.53	0.55		0.538
Times interest earned	4.73	7.96	3.89	–
Operating margin	3.6%	7.9%	3.17%	7.62%
Net margin	1.7%	10.9%	4.4%	7.36%
Return on assets	2.3%	12.7%	4.3%	6.04%

Sources: Data from CSIMarket.com (2017), Merritt Research Services (2017), Office of Statewide Health Planning and Development (2017a).

Comparing Alternative Investments

Strategy formulation regularly requires organizations to decide whether to pursue an option or to choose between alternative investments. All organizations have a finite supply of resources that should be allocated to maximize achievement of the organization's mission and vision. Leaders use three common financial measures to determine the financial impact and value of potential investments: net present value, internal rate of return, and payback. The following discussion only presents essential principles. To gain a more in-depth understanding, readers should explore other finance literature.

Present value The value of future earnings in today's terms, calculated by multiplying future earnings by $[1/(1 + i)^n]$, where i equals the interest or discount rate and n equals the number of years in the future.

Net Present Value

The value of money changes over time. A dollar today is not worth the same as a dollar 5, 10, or 50 years from now. Inflation, risk, and uncertainty of returns from investments diminish the future value of money. The **present value** of projected cash flows takes into account the **time value of money** by discounting future years' earnings back to today's value.

One project may produce immediate and consistent returns, while another might lose money for the first two years and then suddenly begin turning a profit. To level out the unevenness and different timing of returns and compare alternative investments in terms of the value of money today, leaders can calculate the alternatives' present value, which reflects the value of a project's future earnings in today's terms:

$$\text{Present value} = \text{Future earnings} \times [1/(1 + i)^n],$$

where i equals the interest or discount rate and n equals the number of years into the future.

Net present value (NPV) extends the time value of money concept by considering the cost of the investment—that is, NPV equals the present value of future earnings less the cost of the investment. In the example calculation in exhibit 9.4, the cost of the investment that generated the earnings was $3,000. If the project returned $1,000 the first year, $2,000 the second year, and $3,000 the third year, and the discount rate is 10 percent, the total present value of future earnings is $4,815.92. NPV is found by subtracting the cost of the investment from this present value: $4,815.92 – $3,000 = $1,815.92.

Calculation of NPV is especially useful for evaluating strategic options. It accounts for all cash flow so that leaders can determine whether a program or project would generate enough future earnings to cover the initial investment and enables them to compare the alternatives on the basis of a common metric—the dollar. As a general rule, if NPV is positive, the investment should be made; if NPV is negative, the option should be rejected. For example, say a healthcare organization is considering building centers of excellence for four product lines: radiology, cardiovascular, surgery, and diabetes. Does it

Time value of money
The concept that money available at the present time is worth more than the same amount in the future because the value of money diminishes over time as a result of inflation, risk, and uncertainty of returns from investments.

Net present value
A measure that extends the concept of time value of money to evaluate the cumulative present value of an investment, which is the difference between the present value of cash inflows and the present value of cash outflows.

EXHIBIT 9.4
Net Present Value Example Calculation

		Future Earnings		
	Present Value	Year 1	Year 2	Year 3
Year 1	$ 909.09	$1,000		
Year 2	$1,652.89		$2,000	
Year 3	$2,253.94			$3,000
Total present value of future earnings	$4,815.92			
Cost of investment	–$3,000.00			
Net present value	$ 1,815.92			

make financial sense to pursue these projects? The following table presents four alternatives:

	NPV	Investment
Radiology center	$5,770,000	$10,000,000
Cardiovascular center	$3,500,000	$ 7,000,000
Surgery center	$3,000,000	$ 6,000,000
Diabetes center	–$1,500,000	$ 5,000,000

All but the diabetes center have a positive NPV. In other words, the future earnings of the radiology, cardiovascular, and surgery centers would be greater than the original investment, whereas the future earnings of the diabetes center would not. On the basis of these financial results and without capital constraints, the organization would proceed with building the radiology, cardiovascular, and surgery centers but would not build a diabetes center. If the organization has limited capital to invest and can build only one center of excellence, it should choose the one with the highest NPV.

The use of NPV presents a few difficulties, however. First, an organization may have many nonfinancial, mission-based reasons for proceeding with an option, and thus the NPV metric may be too simplistic as a basis for decision making. For example, the University of Chicago Medicine decided to build a Level 1 adult trauma center at its Hyde Park campus to serve the South Side community, although the center will certainly be an expensive drain on the university's financial resources and would probably produce a negative net present value. However, after decades of citizens' insistence that the university had a civic duty to provide trauma services to residents of this community, who experience a very high level of gun violence, the university agreed to add the service (Glanton and Boweau 2015).

Second, the results of NPV calculations can be highly sensitive to the discount rate (also known as the *cost of capital* or *hurdle rate*) used. For instance, the results can change dramatically if a high discount rate rather than a low one is used. The discount rate should account for the time value of money and project risk, which in many cases can be difficult to determine accurately (Zelman et al. 2014). Last, if the organization has capital constraints, the NPV calculation may not provide enough information for decision making. For example, if the organization in the previous example has $15 million to invest in the initiative, which centers should it choose to build? It could invest in the radiology and diabetes centers or the cardiovascular and surgery centers. Which combination would be the better alternative? Additional information is needed to make an appropriate decision in this case.

Internal Rate of Return

Another metric commonly used to better understand and compare alternative projects is *internal rate of return (IRR)*. IRR is the discount rate at which a project's future cash flows exactly equal the initial investment so that the NPV is zero. When deciding which option to pursue or reject, an organization approves any option whose IRR is greater than its established cost of capital. Calculation of IRR, represented by *r* in the following formula, is complicated:

$$\text{NPV} = \sum_{n=0}^{N} \frac{C_n}{(1+r)^n} = 0,$$

where N equals the total number of periods of cash flows and n and $C\,n$ are the cash flow for a specific period.

Mathematically, r cannot be isolated, so the formula must be iteratively solved. Use of a spreadsheet or a financial calculator simplifies this calculation.

For instance, if the cost of capital for the organization is 10 percent and the IRRs for the centers of excellence are those given in the following table, again the organization should approve all but the diabetes center, whose IRR is lower than 10 percent.

	NPV	IRR (%)	Investment
Radiology center	$5,770,000	15	$10,000,000
Cardiovascular center	$3,500,000	18	$ 7,000,000
Surgery center	$3,000,000	19	$ 6,000,000
Diabetes center	–$1,500,000	7	$ 5,000,000

Calculation of IRR also provides other information helpful for decision making. The IRRs on the cardiovascular and surgery centers are higher than the IRR on the radiology center. Therefore, if the organization had a capital constraint of $15 million, the IRRs would suggest that the cardiovascular and surgery centers should be chosen over the other projects.

Payback Period

A simplistic tool called *payback period*, also often used for decision making, examines the amount of time needed to recover an initial investment. Payback period is easy to calculate, but unlike NPV and IRR, it fails to account for the time value of money—that is, the value of each year's earnings is not discounted. The formula for determining the payback period is

$$\text{Payback period} = x + (y/z),$$

where x is the number of years with negative cumulative cash flow (the next year has a positive cumulative cash flow), y is the absolute (positive) value of cumulative cash flows at the end of year x, and z is the yearly cash flow in the year after year x.

According to the example in the following table, the cost of the investment was \$9,000. The organization earned \$1,000 in the first year, \$2,000 in the second year, \$3,000 in the third year, and \$8,000 in both the fourth and fifth years. In the payback period formula, x is 3 (the number of years before the cumulative cash flows became positive), y is \$3,000 (the absolute value of the cumulative cash flow in year 3), and z is \$8,000 (the yearly cash flow in year 4).

	Year	Yearly Cash Flow	Cumulative Cash Flow
Initial investment	0	(\$9,000)	(\$ 9,000)
	1	\$ 1,000	(\$ 8,000)
	2	\$2,000	(\$ 6,000)
	3	\$3,000	(\$ 3,000)
	4	\$8,000	\$ 5,000
	5	\$8,000	\$13,000

Therefore, payback period = 3 + (\$3,000/\$8,000) = 3.375. It would take the organization a little more than three years and four months to recoup its initial investment.

Breakeven Analysis

Breakeven analysis determines the volume point at which a project will cover its costs. This analysis can be helpful to organizations considering new projects, developing a business plan, or formulating a pricing strategy.

The core concept of breakeven analysis is that a business generally has two types of costs: fixed and variable. *Fixed costs* do not vary with volume increases and decreases over a specific time frame. For instance, the monthly rent a physician pays for her office space is a fixed cost. This cost does not vary if she sees 100 or 500 patients per month. On the other hand, *variable costs* change as the business's volume changes. In the same physician's office, variable costs might include the cost of medical and office supplies. As the physician sees more and more patients, she needs more and more supplies, and thus her costs increase.

The formula for finding the volume at which the physician will cover her costs is

Breakeven volume = Total fixed costs ÷
(Average charge per patient – Average variable cost per patient).

To determine a breakeven volume, one first decides which costs are fixed and which are variable. The division of costs into these categories may differ depending on management decisions. For instance, personnel may be required to be present on the job regardless of patient volume (fixed wages) or may be called in as needed (variable wages).

For example, say the physician has three office personnel and two nurses on staff no matter what the patient volume is. The office wishes to use the X-ray equipment and laboratory of an adjoining office on a price-per-use basis. The average cost per use of the X-ray equipment is $66.67. The average cost per use of the laboratory services is $23.34. The physician has determined that she will use the X-ray equipment for 30 percent of her patients and will use the laboratory for 60 percent. The average price she charges per patient is estimated at $100. The average cost per patient and the physician's fixed and variable costs are shown in the following table:

	Monthly Fixed Costs	Variable Costs/Visit
Lease	$ 5,000	
Utilities	$ 800	
Front office staff	$ 6,000	
Nursing staff	$ 5,000	
Supplies		$6
X-ray		30% × $66.67 = $20
Laboratory		60% × $23.34 = $14
TOTAL	$16,800	$40

The breakeven analysis can now be performed:

Fixed costs ÷ (Average charge per patient – Average variable cost per patient) =	$16,800 ÷ ($100 – $40) =
Breakeven	280

The office would need to generate 280 visits per month to pay for its expenses. The physician can then examine the probability of achieving this outcome. If the office is open 20 days per month, an average of 14 visits per day would be required just to pay expenses. The physician can also determine the additional volume required to pay herself a salary of $10,000 per month. Fixed costs therefore increase to $26,800, and the breakeven increases to 447 visits per month or 22 to 23 visits per day.

To evaluate the potential success of a venture more fully, organizations can perform a sensitivity analysis. *Sensitivity analysis* changes key assumptions upward and downward to ascertain the effects on breakeven. Key assumptions are those that could significantly affect results or are most uncertain.

Say the physician in the previous example believes that the most critical assumptions are pending cuts in Medicare and Medicaid, which could lower the average receipts (charges) per patient (i.e., price per unit). She suspects that this change will significantly affect her breakeven analysis, so she performs a sensitivity analysis based on a probable payment range from $82 to $92 per visit:

	Current	Middling	Low
Fixed costs	$26,800	$26,800	$26,800
Average receipts (charges) per patient	$100	$92	$82
Variable cost per patient	$40	$40	$40
Breakeven	447	515	638
Visits needed per day	22	26	32

In this case, if average reimbursement dropped to $82 per visit, the patient volume would need to increase to 638 visits per month, or an increase of about 10 visits per day, for the physician to be able to cover her costs and pay herself a salary of $10,000 per month.

Chapter Summary

Understanding the basics of finance is critical to effective strategic thinking. This chapter briefly examines the principles of operating statements, balance sheets, ratio analysis, other financial tools for capital allocation, and breakeven analysis. Readers are encouraged to explore other financial literature to develop a deeper understanding of these topics.

Operating statements display organizations' financial activities over a defined period (e.g., expenditures made and revenue earned during a particular month). Balance sheets show organizations' financial condition and display their liabilities and assets at one point in time. Both provide data that are critical to evaluating the financial health and value of an organization.

Ratio analyses use data from balance sheets and operating statements to provide more comprehensible information. Ratio analysis can be used to determine an organization's strategic position, analyze possible acquisitions, and compare competitors. The ratios discussed in this chapter are divided into four categories: liquidity ratios, activity ratios, debt ratios, and profitability ratios. Liquidity ratios demonstrate an organization's ability to pay its obligations (liabilities), including debt, interest, and other expenses. Activity ratios (such as asset turnover, inventory turnover, and average payment period) measure how efficiently an organization is using its resources. Debt ratios determine the debt load an organization is carrying and its capacity to take on additional debt. Organizations with too much debt may have difficulty paying principal and interest and may have fewer opportunities for improvement and expansion. Profitability ratios display an organization's profits. In general, the word *profit* refers to the excess of revenues over expenses; however, not-for-profit organizations describe their "profit" in different terms. Operating and net margins examine the percentage of revenue that becomes profit, while return on assets shows the profits earned on each dollar of invested assets.

Another important set of tools used to compare strategic alternatives includes net present value (NPV), internal rate of return (IRR), and payback period. NPV incorporates the time value of money to determine the current value of future projects. It is calculated by discounting future cash flows from a project back to today's value and then subtracting the project's investment costs. On the basis of financial criteria only, projects with a positive NPV should be pursued and projects with a negative NPV should be rejected. Projects also can be compared on the basis of their IRR. Projects whose IRR is higher than the organization's established cost of capital should be pursued, and projects whose IRR is lower than the established cost of capital should be rejected. Payback period, the simplest tool among the three, is the time (usually expressed in years) needed to recover the initial investment made in a project. Unlike NPV and IRR, this tool ignores the time value of money.

The last financial tool explored in this chapter is breakeven analysis. Breakeven analysis identifies the volume at which revenues are equal to expenses. Key concepts in breakeven analysis are fixed and variable costs. Fixed costs do not change as volume changes, whereas variable costs increase as volume increases and decrease as volume decreases. Sensitivity analysis evaluates how breakeven is affected when key assumptions are changed.

Chapter Questions

1. Why do healthcare leaders need to understand finances and learn to use financial tools?

2. How do operating statements and balance sheets differ? How are they similar?
3. How do ratios offer more information than balance sheet data do?
4. What organizational aspect do liquidity ratios demonstrate?
5. To which type of healthcare company would the acid test ratio likely be more applicable than the current ratio? Why?
6. Why would an organization have a large number of days cash on hand? How could its strategic plans influence this number?
7. How does inventory reduction affect the cash position of an organization?
8. How does debt benefit an organization? What load of debt is considered too great?
9. How can a public hospital have a low or negative operating margin yet have enough funds to survive and prosper?
10. What factors affect the magnitude of the time value of money?
11. What are the advantages and disadvantages of basing strategic decisions on NPV?
12. How can the use of NPV and IRR together help leaders make better capital allocation decisions?
13. What is the benefit of basing strategic decisions on payback period? What problems does use of this metric present?
14. In what situations could breakeven analysis be used effectively?
15. What is the advantage of performing sensitivity analysis along with breakeven analysis?

Chapter Cases

Quality Home Health

Quality Home Health (QHH) has been expanding rapidly over the past five years. Although paper profits (i.e., earnings that are shown on reports but may not translate into actual cash in the bank) have been stable at about 3.5 percent of operating revenues, the liquidity of the company has become a concern. You, the CFO, have noted that days cash on hand has dropped to 12 and that the current ratio has decreased to 0.4, while days in accounts receivable has increased to 122 and inventory turnover has decreased substantially. The CEO would like you to answer the following questions:

1. Why does cash flow and liquidity become a problem during company growth?

2. How can a company have healthy profits but lack funds to pay basic expenses?
3. What is the relationship between liquidity and accounts receivable?
4. What could QHH do to improve its liquidity?

Moab Regional Hospital

Many said a small, rural, unaffiliated hospital could not survive. Many such institutions have not. The Moab Regional Hospital was a 17-bed acute care facility located in Moab, Utah. The community consisted of only 9,000 permanent residents, but millions of tourists visited the area annually. The hospital had experienced a high turnover of personnel and struggled with a low census (averaged about four inpatients).

The hospital, opened in 1957, was originally known as the Allen Memorial Hospital. It was operated by a local board and funded by a hospital special service district. This situation continued until 1995, when voters turned down the reapproval of a property tax to support the hospital. The hospital plant was then almost 50 years old and badly needed replacement. Seeking to improve efficiency, a 501(c)(3) nonprofit was created to run the hospital with the special district still owning the old hospital. Drawing on donations and large loans, the new hospital organization designed and built a facility that opened in 2011.

The new building was a great improvement, but long-standing management problems remained. The CEO and the CFO feuded and rarely spoke. Billings were not done on a timely basis, and the hospital's cash flow dissolved. Finally, in 2011, both the CEO and CFO quit and new management was brought in. The new CFO had a long history of turning around hospitals. Moab Regional Hospital went another year without a permanent CEO. The financial results from 2011 to 2015 follow:

Income Statement					
Period ending date	12/31/2015	12/31/2014	12/31/2013	12/31/2012	12/31/2011
Inpatient revenue	$ 12,221,479	$10,969,949	$ 10,031,442	$ 8,429,060	$ 7,337,909
Outpatient revenue	$ 31,000,073	$29,817,093	$ 26,377,807	$ 27,143,672	$ 19,993,503
Total patient revenue	$ 43,221,552	$40,787,042	$36,409,249	$35,572,732	$ 27,331,412
Contractual allowance (discounts)	$ 16,726,220	$14,600,346	$ 14,232,265	$ 13,488,251	$ 7,096,046
Net patient revenues	$26,495,332	$26,186,696	$ 22,176,984	$22,084,481	$20,235,366
Total operating expense	$24,048,564	$23,546,759	$ 21,884,181	$23,060,846	$ 22,477,512
Operating income	**$ 2,446,768**	**$ 2,639,937**	**$ 292,803**	**–$ 976,365**	**–$ 2,242,146**

(continued)

Other income (contributions, bequests)	$ 52,405	$ 238,074	$ 6,463	$ 188,486	$ 1,979
Income from investments	$ 133,148	$ 22,852	$ 75,166	$ 24,278	$ 321
Governmental appropriations	$ 0	$ 0	$ 0	$ 0	$ 0
Miscellaneous nonpatient revenue	$ 890,792	$ 1,047,414	$ 1,181,493	$ 1,083,516	$1,167,274
Total nonpatient revenue	$ 1,076,345	$1,308,340	$1,263,122	$1,296,280	$1,169,574
Total other expenses	$ 5,062	$ 100,861	$ 0	$ 0	$ 0
Net income	**$ 3,518,051**	**$3,847,416**	**$1,555,925**	**$ 319,915**	**–$1,072,572**

Source: Data from American Hospital Directory (2017).

Balance Sheet					
Period ending date	12/31/2015	12/31/2014	12/31/2013	12/31/2012	12/31/2011
Assets					
Current assets	$19,807,244	$16,355,826	$ 13,620,869	$ 8,576,542	$ 8,398,854
Fixed assets	$23,246,503	$25,226,195	$ 27,585,630	$29,295,953	$ 31,397,655
Other assets	$ 4,001,006	$ 3,861,131	$ 1,895,151	$ 3,071,023	$ 0
Total assets	**$ 47,054,753**	**$ 45,443,152**	**$ 43,101,650**	**$40,943,518**	**$ 39,796,509**
Liabilities and fund balances					
Current liabilities	$ 3,227,209	$ 3,998,466	$ 4,500,959	$ 4,331,291	$ 3,668,477
Long-term liabilities	$27,580,010	$28,635,764	$ 29,496,033	$29,093,346	$ 28,901,011
Total liabilities	**$30,807,219**	**$32,634,230**	**$33,996,992**	**$33,424,637**	**$32,569,488**
Total fund balances	$16,247,534	$12,808,922	$ 9,104,658	$ 7,518,881	$ 7,227,021
Total liabilities and fund balances	**$ 47,054,753**	**$ 45,443,152**	**$ 43,101,650**	**$40,943,518**	**$ 39,796,509**

Source: Data from American Hospital Directory (2017).

The chair of the board's performance committee has been asked to evaluate the progress of the hospital. He remembered a few years ago when suppliers would only deliver if paid by cash and short-term loans were used to make payroll. Given this situation, he began by computing the days of cash on hand and found that the hospital had made excellent progress:

Period ending date	12/31/2015	12/31/2014	12/31/2013	12/31/2012	12/31/2011
Days Cash on Hand	260.7	191.4	151.1	48.4	27.4
Definition: (Cash on hand + Market securities) ÷ (Total operating expenses – Depreciation) ÷ 365					

Source: Data from American Hospital Directory (2017).

He now wanted to continue to analyze the rest of the operation. Using both raw numbers and ratios, complete the following tasks:

1. Identify which areas have improved and attempt to explain why these changes have occurred.
2. Compare the ratios to the national financial ratios in the chapter and discuss which are excellent or good, and which ones need improvement.
3. Identify what additional information you might request to understand what has and is occurring at the hospital more thoroughly.

Chapter Assignments

1. Read the 1987 article by Gerald L. Glandon and colleagues titled "An Analytical Review of Hospital Financial Performance Measures" from *Hospital and Health Services Administration*, volume 32, issue 4, pages 439–55, and answer the following questions:
   a. What are the advantages of creating "viability" measures for hospitals? What problems does it present?
   b. What problems are inherent in the use of financial ratios for US hospitals?
   c. How are financial ratios used in relation to bond ratings?
2. Read the Pennsylvania Health Care Cost Containment Council's April 2017 report at www.phc4.org/reports/fin/16/docs/fin2016report_volumeone.pdf, and answer the following questions:
   a. What do the changes in operating and total margins suggest?
   b. Why might total margin have increased in 2016?
   c. What has happened to average days in patient accounts receivable? Why?

3. Access the Indiana State Department of Health's website at www.in.gov/isdh/27224.htm. Look at the 2016 financial reports for Indiana Orthopaedic Hospital, Methodist Hospitals, and St. Vincent Health. Determine the financial ratios discussed in this chapter for each organization and compare them. What are your findings?

PART

V

PLANS FOR ACHIEVING MISSION AND VISION

Organizations commonly develop written plans to establish and communicate strategic direction, time frames, and responsibility. Plans articulate an organization's mission and vision and the goals and objectives an organization has established to fulfill them. Chapter 10 explores the development of strategic and marketing plans and discusses their key components. Chapter 11 introduces business plans, their purpose, and their structure and explains how they are different from strategic plans. An understanding of these plans and their development is important for healthcare leaders.

CHAPTER

10

DEVELOPMENT AND EXECUTION OF A STRATEGIC PLAN

> You don't need a strategy. You need strategies.
>
> "What is your strategy?" is the wrong question. The right question is, "What are your strategies?" No organization can get by with one strategy. You need a handful.
>
> Thomas Aquinas advised, "Beware the man of one book." The same advice applies to strategies. That handful of "driving strategies" should be synergistic. They should strengthen and feed on one another. Each is a linchpin. Remove one driving strategy, and the others suffer; that one strategy is often reduced to impotence.
>
> A handful of strategies persistently and consistently pursued in support of a compelling vision unifies, integrates and coordinates the daily work of the organization. According to Rumelt: "The idea that coordination, by itself, can be a source of advantage is a very deep principle. It is often underappreciated because people tend to think of coordination in terms of continuing mutual adjustments among agents. Strategic coordination, or coherence, is not ad hoc mutual adjustment. It is coherence imposed on a system by policy and design. More specifically, design is the engineering of fit among parts, specifying how actions and resources will be combined.'"
>
> —Dan Beckham, "10 Surprising Keys to Strategic Thinking for Health Care CEOs," 2016b

Learning Objectives

After reading this chapter, you will

- understand the basic principles of strategic plan development;
- be able to describe the process involved in creating a strategic plan;
- have learned how environmental and gap analyses help leaders set strategic priorities;
- perceive the importance of stakeholder alignment and the role of communication in achieving stakeholder buy-in and support;

- be aware of various sources of data;
- comprehend the basics of effective goal setting;
- know how to use project charters; and
- recognize strategic planning structures, including personnel responsibilities and governing body roles.

For most organizations, the principal representation of their strategic direction is their written strategic plan. The plan articulates the organization's mission, vision, values, goals, and objectives and the motives behind its decisions and actions. Most organizations use an annual planning process to formulate written strategies and budgets documents that allocate resources for the upcoming 12 to 18 months, establish financial and operating metrics, and align management's efforts on key strategic priorities. However, as discussed in the quote at the opening of this chapter, strategies, not a strategy, should be developed into written plans that should be used as a guideline, not as a blueprint that has to be followed. Strategic plans ultimately should provide value to their organization by

- defining, developing, and sustaining a clear strategic advantage;
- producing meaningful differences from competitors;
- appropriately allocating and aligning resources;
- creating understanding and commitment; and
- driving accountability and implementation (Beckham 2016b).

Although there are many ways to construct a strategic plan, to be useful and effective it must answer the following questions:

- Where is the organization now?
- What needs to be done to achieve the organization's mission and vision more completely?
- What avenues might the organization take to accomplish the mission and vision?
- What specific actions should be taken?
- How do we translate the strategic plan into action?
- How do we know if we have achieved our objectives?

Strategic plan
A formal, written document that guides an organization's actions and informs stakeholders about the organization's direction and future activities.

This chapter builds on the environmental analyses discussed in previous chapters and examines these questions to provide concrete suggestions on how to create a **strategic plan** that helps an organization achieve its mission. As shown in exhibit 10.1, the environmental analyses inform the organization of

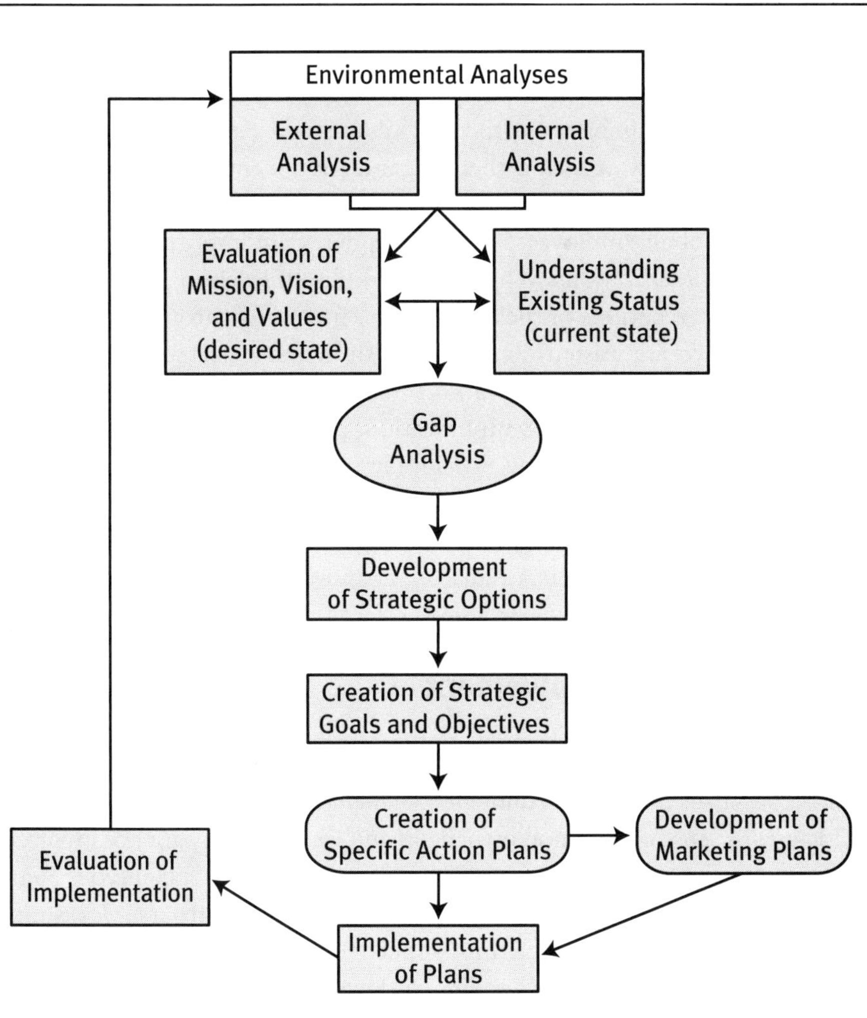

EXHIBIT 10.1 The Strategic Plan Development Cycle

its existing status and the progress it has made toward fulfilling its mission and vision. The gap between an organization's current and desired states inspires objectives and action plans. Once the plans are implemented and outcomes are evaluated, the cycle begins anew.

Understanding an Organization's Current Status

It is critical that examination of the current status of an organization be based on observed and recorded data. Leaders must rely on periodic evaluations of their environment, not just on their "gut feelings." An organized approach to examining the organizational environment involves routine collection of both quantitative and qualitative information to determine whether the organization's strategic plans are working to achieve its mission. As discussed in chapters 7 and 8, environments change, so organizations must reanalyze their circumstances and situation and update their plans accordingly. If they fail to do so, their plans may become misaligned with their mission and vision.

By periodically assessing their organization's environment and communicating the results to all staff, leaders update not only their perspectives but also those of all employees. Periodic updates are important to aligning perceptions in organizations. When staff at different levels in an organization have different perceptions of their external or internal environment, progress derails and efforts are wasted. Research has shown that strategic efforts often (Walston and Chou 2006, 879) "'go off track' as a result of misaligned goals, created in part by inaccurate communication, poor feedback, confused goals, and uncertain strategic directions. Specifically, perceptions of the change efforts may differ along organizational hierarchy and create conflicting perceptions of goals, outcomes, and strategic directions, leading to misappropriations of resources, inconsistent efforts, premature abandonment, and poor results."

Key Stakeholder Involvement

Proper involvement of stakeholder groups in the planning process helps them reach a consensus on the environmental challenges and motivation for change and develop a sense of common ownership and vision. If they are not involved, conflicting positions may arise among stakeholder groups. Stakeholder alignment must be measured periodically through surveys, focus groups, workshops, and interviews. The degree of alignment between stakeholders and leaders can greatly affect an organization's ability to develop and implement strategies. The critical aspect is engaging key stakeholders. A consultant from internationally famous strategy firm McKinsey & Company provides an example of "one large health care company [that] asks the leaders of each business unit to imagine how a set of specific economic, social, and business trends will affect their businesses, as well as ways to capture the opportunities—or counter the threats—that these trends pose. Only after such an analysis and discussion do the leaders settle into the more typical planning exercises of financial forecasting and identifying strategic initiatives" (Dye and Sibony 2007).

Engagement efforts or neglect can cause stakeholders and executives to become aligned or misaligned in various ways. Exhibit 10.2 demonstrates the different opinions stakeholders and executives can have regarding the need to make a major change, along with probable outcomes. If a proper environmental analysis has been conducted and communicated appropriately, a consensus of either negative–negative (indicating a need for change) or positive–positive (indicating agreement that existing practices and programs

EXHIBIT 10.2
Effects of Stakeholders' and Executives' Perceptions on Alignment

		Stakeholder Perception: Negative	Stakeholder Perception: Positive
Executive Perception	Negative	**Joint Negative Perception of Situation** Both executives and stakeholders seek change. Consensus is reached.	**Misaligned Perceptions of Situation** Executives seek change, while stakeholders seek to institutionalize status quo. Conflict results.
Executive Perception	Positive	**Misaligned Perceptions of Situation** Executives seek to institutionalize status quo, while stakeholders seek change. Conflict results.	**Joint Positive Perception of Situation** Both executives and stakeholders seek to institutionalize status quo. Consensus is reached.

Source: Adapted from Walston and Chou (2011).

should be institutionalized) will be reached. If the executive team does not involve stakeholders in strategic planning or communicates poorly with them, the perceptions of the two groups can quickly become misaligned. In these situations, one group has a negative perception, indicating a desire for change, while the other has a positive perception, indicating resistance to change. Therefore, stakeholder involvement, communication, and transparency of organizational issues are critical components of strategic planning. Involving and interacting with employees and other stakeholders promote both emotional and cognitive alignment.

Often the process of discovery and communication during planning is as important (or perhaps more important) than the creation of the ultimate written plan. Prominent football coach Bill Belichick agreed with former president Dwight D. Eisenhower, who, as supreme commander during World War II, said, "In preparing for battle I have always found plans are useless, but planning is indispensable" (Mihoces 2015). The planning process brings stakeholders together; reinforces the organization's mission, vision, and strategic direction; and unites the work effort.

Leaders earn buy-in by involving critical stakeholders early in the strategic planning process. Especially in large organizations, involvement of all employees is impossible. As discussed in chapter 6, influential representatives from key stakeholder groups are chosen to participate on boards, committees, task forces, and subcommittees concerning the strategic planning process.

Organizations should appoint key stakeholders who act as spokespersons for the groups in which they participate and serve as ambassadors or liaisons between their groups and the organization.

The initial steps of strategic planning therefore are to identify, communicate with, and involve key stakeholders. These steps are facilitated by early development of a communication plan. Key milestones in the planning process and the mechanisms to be used to communicate with key stakeholders are specified in this plan. Key milestones might include presentation of a summary of the environmental analyses, including significant challenges facing the organization; a revised mission or vision; the overall strategic goals; and other components of the strategic plan and planning process. Venues through which information and progress can be shared include departmental or companywide meetings, intranet postings, newsletters, bulletin boards, e-mail, Twitter, and Facebook, among others. An established public relations department can implement the communication plan, or a subcommittee of the strategic planning committee may be tasked with managing the communication effort.

Consensus is reached more often in organizations that focus on learning and innovation than in companies that emphasize adherence to rules, budgets, and avoidance of failure. A culture of learning and innovation increases stakeholders' openness to change. On the other hand, organizations that exercise control, focus on rules and policies, and tie budget outcomes to rewards are less likely to engender intraorganizational consensus (Walston and Chou 2011).

Environmental Analysis

Chapters 7 and 8 describe the components of the internal and external environment and types of analyses that may be used to clarify an organization's market status. If too many data are analyzed, however, "analysis paralysis" may result. Therefore, only critical factors should be analyzed. As indicated in chapter 8, key internal data include factors that help measure achievement of the organization's mission and progress toward the vision and reflect important stakeholder needs. These data may be drawn from documentation of volume activity, financial statements, employee opinion surveys, and research. Past successes and failures should likewise be examined. Leaders should identify key factors contributing to both successes and failures and use these to inform the planning process. Areas reviewed should be restricted to a manageable number.

Key external data also include factors that could significantly affect the organization's direction and ability to fulfill its mission and vision. Data on competitors, industry data, community and customer perceptions, market share, and information on customer origin (e.g., from hospital patient origin studies) are some examples. SWOT analysis may be used but should never be an exclusive source of information.

The Affordable Care Act included an interesting provision that requires all tax-exempt hospitals (i.e., those with the 501(c)(3) designation) to assess the health needs of the community and design a plan to meet those needs at least once every three years. The assessment must consider input from individuals representing the "broad interests of the community served by the hospital facility" and must be made publicly available (Internal Revenue Service [IRS] 2010). Information required in the implementation plan appears very similar to that commonly included in a strategic plan, including (IRS 2011)

- a description of the community served;
- community demographics;
- other community healthcare facilities and services;
- the health needs of the community;
- the health needs of uninsured, low-income, and minority groups;
- prioritized community health needs; and
- an implementation strategy.

Strategic planning must be a data-driven process in which decisions are based on current, reliable information. If planning is not data driven, it devolves into decision making based on opinion and conjecture. While there is never only one right decision, relevant and accurate data improve the quality of decision making.

Sources of Data

Finding accurate, timely data can be extremely difficult. Public data commonly take one or more years to be published and often are incomplete or contain errors. Private data tend to be more accurate and timely but are often costly to buy.

The following sites are good sources of healthcare data:

- www.healthdata.gov: This governmental site contains access to many different data sets, including those from the Centers for Medicare & Medicaid Services (CMS), Centers for Disease Control and Prevention (CDC), Food and Drug Administration, and National Institutes of Health.
- www.data.gov/health/: The federal government has organized information from multiple departments dedicated to improving the health and lives of all Americans. These resources include data sets, tools, and applications related to health and healthcare.
- www.cdc.gov/nchs/ahcd/: The National Ambulatory Medical Care Survey is a national survey designed to meet the need for objective, reliable information about the provision and use of ambulatory

medical care services in the United States. Findings are based on a sample of visits to nonfederally employed, office-based physicians who are primarily engaged in direct patient care. The National Hospital Ambulatory Medical Care Survey is designed to collect data on the utilization and provision of ambulatory care services in hospital emergency and outpatient departments.

- www.nahdo.org: The National Association of Health Data Organizations (NAHDO) is a nonprofit educational association dedicated to improving healthcare data collection and use. NAHDO's members include state and private organizations that maintain healthcare databases as well as stakeholders of these databases in the public and private sectors.
- www.ahrq.gov: The Agency for Healthcare Research and Quality maintains a large sample of data on hospitalized patients, including the Healthcare Cost and Utilization Project, a national inpatient sample of about a thousand hospitals.
- www.cms.gov: CMS maintains Medicaid and Medicare inpatient and outpatient claims data.
- www.mgma.org: The Medical Group Management Association collects data on physician productivity in group practices by visits and costs.
- www.imshealth.com: IMS Health maintains data on pharmaceutical agents, diseases, and medical conditions.
- www.cancer.gov/statistics: The National Cancer Institute provides cancer statistics by type, geographic area, and demographic subgroups.
- http://ahd.com: The American Hospital Directory provides data and statistics on more than 6,000 hospitals nationwide.
- www.ahadata.com: The American Hospital Association collects detailed annual hospital statistics.
- www.dartmouthatlas.org: The Dartmouth Atlas of Health Care provides data on variation of care across the United States.

Gap Analysis

Gap analysis A method of identifying the distance between the organization's current position and its desired position with regard to its mission, vision, and values.

An organization's environmental analysis includes examining its mission, vision, and values (if they have been established) to ensure that they are still appropriate. As discussed in chapter 6, the values, mission, and vision express an organization's ideal position and strategic intent. A **gap analysis** identifies the distance between the organization's current position and where it wants to be. The following questions can help leaders measure this distance:

- Which stakeholder groups' needs are not being met?
- What key actions must be taken to attain the vision?

- Which past goals were not achieved? How did this nonachievement affect the mission?
- How is the organization living its values? What can be done to emphasize and more fully incorporate the values into daily work life?
- What core weaknesses may be preventing the organization from living its mission?
- What external threats have to be addressed to be able to continue providing mission-based products and services?
- What is the organization's financial health, and how does it affect the organization's strategic position?

Some of the methods discussed in chapters 7 and 8, such as PEST (political, economic, social, technological) and SWOT (strengths, weaknesses, opportunities, threats) analysis, also can help leaders identify challenges and issues that are impeding mission achievement.

The number of challenges should be narrowed to four or five that are most prominent and most likely to impede the organization from accomplishing its mission and vision. Some key challenges posed by today's healthcare environment include

- availability of technical personnel;
- new technology;
- new or potential regulations;
- financial capabilities;
- market and competitive changes;
- customer satisfaction, preferences, and demands;
- capacity issues (excess or constraints);
- cost pressures;
- relationships and affiliations with partners;
- employee engagement and retention; and
- access to capital.

The following questions can be used to determine which issues are most critical:

- Could this force seriously affect the organization's ability to achieve its mission?
- How significantly could the force affect the organization? What impact may the force have on key stakeholders?
- What effect could the force have on the organization's reputation?

- Could the force significantly change the organization's customer base?
- Could the force have a substantial impact on the organization's finances?

The challenges culled from this analysis form the foundation on which organizations build strategic plans.

Preparing for Planning

Organizations need to prepare for their planning processes. A governing body can examine its preparedness for strategic planning by asking the following questions:

- Is there a written policy for the process and activities of strategic planning?
  - Does it spell out who is responsible for which activities and how the different groups interact and coordinate with the governing body?
  - Are specific time frames established for each strategic planning component?
- Does the organization have a plan for communicating the development of the annual strategic plan and its results?
- Does the governing board use the strategic plan appropriately to set realistic, challenging goals?
- Do strategic or tactical issues dominate board discussions? If strategic issues are not addressed the majority of the time, what can be done to increase the board's focus on them?
- Is there a proper planning structure whose members appropriately represent the key stakeholders? If not, is there a means of obtaining periodic input from other stakeholders (e.g., task groups, focus groups, surveys)?

Planning Structures

Planning structure The person(s) or unit with responsibility for strategic planning.

Organizations use various **planning structures** to organize and facilitate their process. The composition of these structures depends on the size, culture, and ownership of an organization, but they typically combine organizational positions, standing committees, and task forces.

Most companies designate a person or a department as their strategic planning coordinator. This person or unit is responsible for gathering and analyzing data and organizing and conducting committee and task force meetings.

Large organizations, such as Kaiser Permanente in California, may employ a specialist, such as the strategic planning analyst described in exhibit 10.3, for this purpose. Almost 45 percent of healthcare systems reported having a chief strategy officer (Health Research & Educational Trust 2014).

Small organizations might expand the duties of the strategic planning director to include business development and public relations. Job descriptions for the vice presidents of business development and strategic planning sometimes blend strategic planning and these related functions. In small organizations, combining these functions streamlines strategic actions. The integration of public relations and business development is essential to communicating strategic direction appropriately (as discussed earlier) and to translating the written plan into implementation (see chapter 15).

Most strategic planning in healthcare is overseen by a healthcare organization's governing board. In this age of increasing emphasis on board accountability, governing bodies have a greater responsibility to engage in strategic

EXHIBIT 10.3
Essential Functions of a Strategic Planning Analyst at Kaiser Permanente

Essential Functions
Leads, makes significant contributions, and/or provides technical leadership to high visibility projects to identify and resolve issues of strategic importance to the organization.

- Interfaces regularly with senior management to produce timely and valuable results.
- Sets the strategic direction of projects.
- Determines goals and priorities with management team sponsors.
- Establishes team membership and negotiates time commitments and resources.
- Develops proposals for clients outlining proposed project structure, approach and work plan.
- Provides staff leadership to project teams, as well as manages work of outside consultants when needed.
- Designs research plans for data gathering and analysis.
- Participates significantly in interpreting analysis and developing action plans accordingly.
- Produces or oversees development of written materials for senior executives and other key clients.
- Plans and facilitates meetings.
- Makes formal presentations to various senior level audiences.
- Assists, as needed, in planning and coordinating with other ongoing teams and projects to maximize effectiveness.
- Participates in the development and management of the department, including coaching, recruiting, conducting performance reviews for consultants/analysts, and other departmental activities.

Source: Excerpt from Kaiser Permanente (2017).

planning. Although the level of board member involvement varies, the full board should view the strategic planning process and final plan as critical to the organization's direction and as groundwork for executive decisions and actions. Therefore, the governing board formulates the plan but does not usurp management's responsibility to implement and execute it.

As mentioned earlier, the board can approach strategic planning in many ways. An important issue for boards to decide is whether the full board will act as the strategic planning body or whether the responsibility will be designated to subcommittees and task forces. Although most hospital boards have standing strategic planning committees, some have questioned this established practice (Bader et al. 2007):

> It may be time to revisit the assumption that a standing strategic planning committee (SPC) is the best method for engaging the board in strategy. There can be a "dark side" to relying on a committee to do the board's strategy work. All too often, it is only the members of the SPC who fully understand the strategic challenges and opportunities facing the organization over the next five to ten years. The rest of the board members may not have been included in the educational sessions on national healthcare trends, in-depth conversations about current and potential competitors in the market, and discussions of alternative strategies for the organization's future.

Some boards choose to form task forces or advisory groups to represent geographic or special constituencies. These groups may report to the full board or to their strategic planning committee. Focused task groups enable a microlevel evaluation of stakeholder needs that have been aggregated by the strategic planning committee. Whatever the approach, the board should develop a written policy that articulates its expected outcomes; the timeline of the strategic planning process; and the functions of the subcommittees, task forces, and full board.

Most organizations update strategic plans annually; therefore, the committees and task groups generally are organized on an annual basis. If task groups are formed, their primary function is to gather stakeholders' perspectives and explore critical issues during the environmental analyses. They may meet as needed or as often as weekly during the environmental analysis period. As shown in exhibit 10.4, task groups meet throughout the early stage of strategic planning—a period of approximately four months—and report their findings to the strategic planning committee, which in turn reports to the board.

Following the environmental analysis period, the strategic planning committee and board formulate strategy and develop goals over the next three to five months. During this time, members of both bodies may be more engaged if they participate in educational sessions on external and internal environmental issues. Education is a vital means of challenging assumptions and promoting understanding. For example, board and strategic planning

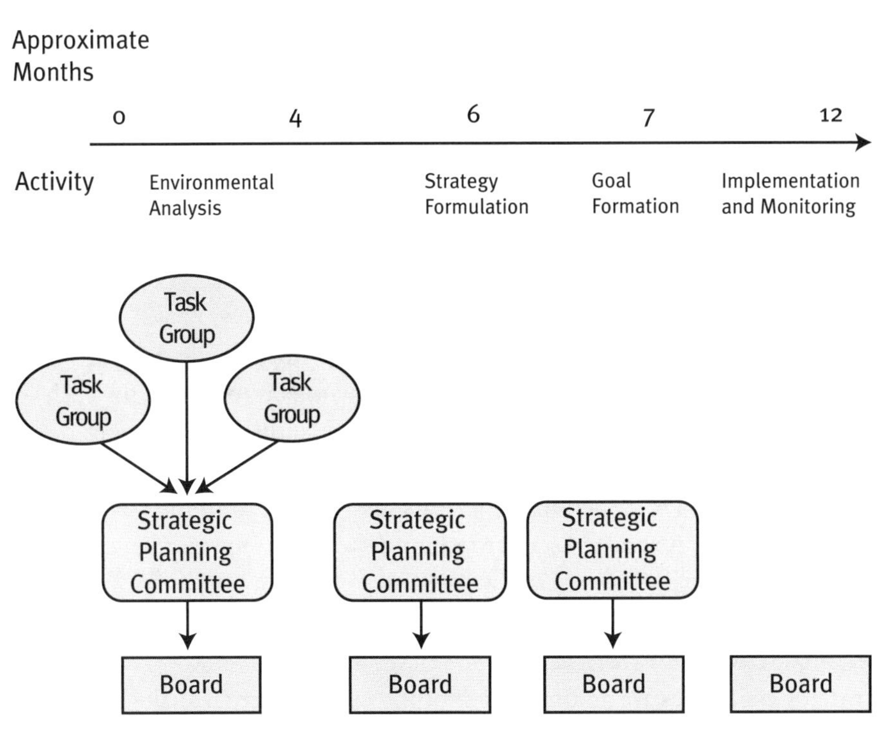

EXHIBIT 10.4 Timeline of Review Bodies' Involvement in Annual Strategic Planning Process

committee members and other key stakeholders can attend retreats organized for educational purposes.

Format of a Strategic Plan

Although strategic plans come in many types and formats and no standard plan exists, the following components are essential to all plans:

- Executive summary: A three- to five-page executive summary of the full plan precedes the plan document.
- Strategic intent: This section expresses the organization's mission, vision, and values and elaborates on these statements.
- Environmental analyses: This section includes subsections on the internal and external analyses. These subsections commonly present the following information:
  - Major market trends and their implications
  - Consumer profiles and demographics
  - Major service line data and analyses by service and payer
  - Competitor analyses

  - Major stakeholder data and analyses
  - Potential technological changes
  - Key quality indicators
  - Critical legal and regulatory issues
  - SWOT analysis
  - Critical factors or driving forces
- Strategic priorities and programs: This section acknowledges and discusses key areas of focus. Environmental analyses, forecasts, and projections are presented as rationales for prioritizing or selecting these areas.
- Strategic goals and objectives: This section delineates the desired outcomes of strategic activities, identifies who is responsible for each activity, presents key performance indicators, and lays out project timetables. Charters for key projects also may be included.
- Appendixes: The appendixes include data referenced in the strategic plan, such as forecasted service volumes, performance targets, expected market shares, and financial projections.

Setting Strategic Priorities

Strategic priorities The most important areas addressed by a strategic plan.

Strategic priorities are an outgrowth of the environmental analyses. Organizations view the gap between where they are and where they want to be and generate options they could pursue to narrow the gap. From these options, a small number of strategic priorities are selected, generally no more than seven. A greater number heightens the complexity of the strategic process and makes it exponentially difficult to manage.

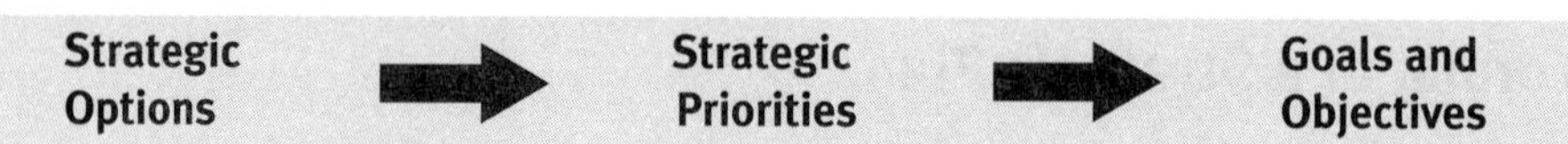

For example, St. Francis Medical Center in the Centura Health network, located in Colorado Springs, Colorado, is a 195-bed acute care hospital (St. Francis and Centura Health 2016). As part of its community assessment and planning process, it identified four strategic priorities:

- Wellness—Healthy babies and children
- Community engagement—Strengthen hospital and clinical behavioral health network
- Behavioral health—Healthy adolescents
- Access to care—Underserved and at-risk population

The next step in the planning process is to create specific strategies and tactics for achieving the key priorities. Centura Health's strategic plan again serves as an excellent example, elaborating on the priorities with goals. Two are shown in the following section (St. Francis and Centura Health 2016):

> **Access to Care:**
> Goals:
> Maximize access to care for underserved and at-risk populations in El Paso County communities through enrollment efforts and more appropriate use of acute care resources . . .
>
> **Wellness—Healthy Babies and Children:**
> Goals :
> Access and evaluate FY 2015 Healthy Babies and Children goal for integration into CHNA future programs
> - Increase opportunities within El Paso Community to directly influence factors tied to babies and children growing up healthy from pregnancy to adolescence

Another example comes from King Faisal Specialist Hospital, a large, international medical center in Riyadh, Saudi Arabia, that made improving its staff selection, recruitment, and retention one of its key priorities. It chose to call its strategies "projects," but their structure is similar to that of St. Francis's strategies. Strategic priority 1 elaborates on the center's need to improve the quality and abilities of its staffing:

> **Strategic Priority 1 (SP1): Staff Selection, Recruitment and Retention**
> To enable the Hospital to compete in the international and regional market in order to select, recruit and retain high quality staff
>
> Problem: The loss of good performers and the difficulty and delays in finding replacements impact efficiency and retention of expertise. Turnover should be reduced. In some areas, staff members work many overtime hours under stressful conditions. Currency fluctuations, limited increase in compensation packages, including the loss of benefits in certain areas, have resulted in a reduced competitiveness of the Hospital in the International and Regional markets.
>
> The candidate projects and initiatives to address SP1 are shown below.
>
> Project 1A: Compensation System
> Project 1B: Career Development
> Project 1C: Performance Management and Review Process
> Project 1D: Staff Support and Satisfaction
> Project 1E: Selection and Recruitment Process
> Project 1F: Identification of Critical, Difficult-to-Fill Positions
> Project 1G: Succession Planning Program
> Project 1H: Education, Training and Scholarship Programs

Goals and Objectives

Goal formulation is perhaps the most difficult aspect of planning. To be effective, organizations must translate each strategy further into specific goals and objectives. **Objectives** are subsets of defined goals and measurable steps that quantifiably support the achievement of goals (Belicove 2013). **Goals** are general intentions; objectives are precise and defined. Goals are broad; objectives are narrow.

Objectives
Objectives are narrow "stepping stones" that quantifiably support and elaborate on goals.

Goals
Broad results that an organization seeks to achieve.

Strategic goals and objectives drive the achievement of the organization's mission and vision. Although directed toward the future, goals and objectives must also fit realistically with short-term budgets and prioritize actions to be achieved in the next fiscal year. Goals, as part of a strategic plan, must not just exist on paper. Rather, they must be integrated with financial control systems and marketing efforts to guide daily decision making.

To be effective, goals and objectives need to be more than just a statement of what should be accomplished. They should also state who will be responsible for them, what actions and events they comprise, when those actions and events should be completed, and the performance metrics that will be used to determine whether they have been achieved.

A popular way to conceptualize goal creation is the SMART method. To be achievable, goals and objectives must have the following characteristics:

- Specific: They must clearly identify what is to be done, who will do it, whom it will be done for, where it will be done, when it will be done, and any related requirements or constraints.
- Measurable: Metrics should be set to know when the goal is accomplished. Key performance indicators should be established for each key goal component. Quantifiable indicators are preferable.
- Attainable: Goals should stretch the organization's capabilities but still be achievable.
- Relevant: Goals should be pertinent and applicable to the organization's mission. Goals should correlate with the strategic priorities and the time frames associated with them.
- Time bound: Target dates should be set for each goal and objective. Target dates should fall in the correct business cycle (e.g., planning and budget cycle). Results should be used to inform the next cycle of strategic planning and goal formation.

When setting objectives, one can use the following questions as a guide:

- What is the outcome I want?
- Why is it important to achieve?
- Who needs to be involved?

- When does it need to be completed?
- How are we going to achieve it?
- How and when am I going to measure the outcome?

For example, St. Francis developed the following tactics for its access-focused and insurance enrollment–focused goals:

FY16 Tactics—

- Tactics/Initiatives:
  - Neighborhood Nurse Centers increase HC access by 5% through collaboratively connecting patients with Centura and community enrollment advocates and enrollment specialists
  - Increase ability to track "Friendly Face visits" through EMR tracking
  - Develop collaborative approach to Educate PSF units and staff 3–4 times/year to determine best practices for uninsured and underinsured common clients
  - Add Personal Health records to data collection at NNC sites and PSF units
  - Meet with team that assesses difficult cases and determine how a bridged practice can be incorporated with the NNC practices to address readmission issues for difficult patients (St. Francis and Centura Health 2016)

A goal is not realistic if one does not have the resources—skills, funding, equipment, and staff—needed to accomplish it. Managers assigned to a particular goal need to ask if they have enough resources to accomplish the supporting objectives and the ability to rearrange priorities to free up time to address those that are most important. The goals and objectives set by US Navy Medicine are reproduced in exhibit 10.5. Note that the objectives are more specific and definitive than the goals.

To make objectives actionable, organizations must write detailed action plans. Each objective should be subdivided into component actions and responsibility and authority for each action driven down the organization to the appropriate level. Action plans translate higher-level aims into specific, narrowly crafted tasks. In large organizations, the development of action plans quickly becomes complex and time consuming. To make this job more manageable, organizations use tools to facilitate it, one of which is the project charter.

The use of a **project charter**, a tool commonly employed for construction management and implementation of information technology, is becoming more frequent in healthcare. Project charters clarify the key components of action plans, including scope, outcomes, participants, resources, time frames, and responsible parties, and ensure that the action plans and the desired outcomes of those action plans coincide with strategic priorities and goals.

Project charter
A tool commonly used in project management that clarifies a project's key components, including scope, desired outcomes, participants, resources, time frames, and responsible parties, and ensures that the project's definition and desired outcomes coincide with the organization's strategic priorities and goals.

EXHIBIT 10.5
Navy Medicine Goals and Objectives, Fiscal Year 2015

Strategic Goals	Strategic Objectives
Readiness We provide agile, adaptable, and scalable capabilities prepared to engage globally across the range of military operations within maritime and other domains in support of the national defense strategy.	**R1 Deliver ready capabilities to the operational commander** Definition: To maximize alignment between requirements, capabilities, and capacities, we will transition our health service support into interoperable adaptive force packages by aligning Navy Medicine's manning, training, and equipping to maintain a medically ready force. **R2 Deliver relevant capability and capacity for Theater Security Engagement operations** Definition: Navy Medicine will lead the Services in defining clinical currency and determining the requirements to maintain currency across the medical force.
Value We will provide exceptional value to those we serve by ensuring the safest and highest quality care through best health care practices, full and efficient utilization of our services, and lower care costs.	**V1 Decrease enrollee network cost/Increase recapture of Purchased Care** Definition: Navy Medicine will decrease network spending, maximize clinical experience of our staff, and optimize resource utilization. We will manage referrals in order to provide our enrollees the best care at the best value. **V2 Realize full benefit from Medical Home Ports and Neighborhoods** Definition: Navy Medicine will strive to achieve full benefit from our MHP and neighborhoods for Fleet, USMC, and MTFs. We will improve the health for our patients, and when they do need care, we will provide the best care possible in a patient-centered care environment.
Jointness We lead Navy Medicine to jointness and improved interoperability by pursuing the most effective ways of mission accomplishment.	**J1 Leverage joint initiatives to optimize performance of Navy Medicine's mission** Definition: We will increase our participation in joint work groups, committees, and nominative positions (MHS, DHA, JS) where essential policy decisions will be determined, and through membership/leadership, we will improve our ability to lead in tri-service initiatives. **J2 Improve Navy Medicine interoperability** Definition: We will improve our ability to respond in a Joint environment by leading in those areas where Navy Medicine has significant expertise and unique capabilities to support our warfighters.

Source: Reprinted from US Navy Bureau of Medicine and Surgery (2015).

Exhibit 10.6 outlines a project charter; the full template used by the CDC is provided in the appendix. Aside from increasing the likelihood of a project's success, project charters identify interdependencies among concurrent projects and place them in proper sequence.

EXHIBIT 10.6
Table of Contents for a Project Charter Template

1. Introduction
   1.1 Purpose of Project Charter
2. Project and Product Overview
3. Justification
   3.1 Business Need
   3.2 Public Health and Business Impact
   3.3 Strategic Alignment
4. Scope
   4.1 Objectives
   4.2 High-Level Requirements
   4.3 Major Deliverables
   4.4 Boundaries
5. Duration
   5.1 Timeline
   5.2 Executive Milestones
6. Budget Estimate
   6.1 Funding Source
   6.2 Estimate
7. High-Level Alternatives Analysis
8. Assumptions, Constraints and Risks
   8.1 Assumptions
   8.2 Constraints
   8.3 Risks
9. Project Organization
   9.1 Roles and Responsibilities
   9.2 Stakeholders (Internal and External)
10. Project Charter approval

APPENDIX A: REFERENCES
APPENDIX B: KEY TERMS
APPENDIX C: GOALS

Source: Reprinted from CDC (2006).

Marketing Plans

An important document supporting the strategic plan is the **marketing plan**. A successful marketing plan builds on the strategic plan and is directed and informed by it. Marketers use the mission and vision along with the market and environmental analyses to determine the right marketing strategies. Marketing's chief role is to generate and retain "preferred customers in defined strategic areas and locations" and to influence and gain buy-in to strategic priorities (Nauert 2005). The

Marketing plan A written document that details an organization's marketing strategies.

Marketing
The activities involved in promoting products and services, including creating, communicating, and delivering offerings that customers value.

American Marketing Association (2016) defines **marketing** as "the activity, set of institutions, and processes for creating, communicating, delivering, and exchanging offerings that have value for customers, clients, partners, and society at large."

In many industries, marketing's key role traditionally has been to initiate transactions or sell more products or services. As suggested by the American Marketing Association's definition, marketing's role has changed. Today, it focuses on building long-term relationships with customers, instilling trust, improving the organization's reputation, creating value, and ensuring satisfaction (Kotler, Shalowitz, and Stevens 2008). As shown in exhibit 10.7, pharmaceutical companies have switched to heavy marketing of prescription drugs through direct-to-consumer advertising, which may not be sustainable in the current healthcare environment.

Marketing in healthcare is complicated by the importance of quality and the dominance of not-for-profit organizations with community service missions. Instead of promoting price, sales, and discounts as in most sectors, healthcare professionals must influence their customers primarily through quality, access, and service advantages.

Marketing builds on strategic planning and incorporates the mission and vision, market analyses, stakeholders, differentiation, and customer value, among other factors. A common approach to marketing plan development consists of three major activities:

1. Segmentation: dividing consumers and stakeholders into defined market segments
2. Targeting: determining which key segments to target
3. Positioning: designing features and images that will occupy a distinctive place in the market's perception

EXHIBIT 10.7
Marketing in the Pharmaceutical Industry

Although pharmaceutical companies traditionally have marketed their drugs by sending salespersons directly to physician offices (a practice known as *detailing*) and advertising in professional journals, they aggressively promoted prescription drugs through direct-to-consumer advertising via broadcast and print media from the late 1990s and into the twenty-first century. Expenditures on direct-to-consumer advertising rose from $150 million in 1993 to $5.2 billion in 2015, with spending on five drugs accounting for one-fourth of these advertising costs. Prescription drugs accounted for almost 17 percent of total US healthcare spending in 2015, up from 7 percent in the 1990s.

Drug advertising remains controversial. Drug companies see it as essential. As Bob Ehrilich, chief executive of the consulting firm DTC Perspectives, noted, "There's no doubt that [direct-to-consumer advertising] is now seen as almost a must-do for a drug that wants to be big," However, about half of drug cost increases may result from the cost of direct advertising, which has prompted calls for regulation. Only the United States and New Zealand permit such advertising.

Sources: Dave and Saffer (2012), Robbins (2016).

Segmentation

Segmentation of the market involves identifying key stakeholders, as discussed in chapter 6. Defining key market segments enables marketers to focus their efforts on consumers most likely to want or need a product or service. Some market segments may be excluded, while others are marketed too heavily. Market segments tend to group stakeholders who have a similar set of needs or wants. These segments can then be further divided into narrowly defined niches and local markets, which has become increasingly important in healthcare organizations. Health systems such as TriHealth, based in Cincinnati, Ohio, and Novant Health, located in Winston-Salem, North Carolina, have embraced market segmentation to improve patient engagement and further their population health management programs (Butcher 2016). Although consumers of healthcare products and services receive primary marketing consideration, other stakeholders (e.g., lawmakers; regulators; referring physicians; hospitals, nursing homes, and home health agencies; insurance companies) may be considered critical market segments.

Segmentation
The division of a market into subsets of consumers with similar needs and wants; enables marketers to focus their marketing efforts on consumers most likely to buy a product or use a service.

Consumer market segmentation can be broken down into four major categories: geographic, demographic, psychographic, and behavioral. **Geographic segmentation** divides customers by political and physical land units. International healthcare organizations may segregate markets by nations. Hospitals and physician clinics may be more concerned with counties, cities, and local neighborhoods. As discussed in chapter 2, patient origin studies help segment geographic markets into primary and secondary markets.

Geographic segmentation
Major category of consumer market segmentation that divides customers by political and physical land units.

Demographic segmentation divides customers into markets on the basis of such factors as age, gender, disease or diagnosis, payer type, and income. Consumer wants, preferences, and rates of product and service use can vary dramatically by these factors. Elderly individuals tend to need products and services different from those needed by young individuals; for example, elderly men have a higher incidence of heart disease, prostate cancer, and erectile dysfunction, while women between the ages of 18 and 40 have dramatically higher needs for obstetric care. People with diabetes require specialized services. Successfully attracting favorable categories of payers (e.g., Medicare, Blue Cross) and discouraging others (e.g., Medicaid, self-pay) may significantly affect an organization's profitability. Families earning high incomes may desire optional services, such as upgraded rooms, cosmetic surgery, and gourmet meals.

Demographic segmentation
Major category of consumer market segmentation that divides customers into markets on the basis of such factors as age, gender, disease or diagnosis, payer type, and income.

Psychographic segmentation categorizes consumers by lifestyle, personality, or values. Often these categories are combined with demographic variables to produce distinct market groups. Strategic Business Insights, a marketing and strategy consulting firm, combines psychographic and demographic data into eight categories: innovators, thinkers, believers, achievers, strivers, experiencers, makers, and survivors (for more information, see Strategic Business Insights 2017). Combinations enable an organization to target its market more precisely in terms of predictable consumer behavior.

Psychographic segmentation
Major category of consumer market segmentation that categorizes consumers by lifestyle, personality, or values.

Behavioral segmentation Major category of consumer market segmentation that divides consumers by their perception and use of a product or service, including their familiarity with it, attitude toward it, and response to it.

Behavioral segmentation divides consumers by their perception and use of a product or service, including their familiarity with it, attitude toward it, and response to it. Marketers may further segregate consumers by occasion of use, benefits gained, user status, usage rates, stage of readiness to buy a product, and loyalty (Kotler, Shalowitz, and Stevens 2008). For example, according to the US Department of Labor (2013), women make approximately 80 percent of healthcare decisions for their families (e.g., when to access care and whom to go to for care).

Targeting

Following market segmentation, an organization must determine the market divisions on which it should focus its efforts. Some market segments are much more important to an organization than others. As illustrated in exhibit 8.9, stakeholders who have high interest and influence are considered important. Interest can be expressed by the stakeholder's use or potential use of the organization's products and services or the stakeholder's affinity for the organization. For example, a religious group might have an affinity for a faith-based organization and have a strong interest in supporting it and using its services. The large Catholic populations in parts of the United States may feel strongly about and have a high interest in their local Catholic hospitals. Stakeholders' influence may be related to the size of their segment or sociodemographic characteristics. For instance, high-income segments may support more profitable services, and females spend 22 percent ($8,315 per capita) more than males ($6,788) (CMS 2017b).

Healthcare organizations should be certain that the market segments they select match their mission and vision. If the mission highlights the importance of charity care, segments of the poor should be present in the target markets. Likewise, if the mission focuses on profits for shareholders, the target segments should include high-income groups.

Five key attributes can be used to determine which market segments to target (Kotler, Shalowitz, and Stevens 2008):

1. Measurability of the segment by size, purchasing power, or other characteristics
2. Substantiality of the market segment that makes it worth pursuing
3. Accessibility of the segment (i.e., it can be effectively reached)
4. Differentiability of the segment
5. Ability to formulate programs that will attract and serve the chosen segments

In healthcare, the primary targeted segments include physicians, payers, and patients (consumers), though the trend "is for healthcare marketers to increasingly target consumers and payers" (Lockard 2017).

Positioning

As discussed in chapter 3, **positioning** means differentiating one's products and services from others in the market. Products and services can be distinguished by their attributes, benefit to customers, or value. Historically, marketers suggested that the **four Ps** established a product's or service's position:

1. Product: the physical features of a product or the intangible aspects of a service
2. Price: the amount paid for the product
3. Promotion: the methods of communication used to inform customers and potential customers
4. Place: the point of access for the consumer

Positioning
Designing and promoting an organization's products and services so that they occupy a distinctive place in the market.

Four Ps
Four attributes that have traditionally been used to establish an organization's market position: (1) product, (2) price, (3) promotion, and (4) place.

Excellently positioned products' and services' unique characteristics, utility, and value are clearly defined.

To these four Ps, consulting groups have added other attributes, proposing five, six, or seven Ps. Organizations can position products and services by many different features and characteristics, including physical form, access, quality, speed, reliability, and performance, among others. These attributes must be significant to consumers, and their difference must be perceived. If an organization highlights attributes that are not perceived as important or as distinct from the attributes of competitors' products or services, it may well have wasted its positioning efforts. For example, in the past, many hospitals launched "We Care" campaigns, seeking—mostly unsuccessfully—to distinguish themselves by their compassion and kindness. Billboards and television advertisements proclaimed that a hospital cared for its patients, which often prompted that hospital's competitors to produce similar advertisements suggesting that they cared even more. Another example of ineffective positioning was a faith-based hospital's attempt to promote its caregivers as "saints in action" via a series of television, print, and billboard advertisements. The dancing saints did little to convince consumers that the hospital provided anything significantly different from its competitors' offerings.

The most critical aspect of positioning is customers' perception of a product or service. As stated a long time ago by the originators of this concept, "Positioning is not what you do to a product. Positioning is what you do to the mind of the prospect. That is, you position the product in the mind of the prospect" (Ries and Trout 2001, 2).

Successful marketers compare and contrast their products and services with those of their competitors to establish their distinct positions.

Healthcare facilities may not advertise as overtly but still seek to position themselves uniquely in the mind of the public. For instance, Cancer Treatment Centers of America (CTCA) has sought to differentiate its services from its competitors by being the company that treats "complex and advanced cancer" through an integrated treatment plan and a personalized approach to care (see www.cancercenter.com). CTCA aggressively acquires state-of-the art equipment and designs its hospitals on the basis of patients' feedback. CTCA selectively targets the market for whom it will provide care, and with its team of communication specialists, determines "the economic viability of prospective client(s)." Its marketing outspends that of all other major cancer centers forming a consistent brand "positioning itself as a destination cancer center on par with the leading major national cancer institutions" (Sabin 2017).

Creation of a Marketing Plan

As mentioned earlier, marketing plans build on strategic plans. Although there are many different formats for marketing plans, the following items are key components:

- Mission and vision: What are the purpose and future of the organization? The answer to this question is first and foremost in any organizational plan.
- Market research and analyses: This part of the plan includes information gathered from the organization's environmental scan. Competitors' positions and strategies, the organization's key products and services, and market segments are identified. A marketing plan may refine the strategic plan's data to provide more detailed direction and plans for the firm's range of products and services.
- Target market: The target market(s) are identified.
- Positioning strategies: This section recognizes the attributes and characteristics to be used to position the organization's products and services.
- Marketing strategies: The marketing and promotion strategies are established. Examples include direct marketing, advertising, training, public service information, direct sales, trade shows, and websites.
- Marketing goals: As discussed previously in this chapter, goals should be quantifiable. This part of the plan assigns responsibility for each goal to an individual or department and sets time frames in which the goals are to be achieved.
- Budget: A reasonable budget is established to accomplish the marketing goals.

Some argue that the traditional practice of targeting products and services to market segments is no longer relevant to healthcare marketing; with advances in information technology and changing consumer demands, healthcare has become more consumer driven, which require new approaches "with usable, transparent, and actionable information" (Krivich 2016). The patient has become a central focus. Modern technology offers many new ways to market to existing and potential patients through patient portals, online videos, social networks, and blogs. As healthcare moves toward accountable care organizations and medical home models, organizations may need to use websites and social media more aggressively to connect with consumers (Ford et al. 2012). Data show how dependent the population has become on the Internet; more than 70 percent of adults in the United States reported using the Internet as a source of information on which to base healthcare decisions (Weaver 2013).

Patient portals are one example of an interactive electronic connection whose use is becoming more common across the world. Through these secure sites, people can view personalized health information and test results, request appointments, query physicians, manage medications, and pay bills. Three growing patient portals in the United States are "MyMercy," sponsored by the Mercy healthcare system; "My Health," provided by Intermountain Health Care; and "My Health Manager" from Kaiser Permanente. In 2015, 70 percent of Kaiser Permanente adult members had registered to use its portal, and e-mails through it represented 33 percent of its primary care physician–patient interactions (Garrido, Raymond, and Wheatley 2016).

Overall, marketing plans will continue to be critically important. Like strategic plans, marketing plans should be periodically reviewed and updated as market conditions change. The quality and effectiveness of an organization's marketing plan directly affect its ability to sustain its strategic direction and accomplish its mission and vision.

Chapter Summary

Strategic plans guide organizations from their existing state to their ideal state (vision). Environmental analyses inform an organization about its existing position and reveal the gap between its existing and ideal positions. Accurate information and effective communication are critical to formulating and maintaining strategic direction. Organizations that fail to appropriately engage their key stakeholders and align perceptions may find that their strategic efforts derail, resulting in conflict and wasted effort.

Strategic priorities are key initiatives that drive achievement of the mission and vision. From these priorities, goals and objectives are formed. Goals and objectives need to be specific, measurable, attainable, relevant to the strategic direction, and tied to time frames.

To facilitate the development of goals and objectives, many organizations institute project charters. These documents elaborate on the scope, outcomes, resource needs, participants, and processes involved. They are especially useful when an organization has many complex, interactive projects to manage.

While strategic planning can be organized in various ways, most organizations assign responsibility for coordinating the strategic planning process to an individual or a department. The duties of this person (unit) can be expanded in smaller organizations to include public relations, communications, and business development. Organizations with boards may designate strategy oversight to a strategic planning subcommittee and use task forces and advisory groups to obtain information from key stakeholders and constituencies.

The strategic planning process generally occurs annually. Organizations commonly set specific time frames for the main components of planning, including the environmental analyses, strategy formulation, goal formation, and implementation. Effective boards spend a significant amount of their time discussing strategic issues.

Marketing plans are derived from strategic plans. The mission, vision, environmental analyses, and strategic goals inform the content of marketing plans. Marketing plans segment the market, target desired customer groups, and position the organization's products and services as distinct from competitors' products and services. Marketing plans should be monitored and updated periodically.

Chapter Questions

1. How does an organization combine its mission and vision with its environmental analyses to develop a strategic plan?
2. Why is alignment of employees' perceptions critical for proper strategic action to take place? Why do you think executives' perceptions might differ from those of other staff?
3. How can an organization better align its employees' perceptions?
4. Why is it not preferable to have more than seven strategic priorities? Would it be better to have fewer?
5. What critical factors do leaders need to consider when setting goals and objectives?
6. What are the advantages of using project charters? What might be some disadvantages?
7. Why might a person or unit in charge of strategic planning also be assigned responsibility for public relations, communications, and business development?
8. When and why might a governance board want to organize a strategic planning subcommittee?
9. What methods can a board or strategic planning committee use to increase communication to stakeholders and better understand their needs and perceptions?
10. Why is it important to have written guidelines for the strategic planning process?

11. What are the differences between strategic plans and marketing plans?
12. How should a company determine which customer segments to focus on?
13. How can a marketing plan help an organization achieve its mission and vision?
14. What critical points should a marketing plan address?

Chapter Cases

Case Studies

Read and discuss "Bozeman Health's Competitive Dilemma" in the case studies section at the end of the book. Answer the questions at the end of the case.

Honnutti Home Healthcare

Honnutti Home Healthcare (HHH) has decided to expand into a new region. It has been successful in its primary market area and is excited to move into a new area. Its primary services include nursing and physical therapy, whose excellent reputation is based on the high caliber of its personnel. HHH has high patient satisfaction scores and secure referral sources. Only one home health agency operates in the new region, and it appears to have a marginal reputation.

To be successful in the new area, HHH must almost recreate itself. New employees, new referral relationships, and a new physical site have to be established. The lead nurse, Sharon, has been tasked with preparing a plan for market entry. She has been told that she can transfer three employees to the new market area. About ten others will need to be hired to begin operations. Sharon's plan must set strategic priorities, goals, and objectives for the first year.

Questions

1. Who are the key stakeholders Sharon needs to coordinate with?
2. What further internal and external data should Sharon try to obtain?
3. What kind of strategic priorities could Sharon set?
4. What goals and objectives might be appropriate?

Setting Meaningful, Measureable Objectives

Ted, the director of strategic initiatives, has been tasked with moving the strategic initiatives established by the board's strategic planning committee to goals and objectives. To accomplish this task, he has been meeting with each divisional chief. He had provided each division with the applicable strategic initiatives and asked each to provide its planned goals and

(continued)

objectives. Most responses have gone well, but a few are requiring more effort to finalize appropriate goals and objectives. His interactions with the head of the Department of Medicine have especially been problematic. Dr. Chou, a prominent physician and the chief of medicine, personally responded with the following "goals and objectives" for his department:

- Strategic Initiative: Improve Patient Satisfaction
  - Medicine Goal: Improve medicine patient satisfaction.
  - Objectives
    1. Make patients more satisfied with nursing care.
    2. Make patients more satisfied with food.
- Strategic Initiative: Improve Clinical Quality
  - Medicine Goal: Improve medicine clinical quality.
  - Objectives
    1. Have high-quality physicians with clinical privileges.
    2. Increase patient safety among clinical care activities.

Ted has to decide how to respond to Dr. Chou's memo.

Questions

1. What is good and bad about the proposed goals and objectives?
2. What form of communication might be best to handle this upcoming interaction?
3. Write an example of better goals and objectives for this area. What did you include?

Chapter Assignments

1. Search the Internet for a healthcare organization's strategic plan. Examine and write a two-page analysis of it. Does it contain all of the components discussed in this chapter? Did the organization involve its key stakeholders in the plan's development? What are the strengths and weaknesses of the plan?
2. Talk to a person responsible for project management. Determine how his role coordinates with strategic planning.
3. Find a marketing plan for a healthcare organization, and look for the key components discussed in this chapter. On what specific features and attributes does the plan focus? Does it identify a target market segment? If so, what is the segment?

CHAPTER

11

BUSINESS PLANS AND STRATEGIC MANAGEMENT

> A strategic plan is primarily used for implementing and managing the strategic direction of an existing organization. A business plan is used to initially start a business, obtain funding, or direct operations. The two plans cover different timeframes as well. According to one resource, a strategic plan generally covers a period between three years to more than five years, whereas a business plan is normally no more than one year. Hence, a strategic plan is a long-term roadmap, and a business plan is utilized to execute the strategic plan on an annual basis.
>
> —Rachel V. Rose, "The Business Plan: A Must for Medical Practices," 2015

Learning Objectives

After reading this chapter, you will

- recognize the differences and similarities between a business plan and a strategic plan,
- comprehend the components and sequence of a business plan,
- understand the purposes and uses of a business plan, and
- know how to create a business plan.

Organizations use different written methods to organize their strategic thinking. As discussed in the previous chapter, a strategic plan is a means of implementing strategy and managing strategic direction. Another commonly used written plan that is similar to a strategic plan is the **business plan**. The creation of business plans also supports strategic thinking and improves operational implementation of strategy. Business plans are critical for all segments in healthcare.

Business plan
A written document that defines, analyzes, and promotes a specific proposal, a line of business, or an innovative concept.

Differences Between Strategic Plans and Business Plans

An organization's strategic plan generally is the foundation of its business plan. Strategic plans provide focus and direction and specify actions an organization needs to take to achieve its mission and vision, whereas business plans define, analyze, and examine a specific proposal, line of business, or innovative concept. Organizations create strategic plans for overall guidance, while business plans are more tactical and often have a narrow purpose—for example, to obtain project funding from corporate governance or an external source of capital (e.g., bank, private entity). For example, Centura Health's strategic priority, access and insurance enrollment (see chapter 10), may translate into various proposals, including mergers, acquisitions, or the creation of new businesses to achieve greater access to care. Business plans analyze the appropriateness, total capital requirements, and feasibility of such projects.

Business plans also differ from strategic plans in terms of the time frame involved. Strategic plans generally cover three to five years but may extend over as many as ten or even twenty years. Business plans generally cover one to three years. Strategic plans aggregate organizational needs, while business plans identify specific resources for a defined entity.

The size of an organization may influence its use of business plans. Small businesses may initially use their business plan as a strategic plan, whereas large companies develop overarching strategic plans and generate business plans as part of their business development process.

Depending on their type and purpose, organizations may use business plans for internal or external audiences. Small entrepreneurial enterprises, such as start-up biomedical companies, may direct their business plans to external financial stakeholders. These plans might make detailed cash flow and profit projections to inform potential investors. Not-for-profit organizations similarly use these documents to procure funding from nongovernmental and governmental agencies and donors (e.g., World Bank, International Monetary Fund). For-profit organizations may use business plans for this purpose as well. For example, in 2008 Ford Motor Company submitted a business plan to Congress to request a $9 billion bridge loan for a proposed restructuring project.

Large firms, such as Clinigen Group, a global specialty pharmaceutical products and services group, may use their business plans for internal purposes. Peter George, chief executive of Clinigen Group, stated, "Creating a consolidated organizational structure is a core part of Clinigen's ambitious five-year business plan to deliver fourfold sales and sixfold profit growth. Two years in, we are well on target" (Business Wire 2012a). Business plans with an internal focus also may be created to evaluate feasibility or for monitoring purposes. For example, organizations might use them to assess the viability of proposed information technology systems, new products, or mergers or be the basis for the development of monitoring systems, such as balanced scorecards.

Like strategic plans, business plans should be considered a work in progress; the creation of the plan is not the desired outcome but a means to an end. The plan should motivate some purpose: obtaining funding, proceeding with a project, establishing better monitoring systems, or some other end. As conditions change, organizations should alter the assumptions and contents of business plans.

Components of a Business Plan

The format and content of business plans are not set in stone; many variations exist. Their content and structure depend on the purpose of the plan and its intended audience. Different organizations highlight different aspects. For example, a not-for-profit organization may emphasize the promotion of its mission, while a for-profit company requesting a bank loan may focus on its ability to repay its loans and generate adequate cash flow.

The US Small Business Administration provides an excellent guide to crafting a business plan for small, profit-driven organizations (select the Business Guide menu, and under Plan Your Business, choose "Write your business plan" at www.sba.gov). It suggests including the following components:

- Executive summary
- Market analysis
- Company description
- Organization and management
- Marketing and sales management
- Description of service or product line
- Funding request
- Financials
- Appendix

Each of these sections is described in the following discussion.

Executive Summary

The *executive summary* is the first (and possibly the only) section read by stakeholders and generally is considered the most important section of a business plan. It generally is kept to one page and contains

- the organization's mission and vision;
- a brief description of the organization;
- growth prospects and projections;
- an explanation of the organization's products and services;

- existing and needed financing and funding, as appropriate; and
- a summary of the organization's future.

Although the authors typically write the executive summary last, after all other sections are completed, it is placed first. Readers form their first impressions of an organization from the content in this section. The organization delivers a short presentation or "elevator pitch" to interest potential funders, customers, or strategic partners quickly. It highlights the organization's strengths and strongly promotes the plan's purpose.

Market Analysis

Market analysis A study that examines competitors and relevant markets, including the market position in which an organization will be placed, relative to other industry competitors.

The **market analysis** is a focused environmental analysis that examines the healthcare organization's sector, competitors, and relevant markets. It defines the organization's current or future market position relative to its competitors. The market analysis typically contains the following information:

- A description of the industry and its prospects, including size, projected growth rates, and other significant trends and characteristics.
- Customer characteristics, including major clusters of customers or potential customers and unmet customer needs. Customers may be broken down by demographics (e.g., age, sex) and location. If the organization is well established, the primary and secondary markets of the organization's existing (if applicable) and projected market share are defined.
- Size of the existing market, including annual purchases, and how its size might change when the organization enters the market.
- A competitive analysis that identifies competitors by product line or service and market segment; their corresponding market shares, strengths and weaknesses, and other factors that might affect the organization's success; and the importance of the organization's target market to competitors. If competitors could expand into the organization's proposed product or service area, the window of opportunity (i.e., time before competitors expand) and the timing needed to succeed are explained.
- Market barriers and impediments to achieving the organization's mission, which might include regulations, technology, and economies of scale, among other factors (as discussed in chapter 7).

Company Description

This section is especially important for new businesses. It describes

- the focus and nature of the business and the marketplace needs the company is seeking to satisfy;

- the consumers the company will serve; and
- the competitive advantages the company will have, which might comprise location, personnel expertise, efficiencies, or any other feature that distinguishes the company from competitors and provides greater value to customers.

Organization and Management

The **organization and management** of the entity, as well as its leadership, ownership, and governance, are discussed in this section. The relationships among personnel, their management expertise, and the experience that qualifies them to lead the proposed company or project are critical details. The description of the governance structure includes the type of board (internal or external), members of the board, and the scope of their authority (advisory or governing). A business plan should provide the following specifics if possible:

Organization and management
The structure, management team, ownership, and governance of an organization.

- An organizational chart that shows the relationships among units, products, and other internal structures
- Ownership information, including legal structure, owners' names, and equity relationships
- Profiles of the members of the management team, including their names, positions, primary responsibilities, education, unique skills and experience, previous employment, community involvement, and number of years with the organization
- Governance structure, including governance type and board members' names, positions, expertise, extent of involvement in the organization, backgrounds, and contributions to the organization's success

Marketing and sales management
An organization's approach to promoting and selling its products or services—the type of marketing to be used (e.g., salespersons, direct mail, media advertising), as well as potential distribution channels and their related advantages (e.g., Internet, distributors, retailers).

Marketing and Sales Management

The **marketing and sales management** section addresses the organization's proposed approach to marketing the new product or service, including its strategy for changing existing customer referral and buying patterns and generating new business. It describes the type of marketing to be used (e.g., salespersons, direct mail, media advertising, promotions), as well as potential distribution channels and their related advantages (e.g., Internet, distributors, retailers).

Description of Service or Product Line

The **service or product line** section specifies the service or product to be offered and clearly delineates the benefits and value customers will derive from it. The life cycle of the product or service (as discussed in chapter 2) is explored, and any existing or forthcoming patents are noted. If applicable, it describes relevant research and development activities.

Service or product line
The particular kind or type of services or products offered by an organization.

Funding Request

If the purpose of the plan is to request funding, the organization discusses its current funding needs and its intended use of the funding. The funder should be made aware of the time at which the capital will be needed; the projected duration it will be needed for; and whether the funds will be used for capital expenditures, operations, working capital, debt retirement, acquisitions, or other purposes. Furthermore, a plan should include the potential for future capital needs as well as any strategic financial plans that may significantly affect the organization, such as buyouts, acquisition by another organization, and debt repayment plans.

Financials

Established organizations should provide historical financial data from the last three to five years. All businesses should provide three- to five-year financial projections. This section presents income statements, balance sheets, cash flow statements, capital expenditure budgets, and ratio and trend analyses of both historical and prospective data. Projected expenditures on the proposed project should match the amount of funding requested.

Appendix

The appendix exhibits confidential data. Enclosures may include

- entrepreneurs' personal and business credit history (if applicable);
- key managers' resumes;
- photos of products;
- letters of reference;
- details of market studies;
- magazine or book references;
- details of licenses, permits, or patents;
- leases, building permits, contracts, and other legal documents; and
- a list of consultants, attorneys, and accountants involved in the business.

Writing an effective business plan requires a skilled presentation. The ability to communicate your business plan professionally is critical to implementation. To achieve this, journalist Patrick Hull (2013) has suggested that a business plan should do the following:

1. Not contain "fluff": Be as concise as possible; delete any nonessential language. Fluff only wastes space. No one wants to read a lengthy business plan.

2. Be realistic: Honestly present both challenges and opportunities. Make credible assumptions.
3. Be conservative: Choose conservative projects and demonstrate how your approach and projections are very reasonable.
4. Contain good visuals: If possible, use meaningful visuals in your business plan. Graphs, charts, and images can improve your presentation. Visuals break up the text, better inform the reader, and improve flow.
5. Be creative: Include creative elements to help your plan stand out, be unique, and seize someone's attention. Make the presentation look original—do not use a template.

Chapter Summary

Business plans are tools that support and organize strategic thinking. They differ from strategic plans in that they typically focus on a specific proposal, a line of business, or an innovative concept. Organizations may create multiple business plans to carry out a strategic plan's goals and objectives. Business plans can be used to ascertain the feasibility of a proposal, obtain funding, or establish monitoring metrics to manage projects better.

The components of a business plan vary according to the issues it addresses and the context. Generally, business plans contain an executive summary; a market analysis; a description of the organization, including its management and governance; marketing and sales strategies; an explanation of the proposed service or product line; funding requests; company financials; and other related documentation. Business plans encourage disciplined thought and provide a mechanism for carrying out strategic decisions.

Make the presentation of your business plan professional. Create a plan that is concise, realistic, and meaningful. Use good visuals that help tell your story and better inform the reader. Ensure that your business plan is creative and stands out.

Chapter Questions

1. How are strategic plans and business plans similar?
2. How are strategic plans and business plans different?
3. In what instances could a business plan be used?
4. How does a business plan encourage disciplined strategic thinking?
5. What factors determine the components included in a business plan?

Chapter Cases

Case Studies

Read and discuss "Bozeman Health's Competitive Dilemma" in the case studies section at the end of the book. Answer the questions at the end of the case.

A Business Plan for New Mobile Ultrasound?

A company is seeking financing for a new mobile ultrasound unit it has developed. The new unit's ultrasound scans are of almost the same quality as those produced in hospitals, and the unit weighs less than 40 pounds. While hospital-based units cost $40,000 to $150,000, the new unit would sell for less than $10,000. The new ultrasound unit would be an ideal means of improving prenatal care in parts of the developing world.

In groups of three or four, design a business plan for the new ultrasound unit. Include all of the elements explained in this chapter. Present your business plan to the class.

Chapter Assignment

Search the Internet for healthcare business plans. Find two plans and write a two-page paper analyzing them. Do they contain all of the components described in this chapter? If the purpose of the plans is to obtain funding, would you be impressed enough to fund the projects they propose? What are the strengths and weaknesses of the plans?

PART

VI

IMPLEMENTING STRATEGIES

Choice of organizational structure can significantly affect an organization's ability to implement its strategies. Strategies commonly catalyze change, which—if not managed appropriately—can seriously impede an organization in pursuit of its goals. Chapter 12 provides an overview of organizational structure and its relationship to strategy and explains how the most appropriate structure for an organization depends on its external and internal environments. Chapter 13 explores strategic organizational change and provides tools for managing the challenges that change presents. Chapter 14 discusses the components of strategic management and introduces methods for improving executives' strategic leadership skills.

CHAPTER

12 ORGANIZATIONAL STRUCTURE AND STRATEGY

> Fast moving global markets and digital disruption have forced companies to innovate rapidly, adapt their products and services, and stay closer than ever to local customers. This has prompted a resurgence in interest in business organization. Our findings in this area are startling: 92 percent of companies believe that redesigning the organization is very important or important, making it No. 1 in ranked importance among this year's respondents. Companies are decentralizing authority, moving toward product- and customer-centric organizations, and forming dynamic networks of highly empowered teams that communicate and coordinate activities in unique and powerful ways.
>
> - Many companies have already moved away from functional structures: Only 38 percent of all companies and 24 percent of large companies (>50,000 employees) are functionally organized today.
> - The growth of the Millennial demographic, the diversity of global teams, and the need to innovate and work more closely with customers are driving new organizational flexibility among high-performing companies. They are operating as a network of teams alongside traditional structures, with people moving from team to team rather than remaining in static formal configurations.
> - Over 80 percent of respondents to this year's global survey report that they are either currently restructuring their organization or have recently completed the process. Only 7 percent say they have no plans to restructure.
>
> —Tiffany McDowell, Dimple Agarwal, Don Miller, Tsutomu Okamoto, and Trevor Page, "Organizational Design: The Rise of Teams," 2016

Learning Objectives

After reading this chapter, you will

- understand the differences among corporate, business, and functional strategies;

- have learned the primary strategic functions of a corporate office;
- know what is meant by *span of control*;
- be able to discuss the benefits and problems of separating an organization's functions into separate departments;
- perceive the advantages and disadvantages of using different organizational structural forms;
- recognize the contexts in which different organizational structures might work best; and
- comprehend the importance of centralization and decentralization of decision making and its relationship to organizational structure.

Strategic focus may differ considerably among an organization's managers, depending on the manager's position and the organization's structure. This chapter builds on the brief discussion of levels of strategy in chapter 1 and elaborates on variation of strategic focus by organizational level and structure. It discusses the key components of organizational structure and factors that affect a structure's applicability to strategy. The construction and implementation of strategy vary substantially between a corporate office and a business or functional unit. Likewise, organizational structure affects the focus and process of strategic thinking and influences the formulation and adaptation of strategy. As stated long ago by Williamson Murray, MacGregor Knox, and Alvin Bernstein (1994, 19) but still very true today, structure influences decision makers' ability to understand the environment and form relevant strategies: "The structure of . . . institutions plays a crucial role in the formulation of strategy and its adaptability to actual conditions. The form . . . affects the ability of decision-makers to analyze and interpret the external environment."

No particular structure is optimal or inherently superior to another. Organizations need to craft their structures to be relevant to the organization's context and mission. As famed management guru Peter Drucker noted, "There is no one right organization . . . . Rather the task . . . is to select the organization for the particular task and mission at hand" (Wolff 1999, 2–4). As the quote at the beginning of the chapter shows, companies across the world are restructuring and redesigning to fit their environments more closely.

Chain of command
The formal channel that defines the line of authority, as well as reporting relationships up and down an organization's hierarchy.

All organizations develop some form of a **chain of command**—the formal channel that defines the line of authority and reporting relationships from top to bottom. A chain of command delineates the direction for formal company communication and decision making. In this manner, each employee knows exactly who is responsible for which personnel and whom to go to for counsel. All of the structures discussed in this chapter integrate a chain of command.

Corporate, Business, and Functional Unit Strategies

Large businesses commonly have a **corporate structure**. In fact, the business community in the United States is often referred to as "corporate America." As healthcare organizations have grown, many have transitioned to an overarching corporate structure. A *corporation* is a legal structure centrally managed by a board that limits its leaders' personal liability.

Corporate structure
An overarching management configuration that controls and supervises divisions or strategic business units. A corporation is a legal structure that can be instituted to limit owners' personal liability and centralize management under a governing board.

Healthcare corporations come in many sizes and degrees of complexity. For instance, the University of Utah Health (UUH), an academic healthcare system that provides care for six US states, runs 4 hospitals and 12 clinics that produce $3 billion in patient revenues per year. As shown in exhibit 12.1, UUH manages its operation in 24 units that report to its CEO, including both academic colleges and operational entities (University of Utah Health 2017). A giant international corporation, Johnson & Johnson, manages more than 250 companies located in more than 60 countries (Johnson & Johnson 2016). For a domestic example, HCA, headquartered in Nashville, Tennessee, operates 164 hospitals and employs more than 230,000 people (HCA 2016). Two of these companies are for-profit, publicly traded organizations that employ corporate structures, divisions, and functional units.

Not-for-profit organizations also can be structured as corporations. They usually are public benefit corporations, mutual benefit corporations, or

EXHIBIT 12.1
University of Utah Health's Organizational Structure

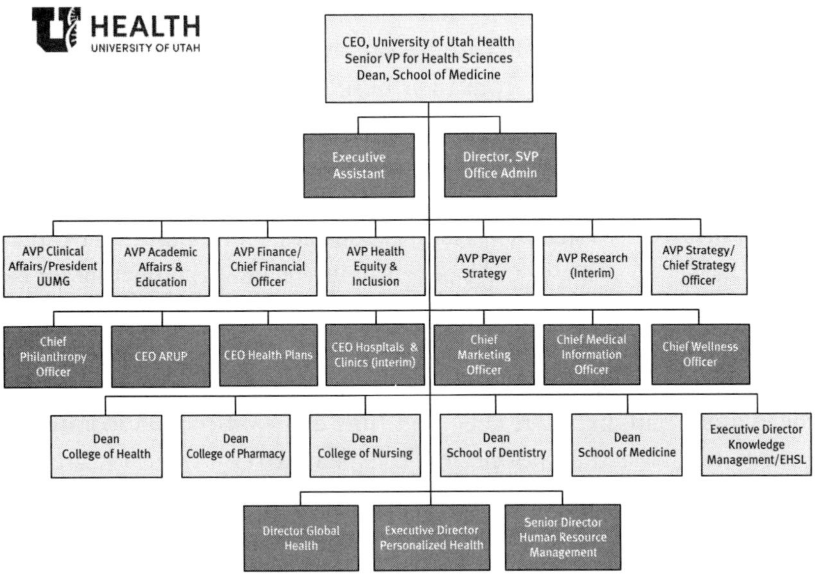

Source: University of Utah Health (2017).

mutual insurance companies. For example, Health Care Service Corporation (HCSC), based in Illinois, is the fourth-largest health insurer in the United States and owns and manages the Blue Cross Blue Shield plans in five states—Illinois, Montana, New Mexico, Oklahoma, and Texas—yet it operates as a not-for-profit, non-investor-owned company. HCSC also has eight subsidiaries that provide related insurance products (HCSC 2016). Similar not-for-profit corporate structures exist and are prominent across the healthcare field.

As shown in exhibit 12.1, corporate offices directly manage business units, and business units manage functional units. Corporate strategy plans for the growth of a portfolio of businesses, while each business unit focuses on a narrow line of products. Although corporations devise competitive strategies, true market competition occurs at the business and functional levels. For example, General Electric, an immense conglomerate, has a division named GE Healthcare. The division's nine primary business units provide a wide range of products and services, including diagnostic imaging, information technology (IT), biopharmaceuticals, surgical tools, and refurbished imaging equipment. The nature of competition for these products varies dramatically. Some units, such as its IT unit, experience much greater competitive pressures than do others, such as its used imaging equipment unit. Corporations have different strategies for their business units by specific product and geographic location and then aggregate these strategies to create an integrated corporate strategy.

When creating and implementing strategy, corporations have three primary concerns: (1) allocating capital across business units, (2) deciding which businesses to compete in, and (3) determining how to integrate and manage those businesses. For capital allocation, corporations have at their disposal the revenues and cash generated from their business units. This capital is one of the most valuable corporate resources, and wise allocation is crucial to strategic success. Strategic allocation of capital entails investment in innovative products, replacement of plant and equipment, recruitment of critical personnel, and payment of dividends to shareholders (if applicable). Corporations have a finite amount of money to allocate, and business units are always competing for capital, making corporate capital allocation both difficult and critically important.

Part of capital allocation involves selecting business and product lines in which to compete. Corporations frequently acquire and divest businesses. On the extreme end, between 1987 and June 2016, Microsoft acquired 198 companies and divested 31 businesses (Wikipedia 2017). In healthcare, managed care organizations completed 291 mergers and acquisitions in this same time frame. The largest—Anthem's acquisition of WellPoint Health Networks in 2003—was worth $16.5 billion (Irving Levin Associates, Inc. 2010). This combination was dwarfed in 2015 by Anthem's proposed merger with Cigna for $48 billion—which the US Department of Justice successfully blocked in 2017 (Kendall and Mathews 2016). As discussed in chapter 8, a company must continually examine and monitor the portfolio of its businesses and, according to its mission and vision, direct its limited capital to appropriately support, acquire, or divest business units and products.

Corporations also are responsible for determining how and to what extent their business units and products will be integrated and managed. Corporate strategies often seek to develop synergies by centralizing appropriate staff and resources and sharing them across business units or by decentralizing resources and placing them inside of business units. Likewise, corporations' governance method and style are determined by the degree of direct corporate intervention and decision making. Decisions and information can be centralized at the corporate level or decentralized to business units. Corporate leadership has ultimate authority on all of these choices.

Strategic business units, on the other hand, are responsible for directing a division, product line, or other revenue (profit) or cost center. Johnson & Johnson, for example, runs three primary units, dividing the company into Consumer Health Care Products, Pharmaceutical Products, and Medical Devices Products substructures (Johnson & Johnson 2017). At the business unit level, strategic issues revolve around developing and sustaining the market advantage of a unit's goods and services. Issues of integration and coordination across the corporation are generally secondary in nature. Business unit strategy deals with positioning the business in its market, anticipating changes in demand and technologies, and influencing the nature of market competition. Many of the strategic applications discussed in chapters 7 and 8 apply directly to formulating and implementing strategy at the business unit level.

Strategic business units
Profit centers in an organization that focus on a product line or market segment.

Depending on the size of the corporation, the functional level may consist of operating divisions, product lines, or departments. The strategic issues that take precedence at this level concern business processes and value chains. Functional units use the resources allocated to them to maximize achievement of the corporation's mission. They may work to integrate with marketing, finance, human resources (HR), and research more thoroughly in an effort to promote their specific products and services and improve business outcomes.

Exhibit 12.2 summarizes this discussion by showing how the different levels in an organization relate to each other. The corporate level provides strategic direction to the business units. It also has primary responsibility for allocating capital and resources and determining which businesses to include and exclude. The business unit level receives strategic direction from the corporate level and translates it into business-level strategies to position the business's products and services more competitively. In turn, the business units provide strategic direction to the functional units, which focus on their value chains and processes and have a more limited scope of responsibility. Feedback and results from the business and functional units cycle back to the corporate office, and strategic planning and actions are modified accordingly.

EXHIBIT 12.2 Strategic Functions by Organizational Level

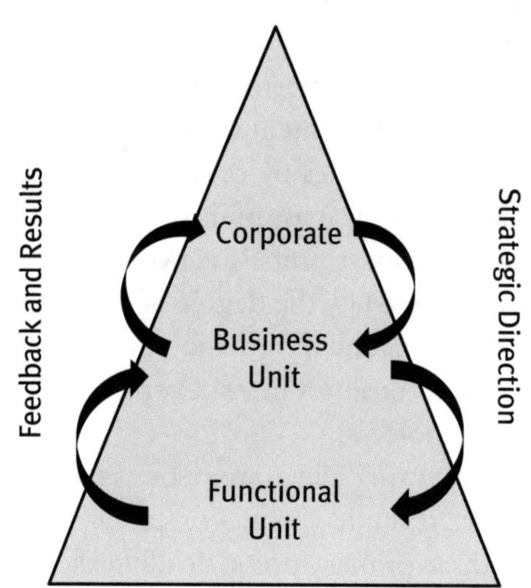

Organizational structure is the manner in which a company arranges its jobs and people to complete its work and achieve its goals. An organization's structure depends on a number of factors, including culture, top management's preferences, number of employees, geographic dispersion, and the range of a company's products and services. Small organizations may lack hierarchical reporting systems, and employees may share common duties. As organizations grow, duties are divided and responsibilities are separated. They segregate employees and units by what they do, whom they report to, and—in managers' case—who reports to them.

Modern organizations and their specialized structures originated with the formation of armies. Almost 2,000 years ago, Roman armies formalized their ranks. Armies were divided into legions—ten cohorts of 5,280 men—and legions were subdivided into centuria of 100 men and contubernia of 8 men. Soldiers had distinct functions and skills; roles included combat medic, heavy infantry and light infantry soldiers, archer, artillery soldier, and cavalryman (Rodgers and Dodge 2005).

Division of labor Specialization of work that breaks down tasks within a production process so that personnel become highly proficient in components of the process.

Until the Industrial Revolution, most businesses were small and dominated by craftspeople. As businesses grew and new technologies were introduced, employers sought greater productivity from their workers through specialization and **division of labor**. Division of labor can significantly affect an organization's ability to think strategically and develop and carry out its strategies. It can impede or facilitate the flow of information and increase or decrease the quality of strategic decisions.

Frederick W. Taylor (1856–1915), a mechanical engineer regarded as the father of scientific management, heavily influenced the structure of today's organizations. His focus on productivity and efficiency prompted businesses to optimize their work through organizational structure (Biography 2014). Many companies spend a great deal of time and effort reorganizing to attain the perfect organizational structure. However, no structure is perfect. Tensions will always be present between forces of **integration** (centralization) and **differentiation** (decentralization). As discussed by midcentury scholars Paul R. Lawrence and Jay W. Lorsch (1967), efforts to gain synergies through integration of organizational functions often seem antagonistic and contrary to efforts to improve quality and gain economies of scale through differentiation.

Integration
Combining, coordinating, and collaborating duties and tasks to facilitate communication and efficiency.

Differentiation
Dividing and separating activities, functions, and products to make them distinct from others.

When companies combine (integrate) duties and tasks to facilitate coordination, they break down silos and may combine multiple job types into one unit. As the number of dissimilar personnel in one area increases, synergies may increase. However, as different positions are grouped together, the overall skill level and efficiency may deteriorate. Likewise, coordination of services becomes much more difficult. As expressed by Karl Albrecht and Ron Zemke (2008) in exhibit 12.3, many hospitals (and other healthcare organizations) divide their departments by functional specialties, which can lead to fragmentation and lack of accountability for overall patient care.

For example, hospital nursing and respiratory therapy services are commonly divided into separate departments. The respiratory therapy department employs experts in neonatal care, pediatrics, and rehabilitation, among other specialties. Training can be better coordinated, and professional standards can be more easily acknowledged and maintained. The departments often can be more efficient (i.e., achieve economies of scale) by sharing personnel

EXHIBIT 12.3
Who Is in Charge of Healthcare?

During a seminar with a group of health care administrators, we asked the participants to diagram the cycle of service that ensues when a patient is wheeled off for, and eventually brought back from, a series of medical tests. After several minutes of discussion about the place of various aides, nurses, doctors, and lab technicians in the cycle, the task was completed. As they sat admiring their handiwork, one of the administrators said aloud—as much to himself as to the group—“My goodness! No one is in charge.” His insight proved to be a valuable one that we have since seen in other organizations. His explanation went like this: Our hospital is organized and managed by professional specialty—by functions like nursing, housekeeping, security, pharmacy, and so on. As a result, no single person or group is really accountable for the overall success and quality of the patient’s experience. The aides are accountable for a part of the experience, the nurses for another, the lab technicians for another, and so on. There are a lot of people accountable for a part of the service cycle, but no one has personal accountability for an entire cycle of service.

—Albrecht and Zemke (2008, 38)

across multiple nursing units and "floating" personnel according to patient need. However, coordination of patient care becomes more difficult by having respiratory therapy as a separate department. Respiratory therapy personnel are not always readily available, so nurses may either provide the services at a lower skill level or wait until respiratory therapists are available.

To rectify the coordination problem, some hospitals have integrated respiratory therapy services into nursing units. If a fixed number of personnel are required to be on each unit regardless of downtime, however, this solution may increase costs and make sharing across units more difficult. Specialization and training similarly may become more difficult. Other organizations use liaisons, case managers, task forces, and other means to bridge the barriers across different functional units.

Span of Control

Span of control The number of subordinates reporting to a supervisor.

A related problem is determining the appropriate span of managers' control. **Span of control** is the number of subordinates who report to a supervisor. In exhibit 12.4, the figure on the right illustrates a narrow span of control; only three vice presidents (VPs) report to the CEO. The figure at the left shows a larger span of control; six VPs report to the CEO. Organizations with narrow spans of control generally have multiple layers of management, and communication is slow between managers at the top and lower-level employees. A tall hierarchy may be more expensive to operate than a flatter one because it includes a greater number of middle managers.

On the other hand, flatter organizations increase executives' span of control by increasing the number of middle managers and decreasing the number

EXHIBIT 12.4 Spans of Control and Levels of Management

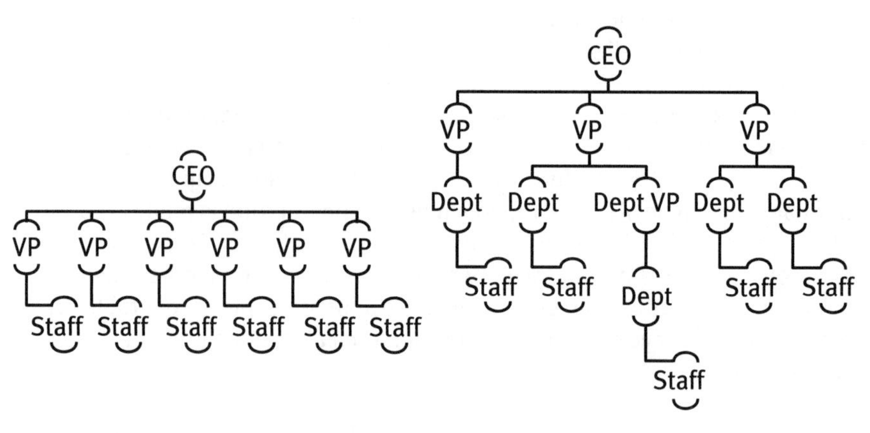

of top management personnel. Executives in this type of structure have more administrative duties, and the number of employees per executive is greater, making coordination of staff more difficult. However, the smaller number of executives may encourage or require employees to take on more responsibility, augmenting their commitment and enabling quicker resolution of problems.

Traditionally, management literature has recommended a span of control of no more than 7 or 8 employees, but in some industries it may exceed 60. However, the spans have averaged 11 in service fields and 16 in healthcare (Davison 2003; Sherman 2013). Aaron Fausz (2014) has found that frontline nursing supervisors (also known as team leaders or patient care leads) can manage approximately 10 staff.

Flat organizations with large spans of control are prevalent in industries and organizations with the following characteristics:

- *A focus on team-based management.* Teams are cross departmental and promote assignment of "process owners."
- *An emphasis on customer satisfaction.* Flat organizations can respond to customer needs quickly.
- *A need for rapid decision making.* Decisions can be made quickly in flat organizations.
- *Large size.* Large organizations tend to have multiple management layers.
- *Effective use of IT.* Flat organizations tend to use IT more effectively than tall organizations do.
- *Culture of trust and excellent delegation skills.* Executives have excellent delegation skills, and organizational culture emphasizes trust.
- *Extensive training, culture of innovation, and excellent job skills.* Organizations that employ highly trained personnel with significant abilities and have an innovative culture tend to be flatter.
- *Low job complexity.* Subordinates' jobs are less complex, less ambiguous, and less complicated than they are in tall organizations.
- *Similar job types.* The greater similarity of subordinate jobs and duties permits a wider span of control.
- *Close geographic presence of subordinates.* Employees are not widely dispersed geographically.

Common Organizational Structures

Although many variations exist, there are three fundamental organizational structures: functional, multidivisional, and matrix.

Functional Organizations

Functional organization
An organizational structure that is divided into subunits based on specialized functional areas such as finance, marketing, and so on.

Functional organizations structure departments by common tasks, services, or roles. In many hospitals, even the C-suite has a functional structure, grouping chief nursing officers, chief financial officers, chief information officers, chief learning officers, and other executive officers, whose primary duties involve managing these specialized areas. Public relations, accounting, the business office, nutrition, housekeeping, pharmacy, laboratory, radiology, emergency services, and every other department each is its own unit.

A typical functional organization in the manufacturing industry is shown in exhibit 12.5. Duties and roles are divided into finance, marketing, manufacturing, research and development (R&D), and HR.

The advantages and disadvantages of the functional structure relative to the other structures were enumerated earlier in the discussion on centralization versus differentiation. As noted, the main advantages are a higher level of expertise and the potential for achieving economies of scale. For example, by segregating IT, the organization can purchase one IT system for the entire corporation rather than have separate systems for each division, and IT roles are centralized, not duplicated in each division across the organization. As a result, IT costs are lower in functional organizations than they would be in organizations with multidivisional structures. A functional organization can more easily standardize processes and products throughout its business because specialized tasks are centralized in units that have responsibility for companywide processes. Therefore, the processes for finance, marketing, manufacturing, and other functions are often standardized across organizations. The greatest disadvantage is the potential for poor communication and coordination among units. Silos form easily, and competition may arise between departments, leading to inefficiencies, conflicting goals, and poor quality.

The problems prompted by a functional structure are heightened in healthcare by its many professions: physicians, nurses, pharmacists, dietitians, and so forth. Each profession has established guidelines. Often professionals place these guidelines before their organizations' directives; promote their own goals; and set their own values, vocabularies, and behavioral norms. At times,

EXHIBIT 12.5
A Functional Organization

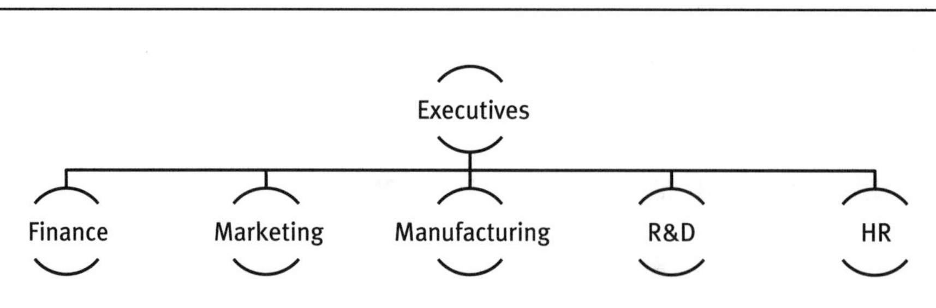

members of one functional unit might feel that personnel in other functional units do not understand them. Workers may withhold information, and inefficiencies and conflict may result (Luke, Walston, and Plummer 2004).

Highly competitive and volatile markets also accentuate the problems inherent in the functional structure. In such environments, the need to coordinate and adapt strategic thinking requires greater coordination and cooperation among organizational units. Uncertain, challenging markets exponentially increase the information that managers must process and understand. A functional structure can delay the transfer of information and retard decision making. Furthermore, the functional structure can impede the strategic planning process. Decades ago Henry Mintzberg, a renowned business author (1994), suggested that functional structures impede the horizontal flow of information and coordination critical to strategic planning, causing the "performance control" activities of strategic planning—establishing objectives and budgets—to be too distant from the "action planning" activities of strategic decision making and program planning.

As an organization diversifies and grows both geographically and in volume, its complexity increases and the information and communication demands on top managers intensify. As firms grow, they may refine and segment their market into many smaller clusters. Some food companies may break their market into more than 650 segments. At some point, these demands exceed executives' capacity, and the organization must restructure. Information overload due to organizational growth has forced many organizations to abandon the functional structure and become multidivisional (Chandler 1962; Galbraith 2012).

Multidivisional Organizations

Multidivisional organizations are broken down into a number of smaller businesses or profit centers (see exhibit 12.6). Functions are not centralized; they are divided and placed in each business unit. For instance, rather than having a centralized marketing function, each division of a multidivisional firm has its own marketing department.

Divisional leaders usually are given sufficient autonomy to manage and organize their business units. Many of the functions performed at the corporate level in functional organizations are performed at the division level in multidivisional organizations. Divisional autonomy encourages innovation and quicker response to localized needs, keeps corporate managers from becoming bogged down in the minutiae of divisional operations, and gives them time to focus on corporate strategic direction. Many global firms have adopted this type of organizational structure.

Because all divisions of a multidivisional organization are profit centers, common outputs from the divisions can be evaluated and compared across

EXHIBIT 12.6
A Multidivisional Organization

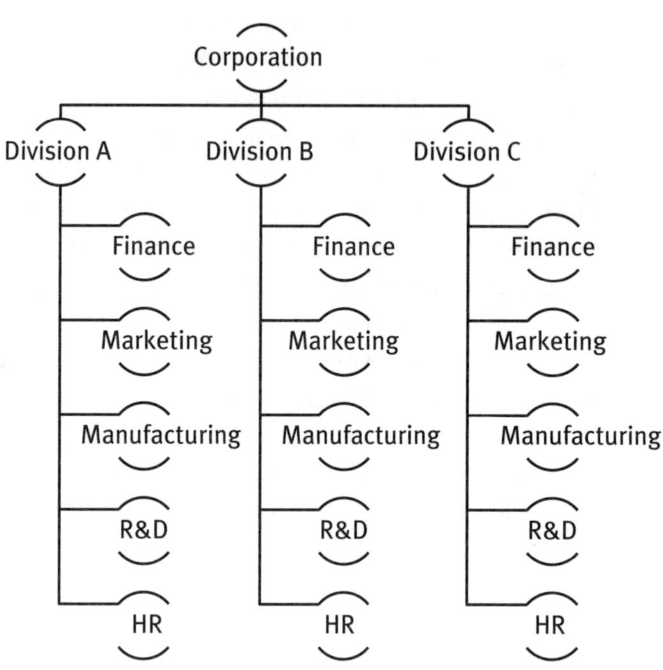

the corporation. Because divisional leaders control and direct their division's resources and operations, divisions can be held responsible for their outcomes. The uniformity of outputs and the facility of comparison help the corporate office make better decisions about the allocation of money and resources to competing divisions. Some have suggested that the corporate office's ability to allocate resources to their best uses is the primary advantage of the multidivisional organization (Williamson 1975, 148): "Investment proposals from the several divisions are solicited and evaluated by the general management . . . this assignment of cash flows to high-yield uses is the most fundamental attribute of the [multidivisional] enterprise."

Organizations generally create divisions on the basis of geography and products. When the cultures, competitive markets, politics, or laws vary significantly among division locations and the distances between offices are great, companies may set up an international, country-specific, or geography-specific division. For example, HCA established an international division in 1973 to manage its ventures in the Middle East, England, and Australia more effectively. Many large pharmaceutical and medical device companies operate international or country-specific divisions.

Organizing divisions by products also may improve management decision making, especially if the customers and foci of products and services differ significantly across divisions. For instance, Johnson & Johnson is segmented into three divisions: consumer healthcare, medical devices and diagnostics, and pharmaceuticals. In addition to different customers and foci, these groups tend to have different competitors and markets. The executives in each division can focus on a specific set of consumer needs and craft strategies for their specific markets.

Healthcare providers have organized multidivisional structures around service lines, such as cardiology, orthopedics, pediatrics, neurology, and women's services. Separate hospitals have been created for heart conditions (cardiology), spine surgery, and sports medicine, among other specialties. Supporters of specialization claim that it lowers costs, improves the quality of patient care and patient satisfaction, and shortens the length of patients' hospital stays. Under these structures, managers have incentives to adapt their facilities and resources to best meet the needs of their distinct customers. Specialists practicing in specialty hospitals treat more patients than they do in general hospitals and therefore are more productive. Furthermore, the larger patient volume provides them with many more opportunities to improve their skills (Barnes et al. 2012; Cook et al. 2014; Koppenheffer 2015).

The allocation of functions to the division level eliminates some coordination problems but creates others. Coordination of functional activities (e.g., finance, marketing, engineering, research and development) is simplified because each division manages its own. However, competition among divisions may increase as each vies for corporate capital. At times, this competition impedes cooperation between divisions and thus increases the corporate office's need to coordinate overall company strategies among divisions. Rivalries can become so intense that divisions stop cooperating with each other. They stop sharing resources and information (e.g., innovative processes, technologies), which may benefit the division but disadvantages the overall firm.

Transfer pricing can also be problematic in multidivisional organizations. As mentioned in chapter 4, establishing a fair transfer price is difficult. If a division that is responsible for its own profits produces components required by another, the price of transferring the goods within the company must be established. When intrafirm competition is high, difficult negotiations can ensue. The selling division may insist on a market price, while the buying division may demand to be charged only the production cost. Also discussed in chapter 4, transfer-pricing problems were one of the primary reasons for the interdivisional challenges at Humana that prompted the divestiture of its hospital division.

The most cited problem of the multidivisional structure concerns costs and quality. As is evident in exhibit 12.6, functions are duplicated across divisions. This duplication poses serious risks of inefficiency, redundancy, and uneven quality. Leaders should frequently evaluate these potential inefficiencies to ascertain whether the benefits of decentralization exceed the costs of duplication.

Matrix Organizations

Matrix organization
An organizational structure that has dual reporting relationships, generally to a functional manager and a product manager.

Matrix structures simultaneously address the issues inherent in functional and multidivisional organizations. **Matrix organizations** incorporate the strengths of the functional and multidivisional structures and compensate for their weaknesses. Their underlying concepts can be applied to all or parts of an organization and even to projects and tasks.

Matrix organizations are common in project-centered industries, such as construction, aerospace, and telecommunications. More than 80 percent of large companies use some version of a matrix structure (Bazigos and Harter 2016). Visible companies such as Procter & Gamble, IBM, Nokia, and Cisco frequently have used matrix structures (Galbraith and Quelle 2009). As shown in exhibit 12.7, a matrix structure organizes employees into functional and project or product groups. Personnel are assigned to a project or product and report to that project's manager as well as directly to their functional department.

Matrix structures have long been used in hospital clinical areas "to promote the coordination and integration of functional department personnel" (Burns and Wholey 1993, 108). Between 1961 and 1978, about one-fourth of all large teaching hospitals used matrix structures, placing administrators on inpatient units to coordinate all functional department employees working in their areas, including nursing, housekeeping, nutrition, and social work personnel. These employees reported to both a unit manager and their functional supervisor (Burns and Wholey 1993). Matrix organizations and multiple reporting relationships are becoming more common. Chief nursing officers especially have emerged with "a matrix of relationships and responsibilities" (Health Research & Educational Trust 2014).

Matrix organizations structure interaction and interchange between personnel from different departments to improve coordination and communication and break down silos. These structures tend to work best in organizations

EXHIBIT 12.7
Matrix Structure

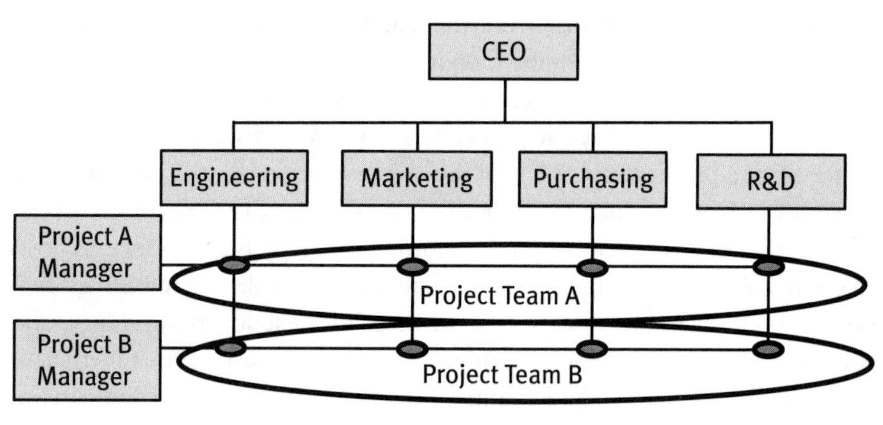

that have novel products or projects. Staff from many disciplines—who normally would not interact closely—may be brought together to develop a new drug or automobile, for instance. Instead of being assigned a task across an organizational boundary and then returning results to the department that assigned it, staff in matrix organizations function as cross departmental teams to jointly and collaboratively accomplish their work. Efforts are focused on completion of a project or product development, not on the specialized duties of functional units.

Many companies have adopted a matrix structure as a result of increasing market complexity. As healthcare transitions toward coordination of care rather than episodic treatment of illness, matrix arrangements may promote cooperative behavior among the many healthcare providers and managers. For example, in 2012, Texas Health Resources appointed an operations leader and a clinical leader to manage each of its three regions jointly (Berdan 2016).

Matrix structures do pose difficulties, however. Engendering cooperative behavior between two bosses who have divergent goals can be taxing. Power struggles can occur and impede performance. Employees also may not know which boss has responsibility for which duties or activities. As a result, many workers involved in matrix organizations are not very engaged in and enthusiastic for their work (Bazigos and Harter 2016). This "two-boss" problem is contrary to traditional command-and-control structures and difficult for many organizations to adopt successfully. Matrix management was popular in the 1970s but fell out of favor with some management experts, who suggested that its complexity could quickly devolve into confusion and become detrimental to innovation (Peters and Waterman 1982).

The manner in which organizations implement matrix structures can dramatically affect their success (North and Coors 2010, 120): "Poorly implemented matrix reporting relationships can misalign goals and mismatch authority and responsibility. Multiple reporting relationships can result in ambiguity and conflict for employees. In the end, dotted lines can simply become blurred lines, allowing performance to suffer."

A significant factor affecting successful use of the matrix structure is the amount of authority given to the project or product manager. In some companies, this manager has no budgetary control or authority over employees and acts more as a liaison and team leader, and the functional manager is ultimately responsible for the performance, expenses, and assessment of employees. The project manager primarily is responsible for documenting milestones and communicating the progress of the project to functional managers. This arrangement may delay project completion.

As an alternative, project managers can be given budgetary control and the authority to recruit resources from multiple business and functional units. Functional managers in a supporting role would still assess the performance of employees assigned to projects and coordinate needs. In this scenario, project managers have more control over completion and implementation of their projects (or products). They can allocate and directly request resources. Their actions, however, can use functional resources, potentially stretching the functional units and creating strain and conflict among them.

A third alternative is for project and functional managers to have shared financial responsibility. For this arrangement to be successful, leaders must be able to collaborate, share decision making, and communicate well. Authors have suggested that in healthcare, outcomes produced by a shared-authority matrix structure are vastly better than the outcomes produced by other matrix structure options (North and Coors 2010).

Comparison of Organizational Structures

Each organizational structure has advantages and disadvantages. No optimal organizational structure exists; trade-offs are inherent in all types. As shown in exhibit 12.8, each structure is suited to different environmental conditions. The functional structure may be best suited for small firms that are centralized geographically and provide a modest number of products and services. Likewise, the functional structure may work best in stable markets.

Adoption of a multidivisional structure may improve the performance of large organizations whose divisions are located in geographically dispersed markets with distinct consumer tastes and preferences. This structure also may work well for conglomerates that own and operate business units that produce diverse products and services (see chapter 4). Matrix structures may work best for firms that develop new products and services for changing markets because they encourage creativity and enable rapid production.

Although often identified as one of the three organizational structures, many organizations actually use a hybrid structure best suited to their strategies, missions, and markets. For example, a functional structure might be used for accounting and finance to maintain consistent, standard oversight across an organization, while a multidivisional geographic structure might be used for product support and customization in different countries.

The locus of decision making or authority affects the success or failure of any structure. Authority—the sanctioned organizational right to make a decision—can be decentralized or centralized, no matter the structural form used. For example, the organizational level at which the decision to hire, fire, and expend funds is independent of the structural form used. However, a high degree of centralized decision making requires increased information flow to top managers, which can accentuate information overload.

Yet, in many cases, organizations that change to a multidivisional or matrix structure to streamline decisions do not concurrently change the

EXHIBIT 12.8 Advantages, Disadvantages, and Best Conditions for Various Common Structures

Structure	Advantages	Disadvantages	Conditions for Which Structure Is Best Suited
Functional	• Specialization and standardization across company	• Growth-induced information overload on top executives • Creation of silos and lack of communication among departments	• Small firms that are geographically centralized and produce a modest number of products and services • Stable markets
Multidivisional	• Adaptability to local conditions • Uniform monitoring and comparisons among divisions • Reduction of information overload on top executives • Focus on allocation of capital and overall strategies	• Duplication of functions • Inefficiency • Less standardization among units	• Large firms with divisions in geographically dispersed, distinct markets that may change independently
Matrix	• Collaboration and interaction among departments	• Two-boss problem • Inefficiency • Difficulty of management	• Firms developing new products and projects • Uncertain markets with changing technology and consumer tastes

authority and locus of decision making. Although the structure may be new, the decision-making process—and thus information flow—remains the same. Adoption of a new structure often does not seem to improve organizational outcomes and lessen the information load on top managers.

Companies struggling with information overload should contemplate decentralization of decision making prior to considering structural change. Decentralization encourages managers to develop their decision-making skills, increases their sense of ownership and responsibility, improves implementation of strategy, and decreases the load on top executives. Decentralization of decision making also can help prepare managers for the greater leadership and cooperation that will be required of them for career advancement or if the organization changes to a multidivisional or matrix structure.

The locus of decision making and organizational structure affect both the quality and timeliness of strategic decisions. Centralized decision making does facilitate the termination of bad products, which otherwise might linger (Joseph and Klingebiel 2016). Similarly, as illustrated in exhibit 12.9 by the Germans' inability to respond strategically to the Allied invasion of France in World War II, Hitler's centralized decision making prevented his generals from taking strategic actions that could have halted the Allies' invasion of the European continent.

Future Structures

Across all sectors, the advance of technology, the rise of smart products, and an increase in customer demands have encouraged the formation of more cross functional collaboration and new business models driven by data (Porter and Heppelmann 2015). The Affordable Care Act (ACA) encouraged many changes to the way healthcare had previously been provided and affected the

EXHIBIT 12.9
How Centralization of Decisions and Organizational Structure Helped the Allies on D-Day

Prior to D-Day, the Allies engaged in subterfuge and convinced Adolf Hitler that the invasion would occur in Pas-de-Calais rather than in Normandy. For the invasion to be successful, the Allies needed German units, especially the panzer groups (tanks), to be absent from the landing sites.

The organizational structures of both armies played a key role in the invasion. The Allies had a unity of command; all troops reported to the supreme commander, General Dwight D. Eisenhower, who coordinated their attacks. In contrast, Hitler, afraid to give too much authority and power to any one general, divided his armies. General Erwin Rommel was placed in charge of Army Group B stationed around Normandy, and General Gerd von Runstedt had overall command of German troops in France—but he had no authority over the powerful panzer groups that Hitler had positioned in Pas-de-Calais in anticipation of an attack.

When the attack hit early in the morning of June 6, 1944, General von Runstedt did not have the authority to move the panzers and had to contact Berlin for permission. Only Hitler could give the order, and he was asleep. No one dared to wake him. When he awoke at noon, he gave the order, and the panzers began to move. However, by then the Allies had established a beachhead in France—and the rest is history.

Source: Duffy (1991).

governmental structure of some organizations. The ACA authorized the creation of **accountable care organizations (ACOs)**—provider networks that can manage the full continuum of network members' care. Becoming an ACO significantly alters relationships among stakeholders and healthcare providers. Among other requirements, to be considered an ACO, the provider network must (Ronning 2010)

Accountable care organization (ACO)
A payment and healthcare delivery model in which a group of healthcare providers work together to coordinate a patient's care, improve quality, and reduce costs.

- be accountable for the quality, cost, and care of the defined ACO population;
- be affiliated with a legal structure that can receive and distribute bundled shared-savings payments;
- include primary care physicians;
- implement clinical and administrative management systems;
- promote evidence-based medicine;
- ensure coordination of care; and
- be patient-centered.

Such organization necessitates a close relationship among all providers, especially physicians and hospitals. For clinical and service value—the goal of patients, payers, and governmental agencies alike—silos need to be broken down and organizational structures formed to facilitate communication, information, and decision making.

Traditionally, healthcare organizations have had functional structures. Hospital acute care, physician office practices, insurance, and suppliers (e.g., pharmaceuticals, devices, equipment) have generally operated independently. To meet the mandates and challenges posed by moving to a population health or value-based orientation, organizational structures of the future will have to be more inclusive and expand to have the authority and ability to better manage and coordinate care. Possibilities include group practice arrangements, networks of individual practices, and partnerships and joint ventures between providers. Although experts predict that hospitals will be at the forefront of value-based organizations, many other providers and groups have an opportunity to form and design these structures (Bennett 2012). As such, integration of the functional and matrix forms of governance will be critical to the success of new structures.

Moving to an approach that requires extensive coordination will be extremely challenging. The transition to an ACO structure will likely be problematic at best and doomed to fail at worst. Scholars Lawton R. Burns and Mark V. Pauly (2012) suggest that many of the structural requirements of ACOs closely resemble features of integrated delivery systems created in the 1990s, which had high rates of failure. Structures that align physicians and hospitals and appropriately coordinate care will be critical to the successful implementation of ACOs (Burns and Pauly 2012). Organizations will need creativity to design structures conducive to such alignment and coordination.

Chapter Summary

Organizational structure can significantly affect an organization's strategic thinking and actions. No single reporting structure is right or correct. There are advantages and disadvantages to the use of all types. The size and complexity of an organization and the nature of its environment and market determine whether the characteristics and features of a structure are beneficial or a hindrance.

Organizational structures consist of three levels: corporate, business unit, and functional unit. At the corporate level, key strategic responsibilities include allocating capital to business units, deciding which fields to compete in, and determining how the organization should be integrated and managed.

The specialization and division of labor became common in business after the Industrial Revolution. To achieve greater productivity and efficiency, organizations segregated jobs into components. However, such partitioning tended to create silos that impeded communication and coordination across departments.

Span of control—the number of subordinates reporting to a manager—has been debated extensively. The number depends on an organization's industry, culture, and type.

There are three common organizational structures: functional, multidivisional, and matrix. The functional structure segments departments by roles and duties. The multidivisional structure breaks down an organization into self-contained business units, each of which contains many of the same functions. The matrix structure combines the functional structure and a project or product focus. Functional employees are assigned to a project or product group and report to both a functional manager and the project or product manager.

Certain market and organizational factors may make the use of one structure more appropriate than another. However, an organization's ability and willingness to centralize or decentralize its decision making can also profoundly affect the successful use of any structure.

Structure significantly affects an organization's ability to formulate and implement strategy and fulfill its mission. Reporting structures and decision-making processes interact, so careful consideration should be given when crafting structures and grouping employees.

Accountable care organizations (ACOs) will need to be structured creatively to meet the coordination-of-care requirement mandated by the

Affordable Care Act (ACA). The success of these new structures will be contingent on appropriate alignment of physicians and hospitals.

Chapter Questions

1. How does organizational structure influence the strategies an organization develops?
2. Why is there no optimal structure?
3. What factors affect the successful use of functional, multidivisional, and matrix structures?
4. Could the three levels of an organization—corporate, business unit, and functional unit—each have a different organizational structure? Why or why not?
5. What are the corporate office's key concerns in creating and implementing strategy? Why?
6. What factors could determine the appropriate span of a manager's control?
7. Could a matrix structure be used across a large corporate organization? Why or why not?
8. What are the advantages and disadvantages of using a functional structure?
9. How could a large, academic hospital use a multidivisional structure?
10. How can transfer pricing affect the successful use of a multidivisional structure?
11. Why might organizations use hybrid organizational structures? How might an organization use part of each of the three structures discussed in this chapter?
12. How could an ACO use a matrix structure to coordinate care?

Chapter Cases

Case Studies

Read and discuss "St. John's Reengineering" or "Deciding on a Population Health Referral Contract Approach" in the case studies section at the end of the book. Answer the questions at the end of the case.

(continued)

Helo Hospital

Helo Hospital is part of a multistate hospital system that has been adding five to ten hospitals per year for the past decade. Originally, three local hospitals made up the company, and the largest hospital's CEO supervised the heads of the other two facilities. When the system grew into 15 hospitals, the organization created a corporate office; when it grew into 30 hospitals, a multidivisional structure based on geography (east and west divisions) was adopted. Currently, disagreements have arisen regarding who should have control of specific services. In particular, the system is debating whether marketing, managed care contracting, strategic planning, business development, purchasing, biomedical maintenance, and recruiting should be centralized or decentralized. The executives from the hospitals and corporate office have scheduled a meeting to decide how these services should be allocated across the system. They have asked you to prepare a report on the advantages and disadvantages of placing these functions in a centralized corporate office, in the divisions, or at the hospital level. What are the problems and possible benefits of each arrangement?

Matrix or Mess

Elizabeth was the chief nursing officer (CNO) of a large health system. Because of the complicated nature of its business in the past, she had led the restructuring of the patient care services across the system. Physicians and staff had expressed concerns that ten of their hospitals often used nonevidence-based practices and were experiencing broad clinical variation. Her restructuring team was asked to create a structure that would facilitate improvements in clinical value, lower costs, decrease complication rates, and cut readmissions across all service lines. Stakeholders in the system perceived the result, which involved nine service lines, to be a great advance, with greater centralization and improved coordinative structures achieved through a modified service line management with clinical comanagement.

According to the design, a chief clinical officer (CCO) responsible for the full system oversaw teams responsible for each service line. Each service line contained several multidisciplinary program committees chaired by doctors and organized by medical condition systemwide. For instance, the cancer service line included subcommittees for breast, colon, and lung cancer clinical care. IT supported the subcommittees and informed them of clinical variation. Subcommittees also included at least one patient and three nurses. Additional support for subcommittees came from data analysts and performance improvement and pharmacy staff. Scorecards were made to show performance data on quality, finances, and patient experience. Those clinicians or service lines in specific hospitals not meeting expectations were referred to their respective administrative and clinical manager.

Nursing services were also grouped into a service line structure, but each hospital also had a CNO who reported to Elizabeth and the hospital CEO. A simplistic view of the structure looks like:

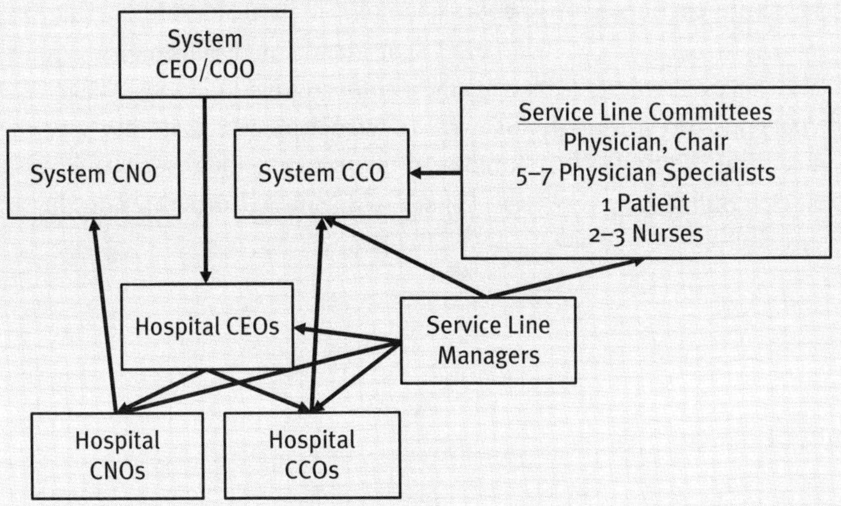

Two years into the reorganization, Elizabeth was pleased with the results from the orthopedic and cardiology service lines. These two had comprehensive quality metrics, and the providers seem to be working well together. However, she had received complaints from some groups, especially nursing, who felt that their authority and input had diminished. Nursing leaders commented that they were often uncertain whom to bring issues to, who was their "real" boss, and how to resolve problems. The service line managers had multiple reporting lines, the importance of which depended on the personalities and management philosophies of the individuals. Coordination was often fragmented and rivalries apparent. In addition, some of the service line committees seemed to lack cohesion and failed to achieve any of the established goals and metrics.

Elizabeth was preparing her thoughts to present to the next system leadership team meeting. She wanted to present both the positives and negatives of the new structure.

Questions

1. According to what you have learned in this chapter, what are some of the structural challenges of implementing such a structure?
2. Why would two of the service lines appear to have success while others fail?
3. What suggestions might you have to improve the success of this organization?

Chapter Assignments

1. Participative management has become a popular concept in business. Write a two-page paper on how the components of organizational structure encourage or discourage employee participation.
2. Matrix structures have been used in academic medical centers to coordinate medical, academic, and administrative functions. What challenges do you think this two-boss structure creates in this healthcare setting? What could be done to overcome those challenges?
3. Search online for two ACOs. What organizational structures do they employ?

CHAPTER

13

STRATEGIC CHANGE MANAGEMENT

> Before making cuts the first step of your change plan, it's important to stop and examine if they'll make the company or its change initiative more efficient. . . .
>
> Take a look at Virginia Mason Medical Center. Their approach to restructuring was surprising. When Dr. Gary Kaplan became CEO in 2002, he was faced with a number of problems that included million-dollar losses and fading staff morale. And when he tackled those problems, he also instituted a no-layoff policy.
>
> . . . 78% of Virginia Mason's costs were attributed to wages and benefits. So leaving those both intact meant serious work needed to be done everywhere else. Part of Kaplan's motivation was to get buy-in from the staff—which is why he didn't want to let anyone go. Employees might not be committed to making the solutions work if, he said, "they might improve themselves right out of a job"—thereby dooming change efforts from the start. Inspired by the Toyota Production System, Kaplan and his team created what eventually became the Virginia Mason Production System (VMPS). Focused on cutting waste and improving process, this philosophy still guides the hospital today.
>
> The VMPS worked. Over two years, Virginia Mason saw savings between $12 and $15 million. Productivity increased, and staff whose positions became redundant (remember, they couldn't be fired) were redeployed within the hospital.
>
> —Dora Wang, "Successful Organizational Change Is Easier Than You Think," 2017

Learning Objectives

After reading this chapter, you will

- know the three phases of organizational change;
- be aware of activities that should be accomplished prior to implementing change;

- be familiar with the use of surveys to identify preparedness for, readiness for, and resistance to change;
- have discovered the nature of resistance to change and methods of minimizing its negative effects on change efforts;
- understand that readiness includes leaders', participants', and the overall organization's level of preparedness for change;
- have learned how short-term wins can be used and their beneficial effect on strategic change; and
- comprehend that change cannot be sustained unless it is anchored in an organization's culture and processes.

Strategic leadership should position an organization to achieve fully its mission and vision. In many cases, significant change is required to do so. Many management theorists have observed that change is an ongoing organizational task; organizations must periodically reinvent themselves and change their products, services, process, and stakeholder value, or they will decline (Drummond-Hay and Bamford 2009; Miller 1990; Romanelli and Tushman 1994; Yip and Johnson 2007). Reinvention impacts an organization's key stakeholders, who are often extremely resistant to change. As a result, only about half of all major change efforts succeed (Aquirre and Alpern 2014). To be effective, change must be more than just cutting staff. As illustrated in the Virginia Mason story at the beginning of the chapter, restructuring without reducing staff in healthcare can be a major challenge, but may be successful.

Organizations need to have the skills and ability to manage change, especially to implement novel and challenging strategies successfully. Change management is a difficult task for most organizations, yet most frequently reorganize and restructure. Globally, an international study showed that more than 80 percent of companies were "either currently restructuring or . . . recently finished the process" (Rigoni and Nelson 2016). The majority of organizations appear to do this multiple times a year, yet 40 percent feel that the changes they make are not successful (Maurer 2009).

As discussed throughout this book, environmental pressures are continuing to mount, forcing healthcare organizations to change their business models and structures significantly to improve quality, lower costs, and meet the needs of key stakeholders. Healthcare leaders frequently engage external consultants to study and identify problems and solutions. In many cases, consultant engagements produce limited results if top executives fail to become champions of the change effort and neglect to prepare and involve important stakeholders. Research has shown that without proper management of the change process, significant resistance often arises among key stakeholders, especially physicians in clinical settings. Their resistance can stop or seriously impede change (Tarantino 2005).

This chapter discusses ways to prepare an organization for implementation of strategic change. It examines methods for identifying potential barriers to change and assessing organizational readiness and describes organizational development efforts that can facilitate and embed change.

Phases of Strategic Change

Change involves three interconnected, sequential phases: (1) prechange preparation, (2) implementation or execution, and (3) sustainment or maintenance. Exhibit 13.1 shows this model, which was introduced by Kurt Lewin (1951). Leaders must appropriately prepare their institution for strategic change (unfreeze), properly implement and execute changes (change), and embed the changes in the fabric and culture of the organization (refreeze).

Failure to address and correctly complete each of these phases puts the strategic change effort at risk. Too often, executives become impatient and implement change without addressing requisite pre- and postchange needs. These change efforts often involve a lot of movement, shuffling, reorganization, and restructuring that fail to improve the organization, meet its goals, and further its mission.

Prechange Preparation

Organizations need to be prepared and ready for strategic change. A critical first step is recognizing the need for change. Key stakeholders must perceive an appropriate rationale for it. The environmental analysis described in chapters 7 and 8 should provide the information and motivation needed to initiate strategic action. If key stakeholders do not understand the basis for action or do not perceive the action's connection with the organization's mission and vision, change may be difficult to implement. Their perceptions can become a barrier to change. With distorted views, key stakeholders can become disengaged from

EXHIBIT 13.1
Lewin's Change Model

Stage	Actions
Unfreeze: prechange preparation	• Recognize need for change • Communicate mission and vision • Instill sense of urgency • Build coalition for change
Change: implementation or execution	• Identify resistance • Remove obstacles • Achieve short-term wins
Refreeze: sustainment or maintenance	• Anchor changes in culture and processes

the change process, strike off in directions that could harm the organization, or even openly fight the change.

Key stakeholders should be dissatisfied with the status quo and perceive the proposed changes as necessary to addressing present and future challenges. If they are not dissatisfied enough, a sense of urgency may be lacking. A leader's role is to generate a case that will motivate key stakeholders to act and participate in the strategic change.

As discussed in chapter 6 and throughout most of this book, top executives must seek to define the mission and vision of the organization and motivate key stakeholders to live the mission and move forward to achieve the vision. A need to adapt to a transformed environment or a desire to improve performance motivates most change (Saebi, Lien, and Foss 2016). The mission, vision, and related strategic objectives should encapsulate the direction in which the organization needs to go and actions needed to prosper in the future. Vision statements can be powerful motivators. Organizational leaders should understand and communicate what must be done differently and how supporting systems, jobs, processes, functions, capabilities, and personnel must be altered to accomplish the vision.

Leaders should also formulate simplified versions of the mission, vision, and strategic direction that can be quickly communicated. The content should be short enough that it could be delivered in five minutes or less as an "elevator speech." It should briefly convey the strategic direction in words that people can easily grasp and remember. Leaders should deliver this speech frequently and powerfully by means of various venues, such as newsletters, intranet, formal speeches, and informal gatherings.

Top executives also need to create a sense of urgency and buy-in across the organization. As discussed in chapter 14, a strong strategic leader is transparent and trusted and engages in honest and convincing dialogue about potential events in the market, in the industry, and among competitors. A lack of transparency and trust often causes employees to abandon their confidence in the strategic direction of their organization and disengage from its goals. This problem is particularly acute with younger workers; though almost 90 percent of executives feel employee engagement is important, only 4 percent feel they proficiently engage millennials (Brown et al. 2016).

Too often, organizations wait until a crisis occurs to engender a sense of urgency. As exhibit 13.2 suggests, the best time to change is during a time of prosperity and strength, when the organization can choose to change. Under threat and pressure, organizations may change, but their options are generally limited and outcomes are not as robust.

A CEO of a large academic medical center once related that he could not motivate his key stakeholders to help him change their organization. After a couple of years of trying to encourage them, he stated that he "engineered" a crisis by not raising prices for two years in a row. As a result, the following year

EXHIBIT 13.2
Time for Change

A CEO had just presented a new program to revitalize and significantly improve the organization's processes and outcomes to his board. The board members were intrigued yet skeptical about the proposed effort. One asked, "Why would you propose to engage in this change process when our organization has done and is doing so well? We already are in the top 15 percent of our peer group for most outcomes and are very profitable." The CEO reflected on this question for only a minute and then talked about the future of their organization. He explained that they were meeting their mission, but to meet their vision, they would have to adapt to the changing environment. He asserted his belief that organizations should begin change from a position of strength—when they have choices—not when they are forced to change. If they initiated the new program, they would do so because they chose to, not because they were forced. When he finished speaking, the board unanimously approved the proposal.

the medical center suffered one of its biggest losses ever, and the stakeholders finally agreed that change was necessary. Unintended consequences arose, however, and two years later the CEO was pressured to resign.

Coalition
An alliance of individuals and groups that support a cause or an effort.

Formation of a **coalition** sufficient to support and embed change is another critical preimplementation step. A core group must fully buy into the strategic change and be cheerleaders, champions, and defenders of the effort. Coalitions facilitate employee empowerment and delegation of authority. Managers who fail to build a coalition early in the change process often fail to implement change efforts successfully (Kelley 2016). Coalitions should include top executives and other influential stakeholders who have necessary status, expertise, and bases of power that can be tapped to support the change effort.

Coalitions do not necessarily need to include members of the upper ranks of the traditional firm hierarchy. Informal leaders or employees with important job titles may be chosen. Informal leaders can be identified by various means. Unit managers usually know who is respected among the staff. Some firms have gone as far as to survey employees for names of respected, informal leaders. In one firm, those mentioned most often were deemed "influence leaders" and invited to participate in the change process.

Organizations should appoint influential employees to committees, steering groups, and task forces. Overall, the coalition should include a representative mix of employees from different departments and different levels of the organization. The important aspect is to bring together a large enough body to influence the organization as a whole.

How does an organization know when it is ready to undertake strategic change? Often this determination is based on leaders' gut feeling and lacks quantitative substance. To better gauge readiness, some organizations use surveys, focus groups, or other methods. Key indicators include

- leaders' preparedness,
- participants' preparedness, and
- overall organizational preparedness.

Leaders' and participants' readiness
The degree of experience leaders and participants have leading change, their skill level, their motivation, and their values.

Leaders' and participants' preparedness can be examined in terms of the amount of experience they have had leading change, their skill level, their motivation, and their values. Overall organizational preparedness includes the degree of organizational learning and appropriateness of its culture. Many books and companies offer survey questions that can be crafted to produce scores based on Likert scales (see Spiro 2011). Generally, organizations determine overall preparedness by asking multiple questions and summing and aggregating the scores.

Often it is helpful to understand the level of ability and preparedness of those tasked with leading organizational change. Surveys of prospective leaders can be tabulated and scored to determine how prepared they are for change. Leadership preparedness surveys could include questions such as the following:

1. How often have you successfully led change in the organization?

   5 Many times   4 Three or four times   3 Twice   2 Once   1 Never

2. What level of skills do you have for enacting strategic change?

   5 All necessary skills   4 Most necessary skills   3 Some necessary skills   2 Few necessary skills   1 None of the necessary skills

3. Are your fellow leaders skillful at leading change?

   5 Very skillful   4 Skillful   3 Somewhat skillful   2 Marginally skillful   1 Not skillful

4. Do you have competing priorities that might seriously distract you from a change effort?

   5 None   4 A few   3 A moderate number   2 Quite a few   1 Far too many

5. Have leaders and participants agreed on the methods by which strategic change will be undertaken?

   5 Definitely   4 Mostly   3 Somewhat   2 Minimally   1 Not at all

Participants would take a different survey; theirs will vary according to the nature of the strategic change. An overall company change may include all employees, while focused change may involve just a segment of the workforce. Although some organizations have their executives complete preparedness surveys for both leaders and participants to conserve time, more accurate information is gathered by directly surveying participants. Depending on the size of the organization, either all or a sample of affected employees can be surveyed. Participant surveys often include questions that have been adapted from questions included in leaders' surveys. Sample participant questions include the following:

1. I understand the goals of the change program.

   5 Completely 4 Mostly 3 Somewhat 2 A little 1 Not at all

2. I believe that the organization has the ability to achieve the strategic goals of the change program.

   5 Completely 4 Mostly 3 Somewhat 2 A little 1 Not at all

3. I trust the leaders in the organization.

   5 Completely 4 Mostly 3 Somewhat 2 A little 1 Not at all

4. The organization achieves the strategic programs it begins.

   5 Always 4 Often 3 Sometimes 2 Seldom 1 Never

5. I agree that the proposed strategic changes will benefit me personally.

   5 Completely 4 Mostly 3 Somewhat 2 A little 1 Not at all

6. I believe that the proposed strategic changes will benefit our customers.

   5 Completely 4 Mostly 3 Somewhat 2 A little 1 Not at all

One can include additional questions so a survey totals between 50 and 100 points.

Organizational preparedness for strategic change can be determined by surveying key stakeholders. Questions on overall organizational readiness might include the following:

1. Has the organization successfully made significant strategic changes in the last five years?

   5 Many times 4 Three or four times 3 Twice 2 Once 1 Never

Organizational preparedness
The degree to which an organization understands planned changes and the rationales behind them, the alignment of an organization's culture with the planned changes, and leaders' and participants' readiness (preparedness) for change.

2. How much does the organization appreciate risk taking?

   5 A great deal 4 Moderately 3 Somewhat 2 A little 1 Not at all

3. How often does organizational learning take place?

   5 Constantly 4 Often 3 Sometimes 2 Seldom 1 Never

4. Does a culture of blame exist when things go wrong?

   5 Never 4 Seldom 3 Sometimes 2 Often 1 Always

5. Does the organization hold ceremonies and events to celebrate its successes?

   5 Always 4 Often 3 Sometimes 2 Seldom 1 Never

6. Are meetings and communications governed by shared behavioral norms?

   5 Completely 4 Mostly 3 Somewhat 2 A little 1 Not at all

7. Do staff believe that the strategic change effort will help achieve the organization's mission and vision?

   5 Completely 4 Mostly 3 Somewhat 2 A little 1 Not at all

8. Do staff believe that the organization can successfully implement the proposed strategic change?

   5 Completely 4 Mostly 3 Somewhat 2 A little 1 Not at all

As in the other two surveys, questions should be added to assess the level of organizational readiness fully.

After the three groups have completed the surveys, the organization can score them and determine each group's level of readiness (from prepared to unprepared). Survey participants are considered prepared if they scored higher than 88 percent. Scores between 60 and 87 percent indicate that they are possibly prepared, and scores below 60 percent signify that they are unprepared (Spiro 2011).

As illustrated in exhibit 13.3, the three groups' combined scores dictate the needed actions in regard to strategic change. Ideally, all three groups should be at least at the "possibly prepared" to "prepared" levels to proceed with strategic change. If any of the groups score less than 50 percent, the organization should seriously analyze the situation and address what is lacking before proceeding with change. Use of a preparedness matrix is a quantitative, systematic

EXHIBIT 13.3
Preparedness Matrix

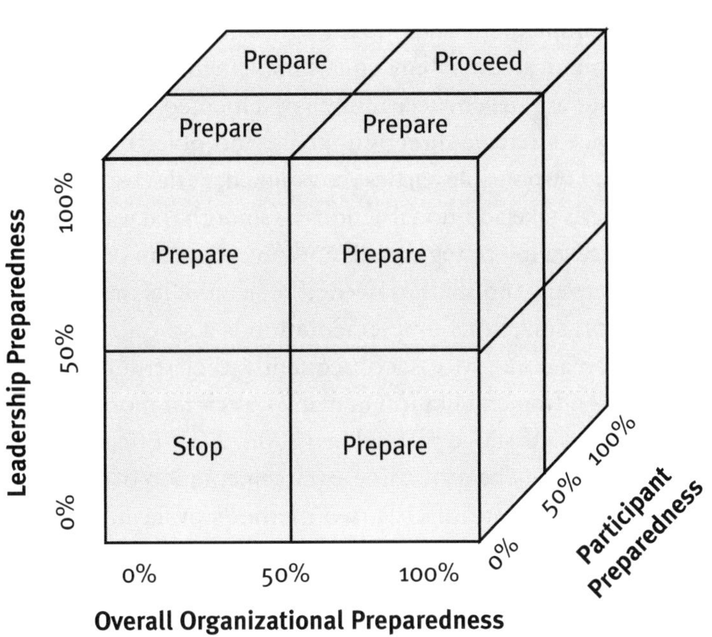

0% = Unprepared
50% = Possible
100% = Prepared

way to assess an organization's level of readiness for change. Organizations that approach change in a systematic, structured manner will be more successful.

Organizations should be concerned about the congruence and alignment of leaders' and participants' opinions. Change programs sustained over time tend to have greater alignment between executives and staff. Efforts should be made to align organizational stakeholders before and during strategic change efforts. For example, leaders might offer stakeholders incentives to develop innovative practices for implementing change, communicate more often and more effectively with them, and encourage them to become more involved in the change program.

Leaders, middle managers, and staff should support the same goals and actions and desire the same outcomes. Although most would think such unity of purpose and vision a given, these groups often do not agree on key issues. Research has demonstrated that in many cases, the outcomes executives perceive are vastly different from those perceived by middle managers and staff (Walston and Chou 2006).

Implementation and Execution

Strategy does not implement itself. Although some may believe that a well-crafted, well-communicated strategy equals implementation, many excellently conceived strategies are never successfully implemented (R. Martin 2010; R. Martin 2015). Once strategic direction, goals, and objectives are established and time frames and responsible parties are assigned, as discussed in chapters 10 and 15, managers can take additional actions to smooth the way through implementation. By meeting its strategic goals and objectives, an organization alters its structures, processes, and skills as needed to achieve its mission and vision.

For many organizations, implementation is a so-called strategic afterthought rather than a core process; consequently, they struggle to implement change (Raps 2004). Implementation in many ways is far more important than having a great strategy. As stated by Sterling (2003, 27), "Effective implementation of an average strategy beats mediocre implementation of a great strategy."

The next two sections discuss two methods of facilitating the implementation process:

1. Identifying resistance and removing obstacles
2. Achieving short-term wins

Identifying Resistance and Removing Obstacles

Managers can identify resistance and remove obstacles to change. Resistance to change is a common impediment to successful strategic implementation. Change almost always affects someone's job security and unsettles organizational norms, power centers, and processes. Stakeholders may perceive business change as a competitive, hostile process that divides communities and fosters resistance from key organizational stakeholders. However, resistance is part of the change process and should be identified and appropriately addressed (Lewis, Romanaggi, and Chapple 2010; Warner 2016).

Resistance does not signify incompetent or disloyal employees; it is a natural reaction to change. Managers need to understand its origins and take corrective actions to address it. Managers who fail to truly understand the roots of resistance may take counterproductive actions, such as enforcing discipline, making threats, showing anger, and enacting other negative communication forms that can reinforce resistance. Executives also can be a source of resistance, especially if they are reluctant to engage lower-level stakeholders appropriately and delegate responsibility.

Organizations should take time to examine the sources and level of resistance. A systematic evaluation can identify its sources and help managers determine a means to reduce it, thereby eliminating potential obstacles to the change effort. Again, stakeholder surveys can be used to identify resistance and measure its intensity. The following statements are examples of survey items that might be used for this purpose:

1. The advantages and disadvantages of the change for organizational stakeholders have been identified and appropriately communicated.

   5 To a great extent 4 Mostly 3 Somewhat 2 A little 1 Not at all

2. Strategies have been developed to better explain to stakeholders the benefits they will accrue from the change.

   5 To a great extent 4 Mostly 3 Somewhat 2 A little 1 Not at all

3. Stakeholders who have resisted strategic change in the past have been teamed with supporters and are now engaged in collaborative planning for the change.

   5 To a great extent 4 Mostly 3 Somewhat 2 A little 1 Not at all

4. Stakeholder groups believe that they are being treated fairly.

   5 To a great extent 4 Mostly 3 Somewhat 2 A little 1 Not at all

5. Stakeholder groups are afraid they will lose their jobs or will not be qualified for their positions following the change.

   5 To a great extent 4 Mostly 3 Somewhat 2 A little 1 Not at all

6. Leaders make efforts to speak with and understand stakeholders who say they agree with the change in public but talk against it in private.

   5 To a great extent 4 Mostly 3 Somewhat 2 A little 1 Not at all

Again, managers should assure that an adequate number of questions are developed to validly determine the level of resistance. The questions should be created to match the company's concerns and situation. Organizations should recognize that resistance cannot be eliminated, but it can be effectively managed. By identifying and understanding the source of resistance, organizations can target communications to those at the source, engage stakeholders to build their trust, and eliminate obstacles to change. Stakeholders may resist change if they lack skills required for the change or are overwhelmed by its scope or pace. In such cases, organizations can provide necessary training or moderate the speed of the change.

Sometimes the obstacle can be a difficult employee. Although it is always best to work with employees and seek their support, at some point the best choice might be to transfer the employee to an area that will not affect or be affected by the change or have the individual seek employment elsewhere. Sometimes the departure of personnel who are resisting change can have a substantial overall benefit and greatly facilitate the change effort.

Leaders should expect and prepare to deal with resistance during any major strategic change. They should predict where in the organization it might originate and what the nature of the resistance might be. In addition, the potential risk posed by resistance should be examined. Could resistance delay or halt projects? Could it alter investments? Pinpointing the root causes of resistance is critical. Leaders who address resistance early and throughout change efforts achieve success more often than those who do not.

Achieving Short-Term Wins

True strategic change can take years to fully implement, yet most managers and stakeholders demand quicker results. To satisfy their demands, most organizations need to achieve short-term wins.

For example, in 2010, the author worked with a Middle Eastern governmental IT organization that crafted an extensive strategic plan calling for the expenditure of more than $1.2 billion to upgrade the country's e-health systems. More than 135 large projects were identified, one of which included installing electronic medical records in 300 hospitals and more than 2,000 physician clinics. The projects were to be implemented over a period of three to seven years. However, the ministry of health leaders wanted to see annual results, beginning in the first year. To address the ministry's request, the e-health leaders grouped the projects into three main categories:

1. Foundational projects:
   - Projects deemed to be essential to implementing countrywide, interoperable, patient-centric clinical systems
   - Projects that provided the necessary tools and infrastructure for mission-critical operations
   - Projects necessary to establish electronic business and clinical support at locations that did not yet have technology
2. Short-term win projects:
   - Projects that required only connectivity and hosting to be implemented
   - Projects that could deliver early, visible value (benefits) to residents or ministry of health employees
   - Projects that were building blocks for later phases of implementation
3. Projects that provided other functions needed to achieve the vision

By dividing the projects into these categories, the e-health leaders scheduled short-term wins, each of which contributed to implementation of the IT strategy. The short-term projects produced annual results, pleasing the ministry leaders and increasing top governmental support of the initiative.

Short-term wins demonstrate success, and nothing motivates an organization more than successes. They keep the longer-term strategic efforts on track and diminish the influence of critics. Short-term wins must be visible, real, and meaningful. They also must be achievable. Only projects that have a 100 percent probability of accomplishment should be chosen. In addition, it is recommended that less expensive projects be selected. Smaller investments often earn proportionally greater returns in less time.

Sustainment or Maintenance

To be sustained over time, strategic change needs to be anchored in organizational culture and processes. If leaders impose change that is not supported by the values, beliefs, and routines of their organization, changes will be superficial and will not last. The Institute of Healthcare Improvement notes that "too often . . . improvements launched by healthcare organizations fail to stick after initial enthusiasm has waned" (Institute for Healthcare Improvement 2017, 66). Strategic change becomes embedded in an organization when the new way becomes the established way.

Just because a change is implemented does not mean it will last or produce predicted outcomes. Leaders should make a continuous effort to ensure that the benefits and results are widely seen and understood. As described in exhibit 13.4, if change is not managed appropriately, it can easily be undone and new practices can revert to prior routines. Leaders need to monitor change efforts periodically to make certain that changes are maintained. They should listen to feedback from staff involved in the effort and allow staff to make alterations if necessary to achieve the desired strategic outcomes.

EXHIBIT 13.4
Strategic Changes

With the help of consultants, a large medical center designed a comprehensive strategic change program to lower its costs and reposition itself to better compete in its market. The changes called for significant alterations to the roles and responsibilities of its clinical staff and the reorganization and reengineering of its nursing units. After extensive efforts, the medical center's executives launched the change program and, within six months, proudly announced that the changes had been accomplished.

They awaited the anticipated results, but after three months the medical center's costs had not decreased. They brought in a consultant to examine the changes and determine what had gone wrong. After visiting the 14 nursing units in which the strategic changes had been implemented, the consultant reported that all of the units had implemented the changes but only 4 units were maintaining them; the other 10 units had abandoned all or some of the changes soon after implementation. In fact, one of the units reversed the changes just 12 hours after they were implemented. The units cited lack of training, new cumbersome processes, and general role confusion as the reasons they reverted to past practices. None of these issues had been reported to the medical center's executives.

Organizational leaders need to use every opportunity they have to tell success stories. One important venue for communicating successes is the training and orientation of new staff. Organizations should highlight their values and vision, and publicly acknowledge their departments and leaders who have excelled in the change process.

Other methods of embedding change and monitoring the progress of a change effort include the use of visual management practices and checklists or audits that can clearly identify important actions and engender accountability. Leaders often are distracted by the many priorities and challenges they face and may forget to focus on anchoring strategic changes. Placing key measures on visual boards or walls can focus attention (Institute for Healthcare Improvement 2017). Likewise, the data generated by the use of checklists or audits engage employees in the change effort and keep managers focused on embedding change. Make checklists or audits simple and easily understood, and make the results public. Exhibit 13.5 presents a checklist that could be used prior to implementation of a change program.

EXHIBIT 13.5
Sample Checklist

Training Questions

1. Does the organization have a documented training program?
2. Has a competency assessment method been documented and established?

Process Questions

1. Are procedures documented at each point of use?
2. Is there documented evidence of compliance with the procedures?

Performance Questions

1. Are performance expectations documented for all staff?
2. Does the organization have a documented process for providing performance feedback?
3. Does the organization have an employee development program?
4. Have visible performance targets been established?
5. Does the organization have a documented process for corrective action?

Benchmarking Questions

1. Does the organization have a documented process for benchmarking?
2. Have the results of benchmarking activities been documented?
3. Have the actions taken to address the benchmarking results been documented?

Communication Questions

1. Does the organization have a documented process for giving directives and asking questions?
2. Does the organization have a documented process for collecting and acting on stakeholders' feedback?

Chapter Summary

Most leaders find organizational change difficult at best. Many organizations spend large sums of money on consultants to generate plans but do not implement them. Even when change is implemented, an organization can easily revert to prior practices and processes. To improve their chances of making change permanent, leaders should divide the change process into three phases—prechange preparation, implementation or execution, and sustainment or maintenance—and plan specific activities for each phase.

Before change can be implemented, stakeholders must recognize that the status quo must be challenged to meet the organization's mission and vision. Information from key stakeholders, the environmental analysis, and other sources can be used to foster the perception that change is needed. Leaders should generate a sense of urgency for change and buy-in to the change effort across the organization.

Coalitions of key stakeholders also need to form prior to implementation. Coalitions may include top executives and stakeholders who have status, expertise, and power. These key stakeholders should contribute extensively to the change process through participation in committees and other activities.

Leaders also should take the time to diagnose their organization's readiness for change. Leaders, participants, and the overall organization should have a reasonable level of preparedness before proceeding with implementation. Diagnostic tools, including surveys, can be used to identify the level of readiness and areas that need to be addressed before initiation of the change effort.

Resistance is a normal reaction to strategic change; it does not signify disloyalty to the organization. The source, extent, and depth of resistance should be identified and barriers to change eliminated.

Many changes take multiple years to implement fully. Short-term wins demonstrate the initial value of the change and keep stakeholders motivated and focused on the change effort.

For change to be sustained, it must be anchored in an organization's culture and processes. Making successes widely known and extensively involving stakeholders help make change permanent. Checklists and audits can be used to validate that change has been implemented and to monitor its maintenance.

Chapter Questions

1. What makes change so difficult for many organizations?
2. Why must an organization prepare for each phase of change?
3. Who might be some of the key stakeholders an organization should address in a change effort?

4. What actions might an organization take if leaders diagnose that it is not prepared for change?
5. Why does resistance to organizational change arise so frequently?
6. Why are short-term wins often necessary?
7. How can change be anchored in an organization's culture and processes?
8. How can checklists and audits help ensure that change has taken place?

Chapter Cases

Case Studies

Read "St. John's Reengineering" in the Case Studies section at the end of this book. What did the administration of this organization do wrong during the implementation of its strategic changes?

Read "Dissolving a Long-Standing Affiliation and Moving On" in the Case Studies section at the end of the book. Review and discuss the questions at the end of the case.

A Shift to a "Value-Based Care" Organization

Jill, the CEO of Redmond Medical Center, and her assistant, Joe, attended the American College of Healthcare Executives' (ACHE) annual Congress last week and, upon comparing notes, they concurred that moving healthcare to "value-based care" appeared to be the direction of most of the country's providers. As defined at the ACHE meeting, value-based care models focus on the value received by patients by rewarding better outcomes, which moves a health provider away from the traditional fee-for-service model that rewards for more volume.

Few systems have moved away from the volume, fee-for-service model to a value-based system. In 2016, only 27 percent of healthcare provider organizations had experimented with or completed value-based pilot programs (Sanicola 2017). However, employers, health insurance companies, and government purchasers have begun to encourage providers to transition to value-based payment models. For example, the Centers for Medicare & Medicaid Services (CMS) had implemented value-based programs primarily for Medicare patients with the goal to link provider performance of quality measures to provider payment. These included the following:

- Hospital Value-Based Purchasing Program
- Hospital Readmission Reduction Program

- Value Modifier Program (also called the Physician Value-Based Modifier, or PVBM)
- Hospital-Acquired Condition Reduction Program
- End-Stage Renal Disease Quality Initiative Program
- Skilled Nursing Facility Value-Based Program
- Home Health Value-Based Program

Until now, the hospital had not put much effort in addressing the requirements of value-based programs, but, as can be seen below, the medical center has seen a great shift in its patient population and profitability. In the past 20 years, the commercial insurance patient market has shrunk by one-third (down 14 percent), while governmental paid patients have gone from 53 percent to 65 percent of all patients. Concurrently, net income decreased by over $4 million and the net margin from 6.8 percent to 2.2 percent.

	1997	2007	2017
Commercial insurance	42%	35%	28%
Medicare	35%	42%	46%
Medicaid	10%	15%	18%
Other government coverage	8%	1%	1%
Uncompensated care	5%	7%	7%
Net income	$10,802,000	$8,932,000	$6,701,300
Net margin	6.8%	4.3%	2.2%

However, Jill expressed concern that they may not have the experience, skills, and abilities to align their physician and hospital rewards and penalties with cost, quality, and outcome measures. Joe has suggested that they consider shared savings or bundled payments.

Yet the last major change they implemented was three years ago, when they installed a medical center–wide electronic health record system, and the shift caused much complaining from the administrative and medical staff. Joe feels that if they do not move forward, they will not be prepared for the shift that is coming. Still—Jill wonders.

(continued)

Questions

1. What could Jill and Joe do to understand their level of preparedness for change more fully?
2. Who would be the key stakeholders for the proposed changes?
3. Why should Jill and Joe expect resistance to this type of change and what could they do to address it?
4. What should they do before they decide to go ahead with this change?

Chapter Assignment

Review a resource such as John Kotter's *Leading Change* (Harvard Business School Press, 1996), Kim Cameron and Robert Quinn's *Diagnosing and Changing Organizational Culture* (Jossey-Bass, 2011), or Robert Quinn's *Deep Change* (Jossey-Bass, 1996). Using the material you have chosen and the information in this chapter, design a 60-question survey that explores preparedness for change among leaders, stakeholders, and the overall organization (20 questions for each group).

CHAPTER

14

STRATEGIC LEADERSHIP

> For a CEO, Strategy is Job 1. A CEO's job is not quality, productivity, finance, human resources or marketing. These are delegated responsibilities. It is the CEO's job to orchestrate competencies and capabilities into a sustainable value advantage. . . . Too many organization-wide strategic planning efforts seem to assume employees will resent and resist efforts by leaders to set overall direction. My experience suggests just the opposite. Generally, employees expect and welcome it when their leaders provide strategic direction. Followers are more likely to follow when they sense insight and depth of commitment at the top of the organization. Making strategy happen requires toughness and resolve.
>
> —Dan Beckham, "10 Surprising Keys to Strategic Thinking for Health Care CEOs," 2016

Learning Objectives

After reading this chapter, you will

- understand that strategic leadership is a combination of strategic thinking and strategic management,
- know the components of strategic thinking,
- comprehend how refusal to question assumptions can cause severe organizational problems,
- realize the importance of feedback to strategic thinking,
- know how strategic management must allocate resources for today's mission and tomorrow's vision,
- be familiar with the components of strategic management, and
- recognize the level of engagement and decision making leaders need to achieve to manage strategically.

Successful strategic efforts are the product of strategic leadership. Too many efforts fail because organizations lack good leaders. Although, as this chapter's opening quote states, the CEO's top job must be strategy, studies show that fewer than 10 percent of leaders demonstrate strategic skills (Beatty 2010). Leaders are integral to the creation and implementation of strategies. They must interpret the organization's internal and external environments and design and guide changes that will better position their organization to meet its mission and vision. Thought leaders have defined strategic leadership as "the ability to influence others to voluntarily make day-to-day decisions that enhance the long-term viability of the organization, while at the same time maintaining its short-term financial stability" (Rowe 2001, 85).

Strategic leadership is made more difficult by the complexity of leaders' demands. Everyday management responsibilities place extreme pressure on executives and distract them from their strategic duties. They are bombarded by meetings, governmental requests, ceremonial commitments, and demands for monthly financial results. Successful strategic leaders are able to balance these short-term, day-to-day demands with long-term strategy development and efforts. Strategic leaders must look ahead to set directions and initiate changes to their organization's structure, strategies, and personnel to drive the organization forward and fulfill its mission and vision—and they must simultaneously maintain the continuity and reliability of the organization's processes and outputs. Successful strategic leaders engender both short-term financial success and long-term growth and viability.

On top of these challenges, multiple difficult barriers stand between the leader and her organizational strategic priorities. These hurdles include the following:

- Physician buy-in and engagement
- Financial constraints
- Organizational barriers to collaboration
- Lack of talent or skill sets for key roles
- Cultural impediments in the organization (Health Research & Educational Trust 2014)

To overcome these and achieve an organization's strategic priorities, leaders must have a balanced combination of skills: the ability to think strategically and the ability to manage strategically (see exhibit 14.1). This chapter considers strategic thinking as a long-term skill and strategic management as a short-term skill. Authors have noted that leaders infrequently demonstrate depth in both areas: "Rare is the business leader who can articulate and instill a long-term vision and manage the day-to-day operations with the requisite obsession for detail" (Rowe and Nejad 2009). Leaders who are able to fulfill both roles are

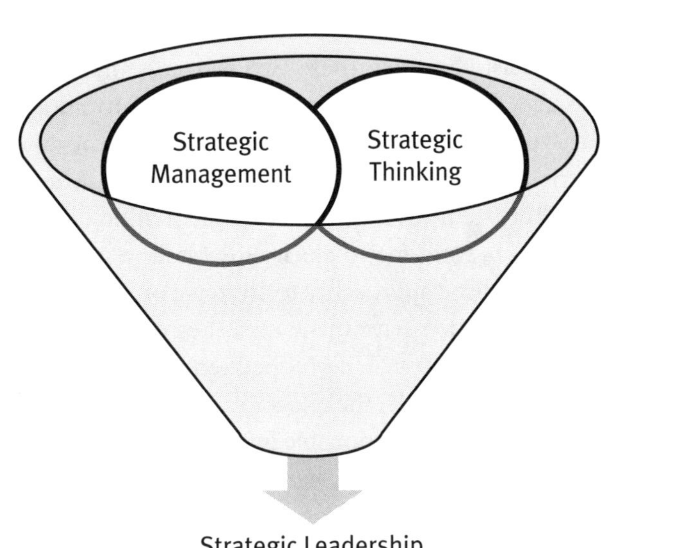

EXHIBIT 14.1
The Components of Strategic Leadership

more likely to increase the organization's value to stakeholders. This chapter discusses critical skills and functions a strategic leader should have to excel in both areas.

Strategic Thinking

Strategic thinking involves collecting, collating, and assembling disparate pieces of information to make decisions. Strategic thinking involves distinctive management activities "whose purpose is to discover novel, imaginative strategies which can rewrite the rules of the competitive game; and to envision potential futures significantly different from the present" (Goldman 2007, 76). Strategic thinkers understand "the complex relationship between the organization and its environment" (Beatty 2010).

Strategic thinking
The generation and application of unique business insights and opportunities intended to create competitive advantage for a firm or an organization.

Successful strategic leaders have an ability to identify critical information, challenge assumptions, collaboratively develop direction with key stakeholders, and communicate the strategic vision through their words and actions. They understand the changing relationship between their organization and the external environment and its relationship with key stakeholders. They are humble enough to learn and strong enough to push for resolutions and results.

Strategies tend to fail when executives do not begin the change initiatives at the top and do not remain fully engaged and committed to that change (Aquirre and Alpern 2014). Executives may be good managers, but past success can make them myopic to the need and desire for change. A related challenge is recognizing that assumptions are changing along with the environment. Leaders' experiences inform their worldviews and the assumptions on which they based their decisions; when these two factors, if inaccurate, can lead to disastrous (McGrath 2016). Many leaders have difficulty adopting a new perspective on the world or new assumptions, especially when old assumptions have served them well. As stated by scholars Williamson Murray, MacGregor Knox, and Alvin Bernstein (1994, 3): "Strategic thinking does not occur in a vacuum . . . cultures, in turn, may make it difficult for a state [organization] to evolve sensible and realistic approaches to strategic problems that confront it."

Across history, leaders have made critical errors by clinging to outdated assumptions. In 1876, Western Union operated the most sophisticated communication technology available, the telegraph, as a monopoly. That year, it was offered the patent on a new, questionable invention—the telephone—for about $2 million in 2017 dollars. Western Union's president, basing his judgement on old assumptions, rejected buying the patent, writing, "After careful consideration of your invention, while it is a very interesting novelty, we have come to the conclusion that it has no commercial possibilities. . . . What use could this company make of an electrical toy?" (Andersen 2013). Likewise, many in the past have assumed the United States has the best healthcare system in the world. Therefore, its structure, processes, and outcomes need not be changed (Kaplan 2012).

Leaders should seek to understand and be open to other opinions. Those who use their management position to enforce their opinion cut off communication and harden assumptions. A detrimental characteristic of many managers is the belief that they are always right. Such managers stand their ground during meetings and refuse to listen to others. They grow red in the face with apoplectic anger if anyone challenges their views and categorize anyone who does not agree with them as a fool or a knave. These people destroy an organization no matter how talented or brilliant they are (Rein 2010).

Strategic leaders also need to evaluate their assumptions on the basis of disparate data. Frequently, they base decisions on anecdotal stories or singular events. Basing assumptions on single data points can be risky, if not dangerous. For instance, managers often make erroneous assumptions about old and young workers, which can lead to stereotypes based on age and discrimination against older employees (exhibit 14.2).

Hubris
Excessive pride and arrogance.

Leaders can similarly allow their past successes to cloud their judgment and induce hubris, excessive pride, and arrogance. **Hubris** often causes leaders to ignore other perspectives and sometimes even to denigrate the opposition. Consider the true story of an assistant administrator at a not-for-profit community hospital. The community had two hospitals but could realistically support only one. Negotiations to merge or share services had been ongoing between the two hospitals for years. The other hospital was somewhat larger, belonged to a religious organization, and was better funded. During a particularly difficult meeting, the CEO of the religious hospital turned to the

EXHIBIT 14.2
Our Assumptions About Old and Young Workers Are Wrong

Many assume that if an employee or potential employee is in his twenties, he must be technologically savvy, fitness oriented, and in search of meaningful work. Conversely, older employees or potential employees in their sixties and seventies are supposedly less interested in work, less focused on fitness, and hoping for leisure time. Although these assumptions are prevalent, they may be more and more wrong today.

A survey found that many of the traits and characteristics attributed to the younger population were shared by the older group. People are working much longer, many into their seventies, and this fact, coupled with influential technological changes, is causing the common life stages (education, work, retirement) to blend across the life span. People of all ages are continually reinvesting in education and improving their skills, looking after their health, and considering career transitions. About 50 percent of both groups are also positive and excited about their work. Some differences between the age groups do exist, but overall, major similarities predominate. This reality means that managers need to carefully consider their assumptions about age categories.

Source: Gratton and Scott (2016).

delegates from the community hospital and told them that they should stop being so difficult—his hospital would win because God was on its side. The discussion and collaboration efforts deteriorated after this point.

Self-righteousness and egos must be left at the door when executives craft the vision of tomorrow and examine the relationship of their choices to outcomes. If a person claims that he is clinging to a decision as a matter of principle, the assumptions behind the principle should be examined. During the American Revolution, many approached King George III with requests to modify England's rigid policies toward the colonists. He cloaked his obstinacy in self-righteousness and stated, "I know I am doing my duty, and therefore can never wish to retreat" (Cook 1995, 14). Instead of fostering trade and a strong alliance with its colonies, Britain spent more than £100 million to lose its 13 colonies in North America (Tuchman 1984, 217). Leaders must have the humility to recognize and change their biases and false assumptions.

Moreover, hubris can develop when leaders isolate themselves from new knowledge and outside thinking. Strategic thinkers should surround themselves with diverse, intelligent people who are willing to challenge the leader's assumptions and bring novel perspectives to the table. Too often leaders surround themselves with like-minded individuals or create an environment in which honest feedback is lacking. In many organizations, followers may be afraid to speak their mind or may say what they believe their boss wants to hear.

Although Niccolò Machiavelli, a famous author in the sixteenth century, proposed a nonethical form of management, his philosophy regarding feedback resonates. He stated that a prince (leader) should always be a greater asker and a patient hearer of the truth but should be most angry if he finds that a subject has scruples about telling him the truth. Strategic thinkers must break through these barriers and open the feedback and learning loops to increase the flow of new knowledge and understanding.

The problem of obtaining good feedback from one's subordinates has existed across the ages. Many centuries ago, a Catholic pope, Alexander, was embroiled in controversy and intrigue after the murder of his eldest surviving son. He expressed his frustration about the lack of honest feedback in a meeting of his cardinals. He said, "The most grievous danger for any Pope lies in the fact that encompassed as he is by flatterers, he never hears the truth about his own person and ends by not wishing to hear it" (Tuchman 1984, 85). Without candid feedback, leaders often fail to learn and to update their assumptions.

An innovative culture fosters learning and is a critical product of strategic thinking. Leaders who fashion a values-driven organization create an environment in which employees make decisions that align with the organization's strategic vision without extensive formal monitors and control mechanisms. Research suggests that organizations that cultivate innovation are better able to motivate their workforce, uniting employees behind a common vision and direction (Walston and Chou 2011). Innovation and invention build new knowledge and tools necessary to managing the dimensions of an organization's future.

Strategic thinking is a skill that both organizations as a whole and individuals can develop, and every leader has the capacity to be a strategic thinker (Beckham 2016b). The following list includes some activities leaders can engage in to encourage strategic thinking in their organization (Goldman et al. 2009; Rein 2010):

- Create personal development plans for key employees. Identify and build needed core competencies. Map career paths.
- Maintain a focus on continuing education for all employees. Educational offerings should include university degrees, certifications, on- and off-site training, and conferences.
- Develop mentoring programs for new and newly promoted employees.
- Establish ground rules for meetings that encourage open conversation and honest feedback.
- Rotate personnel into different job functions. Allow different people to engage in strategic planning, task forces, and initiatives.
- Network with outside professional organizations and peers in the same industry and other industries.
- Constantly question and examine one's own opinions and assumptions.
- Surround themselves with people who look at the world differently than they do.

- Be concerned with ideas, ethics, and values and how they are communicated to and lived by all personnel.
- Base decisions on organizational values and ethics.

Texas Health Resources (THR) has been an excellent example of an organization that promotes strategic thinking. THR's ten-year strategic focus is the development of visionary leaders who live their values, demonstrate decisive action, and promote excellence. The organization selected six core leadership behaviors that all executives should emulate:

1. Values-based leadership
2. Focus on excellence
3. Action orientation
4. Managerial courage
5. Visionary thinking
6. Sound decision making

To embed these behaviors, THR implemented comprehensive 360-degree feedback processes for all senior leaders, directors, and selected managers every three years, as well as annual individualized development plans. It also invested heavily in a center for learning and career development that provides leadership training, coaching, mentoring, and a leadership academy for prospective leaders.

Strategic management
Overseeing and directing daily activities in an organization to ensure they support achievement of the organization's mission and vision. Responsibilities may include designing organizational structures, policies, and procedures; evaluating budgets and progress toward goals; and coordinating staff training.

Strategic Management

In addition to strategic thinking, strategic leaders must exercise strategic management. Strategic leaders are required to produce results on a day-to-day basis while concurrently aligning the organization with its long-term strategies and vision. Time management is essential to fulfilling the myriad roles of a leader. Daily activities include designing organizational structures, policies, and procedures and evaluating budgets, goals, and training. Leaders manage multiple stakeholder groups, select and hire key managers, and foster a culture that sustains the organization's values.

Strategic management involves building and allocating resources both to meet the needs of today and to fulfill the vision of the future. Allocation of resources is one of the most demanding and important decisions a leader makes. Resources are always finite, while demands are seemingly infinite.

Likewise, leaders must develop internal core competencies to meet goals. **Competencies** have been defined as activities "that a company has learned to perform with proficiency." **Core competencies** have been described as activities "that a company performs proficiently that [are] also central to its strategy

Competencies
Activities "that a company has learned to perform with proficiency." (Thompson et al. 2016, 93)

Core competencies
Activities "that a company performs proficiently that [are] also central to its strategy and competitive success." (Thompson et al. 2016, 93)

and competitive success" (Thompson et al. 2016, 93). Organizations that do not take the time and effort to develop core competencies to meet changing circumstances may not be prepared for the future. Leaders exhibiting expertise in strategic management allocate resources to encourage, create, and maintain competencies and behaviors to exact both short- and long-term success.

Studies have shown that hospitals that do not have the active, consistent support of senior executives are more likely to perform poorly in clinical care. On the other hand, high-performing hospitals have highly involved executives who empower and engage their employees (Curry et al. 2011).

Strategic leaders must be accessible so that they can make timely decisions, organizing their work life effectively to allot time for strategic consultation, advisement, and decision making. They must attend to daily details but delegate appropriately to free up time to deal with the big picture and strategic issues. Subordinates should not have to wait long periods to meet with their manager.

Prompt decisions can be made through a mix of informal and formal meetings. Informal meetings place leaders in work settings where they can interact with employees. Leaders may want to eat in common dining areas, visit departments, and meet with small groups of staff, among other activities. Leaders should regularly schedule formal meetings. Periodic meetings in neutral locations or in subordinates' offices encourage greater participation and openness among employees.

Leaders should be actively engaged in strategic planning from the beginning of the process. Those who delegate strategic planning and implementation to others often fail to obtain value from these efforts. Top leaders should be highly visible and coordinate the work of everyone engaged in developing plans and strategies. Their actions reflect desired employee behaviors. They need to walk the talk and lead by example. As shown in exhibit 14.3, if leaders disengage from the process, strategic planning can easily derail, wasting effort, time, and money.

EXHIBIT 14.3
The Consequences of Delegating Strategic Planning

Hospital A was a large, complex teaching hospital. Initially established in 1972 by a western US hospital company, the organization grew and prospered over the next 30 years. It grew to almost 800 hospital beds and received $900 million in funding per year. Yet, the hospital never established a formal strategic plan or planning process. The government, which provided most of the $900 million in funding, appointed the CEO. This dependency created a certain level of caution in management's actions and made the hospital's top executives sensitive and reactive to governmental pressures and whims.

A new CEO—a general surgeon—was appointed five years ago. Aside from serving as a chair of a university department of surgery and as a deputy minister of health, he had little administrative experience. However, he wanted to address the many challenges facing the hospital, including long

EXHIBIT 14.3
The Consequences of Delegating Strategic Planning *(continued)*

wait times, complaints about quality, and increasing local and regional competition, and he was pleased that the outgoing CEO had hired a prominent strategic planning firm to craft the hospital's first written strategic plan. He met with the firm's consultants and assigned the strategic planning process to one of his subordinates, Jack, directing him to move the planning process forward and to let him know when he needed his input.

Jack wanted to make a name for himself and be the author of the best strategic plan in the country. First, he and the consultants examined the strategic intent of the organization. Creating a mission and vision was easy; they simply adopted the governmental charter. The charter consisted of two pages of directives written 30 years earlier. Points of focus included the following:

- Provide the best specialized medical care services.
- Contribute to increasing the standards of healthcare quality in the country.
- Conduct scientific and applied healthcare research, and implement collaborative efforts to advance and improve healthcare processes and procedures in general and medical subspecialties.
- Contribute to enhancing the level of awareness and health education in the community.
- Contribute to educating and qualifying staff in healthcare and health education programs.
- Issue medical and scientific journals and other publications.

As these directives demonstrate, the governmental charter did not specify actual services or practices and was extremely general in nature.

Despite the fact that none of the directives mentioned cost efficiency, the consultants decided that saving money was most important and went about collecting financial data. They found that the hospital was spending far too much money per patient. The average cost per patient was almost double that spent by other governmental hospitals. The consulting firm and Jack began devising specific, detailed plans on how to reduce costs.

After almost two years of intense work, the consulting firm and Jack presented their findings to the CEO. Their research showed that the hospital could save about 20 percent of its budget by being more efficient. The plan called for various cost reduction initiatives that would streamline hospital services and eliminate waste. Jack was surprised by the CEO's reaction. The CEO was upset that costs had been their focus. He had expected that they would focus on improving specialized care and national and regional reputation. He could not imagine why they had spent so much money and time focusing on costs. Jack became defensive and engaged in a nasty argument with the CEO. The CEO reassigned Jack to other work, and a year later, Jack resigned.

The consultants also were negatively affected. After the hospital paid them almost $3 million for their services, the CEO terminated their contract, tarnishing the firm's reputation. The hospital ended up with two large binders filled with PowerPoint slides and cost data, which it never used. Eventually, the hospital hired staff and restarted the planning process. Another two years passed before its first acceptable strategic plan was completed.

Another mechanism for engendering good strategic management is effective meetings. Much of a manager's work life seems to be spent in long, unproductive meetings, and employees spend almost four hours a week in such worthless meetings, which is one of the top reasons employees become unmotivated (Koort 2014). Committee meetings in particular are often ineffective. Healthcare organizations often organize too many committees, do not manage them well, and gain little value for the time spent on them. Leaders should seek to improve the caliber of meetings by making certain that all committees have specific purposes and desired outcomes. Furthermore, the correct people should participate. Remove people from committees who are not contributing or have little interest in the meetings. Agendas and ground rules must be set for every meeting, and meetings must start and stop on time. A meeting coordinator should be appointed and appropriately involve all attendees. Effective use of meetings greatly facilitates strategic management.

The following list recaps the advice given in this chapter for leaders who want to become strategic managers:

- Allocate resources appropriately, efficiently, and effectively to fulfill today's mission and tomorrow's vision.
- Identify and develop key organizational competencies to meet the organization's mission and fulfill its vision.
- Organize time appropriately to ensure adequate consultation and timely decision making in both formal and informal settings.
- Engage top executives throughout the strategic planning process.
- Manage meetings effectively.
- Lead from the front—be actively involved in the strategic effort.

Chapter Summary

Strategic leadership consists of strategic thinking and strategic management. Strategic efforts often fail because leaders lack one or both of these skills. Strategic thinking drives an organization forward to fulfill its vision, while strategic management addresses current demands to achieve an organization's mission. Strategic efforts are more likely to be successful when leaders have both skills.

Strategic thinking involves understanding and perceiving different ways to organize and compete. Leaders must exhibit behaviors that imbue employees with the values of their organization. Innovation and learning enhance strategic thinking.

Strategic management involves ensuring successful short-term outcomes while investing for the future. Resources must be allocated to maximize mission achievement and, at the same time, prepare the organization for the future.

Leaders who are successful at strategic management develop core competencies to meet challenges, use their time wisely, are engaged throughout strategic planning, and make meetings productive.

Chapter Questions

1. What is the relationship between strategic thinking and strategic management? How do they complement each other? How do they contrast?
2. Why might it be difficult to possess both strategic thinking and strategic management skills?
3. How do learning and innovation encourage strategic thinking?
4. What is the relationship between an organization's mission and vision and strategic thinking and strategic management?
5. As environments change, why must assumptions behind decisions likewise change?
6. How can hubris impede strategic thinking?
7. How does feedback improve strategic thinking?
8. What might be some of the core competencies leaders need to practice strategic management?
9. How is meeting and committee management a core function of strategic management?
10. Why is it necessary for a leader to be involved in all phases of strategic planning?

Chapter Cases

Case Studies

Read "Deciding on a Population Health Referral Contract Approach" in the case studies section at the end of the book and answer the related questions.

Halburt Hospital Need for Change

Stephanie Short, CEO of Halburt Hospital, just got a promotion. She previously worked in a consulting firm that had done turnaround consulting at struggling hospitals. Her work was recognized in many journals, and when Halburt Hospital's board of trustees needed a new CEO to bring about radical change, it offered the job to Stephanie.

(continued)

Halburt Hospital is a 500-bed acute care hospital in the southeastern region of the United States. Its mission is to provide care for the poor and underprivileged. However, in the past two decades, the hospital constructed a new facility and feeder clinics around one of its affluent suburban areas. The hospital had been run by an ex–military officer for the past 15 years, and decisions were highly centralized. He authorized all new hires and replacements and nonroutine purchases of more than $10,000. The centralization of decisions slowed actions and inhibited innovation. However, until recently, the hospital prospered and consistently earned high returns.

In the past few years, new organizations entering Halburt's market have been eroding the hospital's profits. Physician specialty hospitals, national physician clinics, surgery centers, and other new services have attracted many of Halburt's patients. The hospital's operating margin dropped to just 1.8 percent in the year before the previous CEO retired.

The board of trustees is concerned about the future of the hospital. In recent years, state legislators have discussed taxing not-for-profit hospitals that earn too much money. The board also is questioning whether Halburt is meeting its mission, given its location in one of the most affluent areas in the region. Recent staff surveys suggest that many employees are not satisfied with their jobs, which may have contributed to recent high turnover. As one employee wrote at the end of the survey, "I thought I was getting out of a dysfunctional culture when I left the Army. Little did I know that yelling, haranguing, and extreme bureaucracies exist outside of the military. Halburt's culture needs an extreme overhaul."

Into this situation walked Stephanie Short. After three months of mostly observing and noting problems, she believes that she is ready to develop a plan of action.

Questions

1. What are the main issues Stephanie is facing?
2. What actions could she take to improve strategic thinking and strategic management at the hospital?
3. What stakeholder issues should she immediately address?
4. What changes could she make over the short term to refocus the organization and achieve quick wins?

Chapter Assignments

1. Write a two-page paper describing the differences and interactions between strategic thinking and strategic management. Address why

many leaders often fail to think strategically. Include experiences you have had with leaders for whom you have worked.

2. Interview a healthcare leader. Ask her what the leader of an organization can do to encourage learning and innovation. Find out how the organization's executives encourage strategic thinking throughout the organization. Ask how involved executives are in strategic planning.
3. Reread exhibit 14.3 and answer the following questions:
   a. How did the CEO fail to integrate strategic management and strategic thinking?
   b. What could Jack have done to help the CEO implement better strategic thinking in the organization?
   c. If you were the CEO, what would you have done differently?

PART

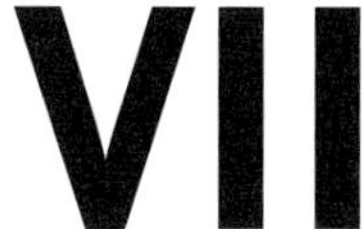

MONITORING STRATEGIC ACHIEVEMENT

This final section presents methods of monitoring and evaluating the status of strategies. Creating a written strategic plan does not ensure achievement of an organization's mission and vision. Once plans are set in place, managers must establish means and processes to monitor performance and determine whether any strategies need to be modified. Chapter 15 discusses methods of evaluating strategic outcomes consistently, including the use of balanced scorecards and budgets.

CHAPTER

15

IMPLEMENTING, MONITORING, AND EVALUATING STRATEGY

> Many hospitals and health systems have strong strategic plans in which they outline long-term goals and tactics to reach those goals. Where organizations tend to fall short is in the execution stage, primarily due to a lack of accountability, according to Scott Becker, CEO of Conemaugh Health System in Johnstown, Pa. "Everybody has a great strategic plan. The organizations that are successful are the ones that effectively operationalize it," he says. . . .
>
> Once goals are set, leaders need to determine the critical success factors [CSF] to meet those goals. . . . Every CSF should have an assigned leader, a set of key performance indicators [KPIs], and action steps or tasks to be completed to achieve the CSF. KPIs track the quantitative progress or effectiveness of a CSF in achieving a measurable target. For example, increased margins may be measured by KPIs such as reduced expenses per adjusted admission, reduced readmission penalties and shorter length of stay. . . . Hospital leaders need to measure KPIs to determine areas for improvement and then create action plans to meet KPI targets. . . . Hospital executives need to work with medical staff leaders and other stakeholders to develop specific plans to reach their objectives. . . . Emphasizing the link between assigned actions and the hospital's overall goals helps employees understand how they personally contribute to the organization's mission and vision, which is essential for employee satisfaction and the hospital's ability to meet its goals.
>
> —Sabrina Rodak, "Creating Accountability in Healthcare Strategic Plan Execution," 2013

Learning Objectives

After reading this chapter, you will

- understand the role of budgets and controls in the strategic planning process;
- have learned methods of implementing strategy;

- be familiar with the various bodies and structures involved in strategic planning, along with their roles;
- have discovered ways in which progress toward strategic goals can be monitored; and
- know what a balanced scorecard is and how it can be used to monitor strategic planning efforts.

Formulating a cogent, meaningful strategy is a critical organizational function. However, even the best plan document is worthless if the organization does not implement it. Sadly, a top strategy consulting firm has found that more than one-quarter of companies having strategic plans lacked an execution plan and 45 percent failed to track the accomplishment of strategic initiatives (Dye and Sibony 2007). Some top executives think that strategy formulation is their primary responsibility and strategic implementation can be delegated downward. As seasoned, successful executives can attest, strategy formulation is only the beginning; the hard work comes after. As Arthur A. Thompson and colleagues (2016, 287) attest, "Experienced managers are well aware that it is a whole lot easier to develop a sound strategic plan than it is to execute the plan and achieve desired outcomes."

Many executives engage outside consultants to stimulate strategic thinking, evaluate their organization's situation, and put their strategic direction into words, thinking they can preserve time for what they consider to be more important tasks. However, as recounted in exhibit 14.3, when consultants depart, many times all they leave are a series of nice PowerPoint slides or a brightly covered, bound document. Leaders who have limited involvement in the planning process may find translating the strategic document into action a challenging and difficult task.

The successful implementation of strategic thought is preceded and followed by critical activities that involve different skills and tools. As shown in exhibit 15.1, the **strategic action cycle** includes strategic planning, budgeting, implementation, and controlling or monitoring. Implementation integrates budgeting, monitoring, and evaluation. Organizations should assign an appropriate mix of internal and external personnel to these various tasks. In addition, performance standards must be established so that progress on implemented strategies can be measured and any problems can be controlled.

Strategic action cycle
The four stages of the strategic action cycle are (1) strategic planning, (2) budgeting, (3) implementing strategy, and (4) controlling problems or monitoring progress.

This chapter discusses methods for transitioning from strategy formulation to implementation to monitoring, identifies those who should be engaged in the cycle, and presents balanced scorecards and budgets as means of monitoring and evaluating strategic progress. We will examine methods for organizing personnel, selecting appropriate budgetary targets, creating critical success factors, and integrating budgets and strategy.

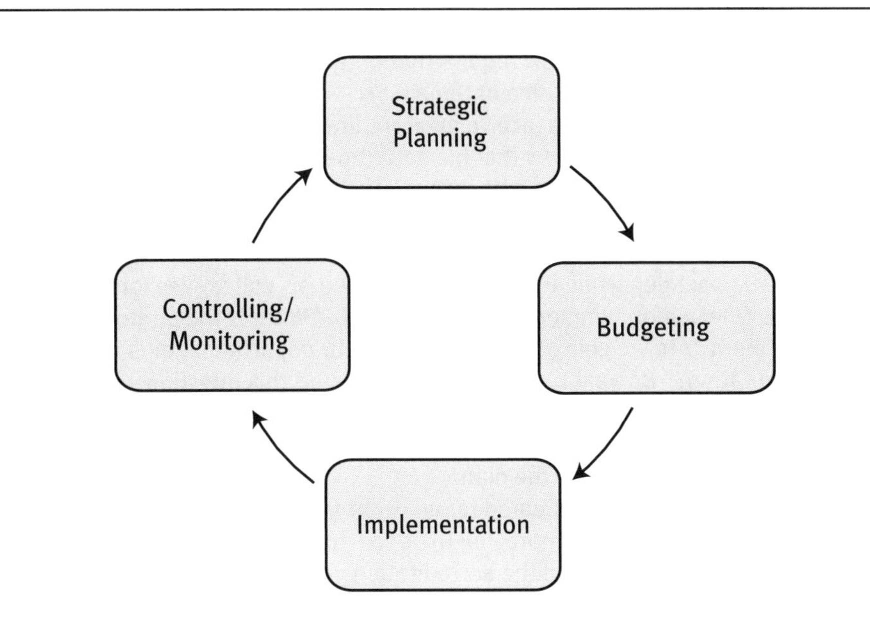

EXHIBIT 15.1
The Strategic Action Cycle

Engaging the Right Structures and the Right People

Ideally, strategic thinking and strategic planning should be infused throughout an organization and drive its actions. As discussed in chapter 12, organizational structure can significantly affect the formulation and implementation of strategy. Just as vital, or even more so, is having the correct people prepare and enact strategy.

For employees to become actively involved in the strategic action cycle, they must perceive it as a process, not an event. If they believe that the strategic plan will be used to change and improve the organization, they will be much more easily engaged. As exhibit 15.2 explains, few will choose to participate when planning is directed at achieving a non-mission-based end.

How to organize the strategic process and whom to involve are critical decisions. Almost all organizations designate someone to be in charge. This person is responsible for facilitating the process, coordinating data and meetings, and ensuring that key tasks are achieved. She does feasibility and planning studies; completes environmental assessments; and develops the plan's format, timetables, and methods for evaluation.

An organization's CEO must direct and be highly involved in overall strategic planning as a strategist, organizer, and tactician, but experts recommend that the person charged with leading the day-to-day strategic process be someone other than the CEO (Zuckerman 2005). Consensus building and visioning discussions are difficult when CEOs have this role because their power and authority can easily inhibit the free flow of dialogue.

EXHIBIT 15.2
Is Strategic Planning a Process or an Event?

Many accreditation bodies now require that organizations produce a strategic plan if they wish to become or remain accredited. Bob, the chair of a department that was soon to receive an accreditation visit, was fully aware of this requirement. He also knew that his department did not have a functioning strategic plan. He carefully gathered past attempts at strategic planning, combined the results into a 20-page plan proposal, and circulated it to the members of his department for comment.

At the next department meeting, Bob asked his colleagues for their feedback. One senior member bluntly asked Bob, "What is the purpose of this document? Are we going to try to improve our department, or is it just for accreditation?" Bob sat back as he contemplated this question and then honestly answered that it was primarily for accreditation purposes. Given this answer, his colleagues commented that what he had written was fine and proposed no changes to the plan.

Clearly, the plan was created for an event (to receive accreditation); it did not detail a process for improving the department. The approved plan sat unopened on Bob's desk until the accreditation visit.

However, the person responsible for facilitating strategic planning generally reports directly to the CEO. Depending on the organization, this person's title might be chief planning and development officer, director of planning, vice president, coordinator, or chair, or—depending on an organization's size, market, expertise, and culture—this person may be responsible for just strategy development or for any or all of the many related duties that follow:

- Strategic formulation
- Business development
- Data generation and analyses
- Marketing
- Public relations
- Change management or organizational development
- Project management

In large systems especially, this person also integrates strategic planning and system or network development (Bhasin 2016).

Although the participants in the process can be organized in various ways, the structures described in the following sections generally are considered core groups.

Governing board
An overarching entity whose principal responsibility is to oversee and direct an organization.

Governing Board

The **governing board** has principal responsibility for the strategic planning process. Under a governing board's direction, organizations have completed strategic plans in as little as one day at a retreat. However, development of a strategic plan typically takes 40 to 120 hours of board and committee meeting time. The duration depends on the availability of needed information, the organization's expertise (or lack thereof), and the type and quality of staff and resources allocated to the process.

The governing board bases the guidelines it sets for the development of a strategic plan on the organization's mission, vision, and values. The board's responsibilities include

- approval of the organization's mission, vision, and goals;
- discussion and approval of key strategic directions;
- final approval of the strategic plan document; and
- periodic monitoring of implemented strategies.

Strategic Planning Committee

The **strategic planning committee** generally reports to the governing board and may consist of both board members and nonmembers. This committee may be either standing (i.e., permanent) or ad hoc. This committee engages key stakeholders who are not represented on the governing board. During the development of the strategic plan, the committee typically meets once every two weeks for two to six hours. The strategic planning committee is responsible for

Strategic planning committee
A standing or ad hoc committee that is responsible for organizing and leading an organization's strategic planning process.

- organizing and facilitating the planning process;
- determining key stakeholders' needs;
- regularly (usually annually) reviewing the organization's mission and vision;
- monitoring trends and periodically reviewing the internal and external environment;
- developing a strategic plan draft, including planning goals and objectives for board consideration; and
- evaluating progress toward strategic objectives.

Medical Staff (in Clinical Organizations)

In the United States, the **medical staff** of a hospital primarily comprises independent practitioners, although the number of doctors employed by medical facilities today is greater than it was in the past. For clinical operations, including hospitals, surgical centers, nursing homes, hospices, and so forth, physicians are key stakeholders and the principal source of referrals. Thus, the involvement of the medical staff in strategic planning is fundamental to properly creating and executing a strategic plan. Key medical staff should serve on the governing board, the strategic planning committee, and other task forces established for

Medical staff
An organized body of licensed professionals who are approved and given privileges to practice medicine at hospitals and other healthcare facilities.

the strategic planning process. The governing board may also enjoin medical staff members to organize their own planning committee and responsibilities. The medical staff committee should report to the strategic planning committee.

Consultants

Organizations often hire planning consultants for their expertise, data resources, extra manpower, and insight regarding future changes and innovative strategies. Conditions that might motivate an organization to bring in outside consultants include a lack of internal staffing or expertise and the need for a neutral facilitator between leaders and key stakeholders who hold strongly vested positions regarding controversial opinions or proposed future directions.

Consultants also can provide an objective view of the organization's strengths and weaknesses. Their outside perspective can help break down departmental barriers that often exist in large, complex organizations. Good consultants bring lessons learned from similar organizations, fresh perspectives, and novel tools and can mediate turf battles. Their involvement also can help an organization maintain strategic momentum and frankly evaluate its past performance (Griffioen 2016).

However, consultants can be very expensive to hire and, if not managed correctly, can create significant problems. The following points are a few recommendations for dealing with consultants:

- Clearly specify up front what you hired the consultants to produce. Define their deliverables in a visible, unmistakable manner.
- A consulting firm, even one with a great international reputation, is only as good as the individuals assigned to the project. Most firms assign junior staff to projects. Prior to the engagement, find out who will be assigned to your project. Review their backgrounds and experience, and insist on working with more senior consultants, especially on critical project aspects.
- Do not turn a project over to a consulting firm. Make time to meet with the consultants on a consistent basis. Meetings keep projects on track and focused on desired results.
- Consider establishing an external advisory board of experts to review and evaluate the consultants' progress. By critiquing the consultants' planning efforts throughout the project, advisory boards improve the quality and functionality of project outcomes.

Monitoring Strategic Efforts

The results of strategic efforts should be regularly monitored so that management can determine what progress is being made and identify strategies that need to be adapted or adjusted. Most healthcare organizations establish metrics for their key strategic goals. However, research has suggested that some organizations begin to make major strategic changes without establishing specific outcome measures beforehand. This oversight can derail change efforts and leave strategic goals unfulfilled (Walston, Lazes, and Sullivan 2004). Most claim to understand the need to quantify their objectives, but what Joseph Grenny, David Maxfield, and Andrew Shimberg (2007, 49) found is regrettably common: "We were stunned at how few of the managers in the 40 companies we interviewed during our research had any reliable information about corporate performance at project execution. In spite of the fact that billions of dollars were spent in the form of strategic projects every year, only a handful could tell us what percentage performed to specifications."

It is imperative that responsible parties set metrics and periodically compare strategic goals to actual results. Monitoring is important for the following reasons:

- It ensures that efforts are following the direction set by strategic planning.
- It helps organizations better achieve their goals and objectives.
- It helps organizations evaluate the progress they are making toward their mission and vision.
- It helps organizations meet the needs of key stakeholders.
- It helps managers to assess whether resources are being used efficiently.
- It encourages ongoing improvement.
- It provides a continuous basis for informed decision making and planning.

Monitoring and review are not inspections focused on catching and punishing nonachievers. They are an ongoing process of learning and embedding positive change that advances organizations toward mission and vision fulfillment. If data suggest that an organization is deviating from the strategic direction it has set, managers should determine why it has derailed and whether environmental shifts or other causes might account for the deviation. If deviations are justified, leaders must adapt their plans to the new circumstances.

Monitoring involves collecting data and assigning **key performance indicators (KPIs)** to each strategic objective. Target metrics set for each KPI should be quantifiable, based on benchmarks, and challenging to achieve. They might be based on external benchmarks, such as market share and patient satisfaction scores of top-performing organizations, or internal benchmarks, such as recruitment of key personnel, patient volume, and service delivery improvements.

Key performance indicators (KPIs) Critical milestones that can be used to measure progress toward an objective or a goal.

As discussed in chapter 8, there are two methods of monitoring and evaluating data: (1) tracking organizational trends and (2) comparing organizational data to data from other firms. Organizations can gather data periodically and note changes.

Consistent, periodic evaluation of the outcomes of their constituent goals and objectives is critical to the success of strategies. An appropriate group of leaders should conduct this evaluation at weekly, monthly, or quarterly meetings. To be able to evaluate outcomes, the group needs to know the following information about each strategy:

- Key objectives and expected results
- Key indicators of successful progress
- Existing status and challenges
- Critical needs
- Time frame for completion
- Recommended actions

Monitoring Tools

Gantt Charts

Gantt charts
Bar charts that lay out the schedules, steps, and time frames of a project or projects.

Gantt charts are a useful tool for monitoring project status. A Gantt chart is a bar chart that displays the schedules of multiple projects, including their start and finish dates and percentage of completion. Gantt charts rapidly communicate the status of projects, critical dependencies, and key start and end points. A simple example of a Gantt chart is presented in exhibit 15.3.

Balanced Scorecards

Balanced scorecard
A monitoring system used to simultaneously evaluate multiple metrics and gather feedback on strategic progress.

Many leading healthcare organizations elaborate on benchmarking and data trending by using an evaluative tool called the **balanced scorecard**. Traditionally, organizations have focused on financial and, perhaps, quality results. In many cases, each domain is reviewed separately without regard for the other. Companies often believe that "their existing control systems and performance-management processes (including budgets and operating reviews) are the sole way to monitor progress on strategy" (Dye and Sibony 2007). This belief results in strategic initiatives translated into budget targets or other financial goals. Although important, such an emphasis is not sufficient. A large portion of the strategic decisions cannot be tracked solely through financial targets but rather require a variety of measures to truly understand the progress on strategic initiatives (Dye and Sibony 2007). Balanced scorecards give leaders a more comprehensive perspective of their organization's strategy. They have been implemented in a wide array of healthcare organizations with diverse "missions, services, products, and clinical settings" (Zelman, Pink, and Mathias 2003, 3).

EXHIBIT 15.3
Sample Gantt Chart

Item	Task	Depen-dencies	Start Date	Days	% Done	Jul 1–15	Jul 16–31	Aug 1–15	Aug 16–31	Sep 1–15	Sep 16–30	Oct 1–15	Oct 16–31
1	Mission and vision	None	Jul 1	31	0								
2	Environmental analysis	None	Jul 1	62	0								
3	Strategic priorities	1 and 2	Sep 1	15	0								
4	Strategic programs	1, 2, and 3	Sep 16	15	0								
5	Strategic plan	1 and 2	Aug 16	60	0								
6	Board evaluation and approval	1, 2, 3, 4, and 5	Oct 16	15	0								

As shown in exhibit 15.4, a balanced scorecard expands monitoring to include at least the following metrics (Kaplan and Norton 2006):

1. Financial: Financial metrics that demonstrate achievement of the organization's mission (e.g., profits, revenue growth, return on investment, expense reductions)
2. Customer or stakeholder: Impacts the organization must make to satisfy customers, funders, and other key stakeholders (e.g., customer acquisition, retention, satisfaction)
3. Internal business processes: Level of excellence that business processes must reach to satisfy customers (e.g., production costs and volumes)
4. Learning and growth: Presence of leadership or managerial skills and infrastructure needed to achieve desired business outcomes (e.g., new services, employee satisfaction and retention)

These four dimensions have been included in the balanced scorecards of a wide range of companies in the healthcare sector. To reflect more accurately the complexity, professionalization, values, industry realities, and organizational realities, however, many organizations modify these dimensions. At times the category "*People*" has been considered separately from *Customers or stakeholders* because healthcare's service ethos and reliance on physicians, nurses, and other professionals makes this category critical to success (Gurd and Gao 2007). Other healthcare organizations have included areas of quality of care, clinical outcomes, and access (Zelman, Pink, and Matthias 2003).

For example, when it established its balanced scorecard, Mayo Clinic increased the number of scorecard dimensions from four to eight to address

EXHIBIT 15.4 Core Dimensions of the Balanced Scorecard

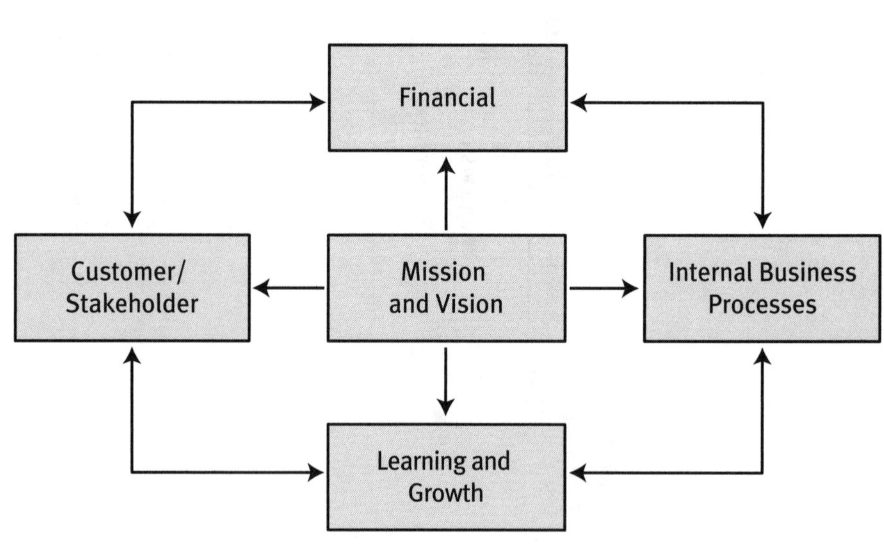

its core principles more effectively (Curtright, Stolp-Smith, and Edell 2000). These included the following.

1. Customer satisfaction: ratings of primary and subspecialty care provided
2. Clinical productivity and efficiency: clinical productivity per physician and outpatient visits per physician per workday
3. Financial: expense per relative value unit
4. Internal operations: average length of stay in days, patient complaints per 1,000 patients, and patient waiting times for appointments
5. Mutual respect and diversity: percentage of staff from underrepresented groups and employee satisfaction
6. Social commitment: Mayo's contribution to society
7. External environmental assessment: environmental scan and market share
8. Patient characteristics: patient mix by geography and payer group

Exhibit 15.5 shows a further elaboration that presents the balanced scorecard of Sunnybrook Health Sciences Centre in Toronto, Ontario, Canada. Like that of Mayo Clinic, Sunnybrook's balanced scorecard includes dimensions that reflect Sunnybrook's key strategic goals, mission, and values.

EXHIBIT 15.5
Sunnybrook's Balanced Scorecard

Sunnybrook Health Sciences Centre is a large tertiary medical center in Toronto with more than 1,000 inpatient beds. Sunnybrook initially crafted a strategic plan in 2006 based on its mission and values; the plan was updated in 2016. The strategists segmented the plan's goals and objectives into three key dimensions and used those dimensions to develop a balanced scorecard. Wishing to be transparent, Sunnybrook makes its balanced scorecard available to the public by posting it online. It has also posted video clips of Sunnybrook staff and physicians explaining the various measurements.

The scorecard's nine critical goals are divided among the three dimensions, each with quantitative metrics. To view the status of its goals quickly, Sunnybrook color-codes each goal's indicators as follows:

- Green = equal or better than the target
- Yellow = moving toward the target
- Orange = moving away from the target
- Red = worse than the baseline and target

Policy requires that any indicator colored red be shared with the public to reinforce Sunnybrook's accountability and focus the organization's efforts. This approach ensures that Sunnybrook's strategic priorities are clear to all stakeholders.

The following partial sample of its balanced scorecard report for 2016 includes goals and objectives in each of the three dimensions. Colors have been translated into gray scale as follows:

(continued)

EXHIBIT 15.5 Sunnybrook's Balanced Scorecard *(continued)*

- ■ = equal or better than the target
- ■ = worse than the baseline and target

Dimension 1: Quality of Care				
Goal 1	Improve the patient experience and outcomes through interprofessional, high-quality care			
Objective 1.1.2	Lead provincially in patient outcomes for select quality-based procedures (QBPs)			

Indicators	Baseline	Target	Previous Score (Jan 2016 – Jun 2016)	Current Report (Jul 2016 – Dec 2016)
1.1 Stroke: 30 day in-hospital mortality (rate)	7.7	< 6.6	8.8	8.7
1.2 COPD: 30 day in-hospital mortality (rate)	7.0	< 7.0	3.6	2.8
Goals 2–5 have been omitted				

Dimension 2: Research and Education	
Goal 6	Lead in the development of innovative methods of teaching and learning
Objective 2.6.1	Enhance utilization of technology-enabled learning throughout Sunnybrook

Indicators	Baseline Previous/ Annual	Target Previous/ Annual	Previous Score (Apr 2016 – Sep 2016)	Current Report (Apr 2016 – Mar 2017)
Simulation encounters of non-Sunnybrook staff learners (*n*)	487/973	≤506/≤1,012	1,118	1,881
Simulation encounters of Sunnybrook staff learners (*n*)	≤ 209/695	≤ 217/ ≤ 723	888	1,632

EXHIBIT 15.5
Sunnybrook's Balanced Scorecard *(continued)*

Goal 7 has been omitted				
Dimension 3: Sustainability and Accountability				
Goal 8	Deliver sustainable performance that meets health systems expectations and commitments			
Objective 3.8.2	To optimize capacity by ensuring patients are cared for in the right place			
Corporate Acute Care Occupancy (%)	99	<95	101	105
Goal 9	Create a culture of engagement, respect, and inclusiveness that attracts and inspires talent to achieve excellence			
Objective 3.9.1	To attract and retain talent			
Indicators	**Baseline**	**Target**	**Previous Score (Jan–Mar 2011)**	**Current Report (Oct 2016–Mar 2017)**
Leadership promotion from within Sunnybrook (%): Directors	62	>50	61	64
Leadership promotion from within Sunnybrook (%): Managers	64	>50	66	68
Leadership promotion from within Sunnybrook (%): Program Chiefs	74	>50	72	74

Source: Sunnybrook Health Sciences Centre (2017).

Balanced scorecards have become, in essence, a prerequisite for receiving international awards, such as the Malcolm Baldrige National Quality Award for high-performing organizations. The Baldrige scorecard for healthcare includes seven criteria that must be met to attain this coveted award: excellence in (1) leadership; (2) strategy; (3) customers; (4) measurement, analysis, and knowledge management; (5) workforce; (6) operations; and (7) results. Only 22 healthcare organizations have been able to achieve this prestigious award since its inception in 2002 (National Institute of Standards and Technology 2016). See http://patapsco.nist.gov/Award_Recipients/index.cfm for more information.

Dashboard
A data visualization tool that displays the statuses of key metrics and performance indicators.

Balanced scorecards are also called **dashboards** because they resemble the display panels in cars. In the same way drivers can quickly examine multiple indicators on a car's dashboard to ensure the vehicle is functioning properly, managers can quickly gather information about the status of a strategic goal from a balanced scorecard. To make scorecards easier to understand, organizations may add colors or grades to show that they have made progress on each goal. For example, as described in exhibit 15.5, Sunnybrook assigns one of four colors to each goal's indicators.

Other organizations use grades (from F to A) instead of colors. Like colors, grades enable managers to visualize the status of scorecard goals rapidly. The use of grades is advantageous because scores can be easily weighted and aggregated. A C grade or lower on a metric goal usually indicates leaders need to develop specific action plans to address the deficiencies and problems in that area. For instance, as one part of its balanced scorecard, a large company in Texas set the metrics in exhibit 15.6 for its employee development goal. Each metric was weighted equally and assigned a grade based on the company's performance in that area. The company scored an A– for its performance on the average training hours per FTE (full-time equivalent) metric, a B for the time of internal hiring metric, and a B+ for the number of internal hires metric. These three grades averaged together equate to an overall grade of B+.

Balanced scorecards identify and highlight critical strategic objectives and enable managers to recognize situations in which areas are not performing according to expectations more quickly. However, to be effective, this monitoring mechanism needs to be used at each level of the organization's hierarchy. The measures and objectives tracked at lower levels may be different from those tracked at higher levels. However, key areas and their representative metrics should be consistent at all levels.

Despite the significant potential benefits of using balanced scorecards, they can present problems. One major issue is a lack of good data. To be useful, measures must be derived from accurate, relevant data. At times, organizations may find that data are unavailable and may have to create primary data. Data also can be expensive to obtain and maintain. For these and other reasons, scorecards should be considered only one indicator of the status of strategic

EXHIBIT 15.6
Employee Development Goal Results

Overall Grade: B+		
Metric	**Weight**	**Grade**
Average training hours/FTE	33%	A–
Time of internal hiring	33%	B
Number of internal hires	34%	B+

achievement. Organizations work in complex, complicated environments, and balanced scorecards provide only a snapshot of an organization's progress. The data raise questions that should prompt further evaluation and investigation.

Whatever method is chosen for monitoring and evaluating strategic efforts, organizations should establish a periodic time frame for a review. Key indicators should be presented to and reviewed by the governing board, executives, and middle managers on a frequent basis.

Integrating Strategy and Budgets

Almost all healthcare organizations use budgets. For strategic actions to be successful, an organization must integrate them into its budget process. Strategic plans provide direction, while budgets provide the resources needed to implement the plans and monitor achievements. Strategic plans that are not connected fiscally to a budget are not based in reality. Conversely, allocation of budgets without strategic thinking would waste valuable assets.

Strategic planning guides the budget process and offers executives an opportunity to reevaluate their allocation of resources. As strategic directions change, budget allocations likewise need to change. Strategies are based on assumptions about available resources. Organizations' resources are finite, and they must frequently make difficult decisions regarding their allocation. This section discusses the integration of budgets and strategies, as well as budgets' role in implementation, monitoring, and evaluation.

Budget Process

Most organizations engage in an **annual budget process** based on a fiscal year. Leaders should incorporate plans for the coming fiscal year into that year's budget. For example, one of a healthcare system's strategic priorities might be opening services in a new market over the next five years, including a new hospital, surgery center, radiology center, home health services, and durable medical equipment services. The healthcare system cannot implement all of these services in one year because the constraints of capital costs, available personnel, and development times would impede such an aggressive schedule. Therefore, an action plan such as the following must be created to prioritize and set time frames for projects:

Annual budget process
Yearly generation of action plans and budgets to drive implementation of strategies and subsequent control of problems and evaluation of progress.

Fiscal Year	Project Implementation
20XX	Radiology center, home health services
20XX	Durable medical equipment, surgery center
20XX	Hospital

Capital budget The estimated dollar amount to be expended on projects in a given fiscal period.

Statistical budget Merger of an organization's capital budget forecasts with estimated statistical projections for an organization's services or products for a given fiscal period.

The segmentation of projects by year enables leaders to translate the projects into budgets. As shown in exhibit 15.7, annual projects and actions directly affect the capital budget, which in turn influences the statistical, operational, and cash budgets.

Adoption of a **capital budget** is an important first step. It includes the cost of major equipment and forecasts the impact that the projects will have on the organization's finances, patients, clinical staff, and community (Zelman et al. 2014). For instance, the capital budget considers projected increases in patient volume resulting from the acquisition of new equipment and the provision of new services. In the earlier example, the healthcare system would determine how many more patient visits would be generated from implementation of the radiology center and home health services.

Managers also make statistical projections for existing services and merge those forecasts with the capital budget forecasts to form a **statistical budget**. Once the statistical budget is established, the organization can form its operating

EXHIBIT 15.7 Relationship Between Strategic Planning and Budgets

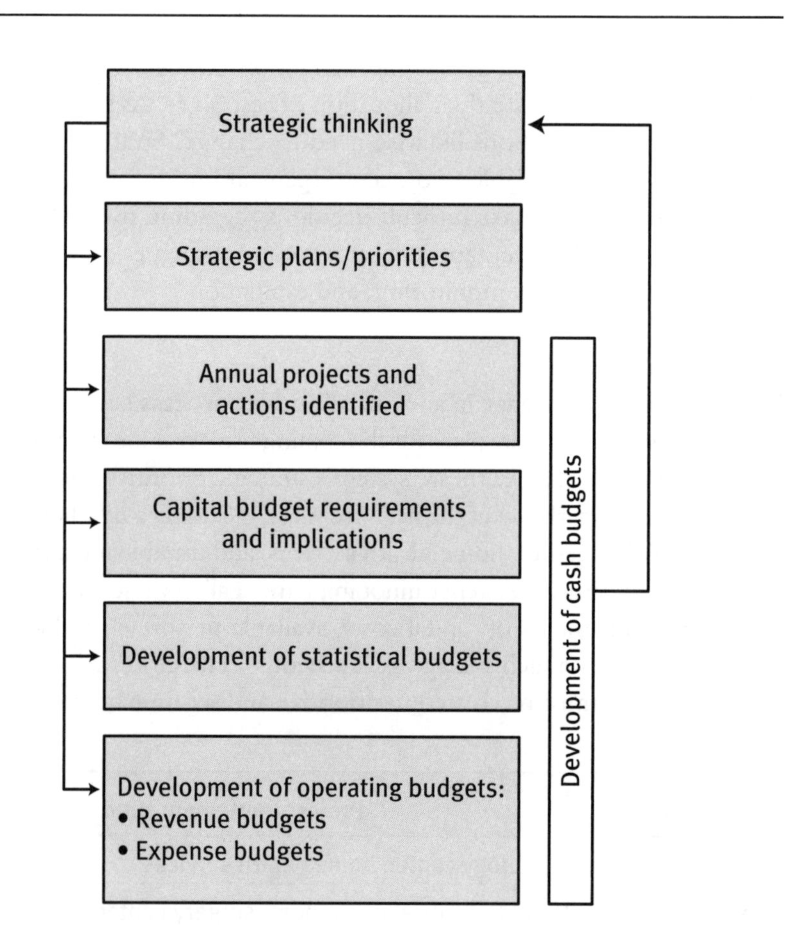

budget, which is generally displayed in the form of an operating statement (see chapter 9). The operating budget consists of two budgets: revenues and expenses. On completion of the operating budget, managers know what profits are expected (excess of revenues over expenses) and are able to complete their cash budgets.

Adherence to budgets is a means of monitoring an organization's strategies. As discussed in the previous section on balanced scorecards, financial performance is one key aspect of control and evaluation.

Budget Variances

Managers control and evaluate strategic efforts by examining the **budget variance** (the difference between budgeted amounts and actual results):

Budget variance The difference between a budgeted amount and actual expenditures.

Budget variance = Budgeted amount – Actual amount.

Exhibit 15.8 shows an example. The small surgical unit is a strategic venture by a healthcare system in a new market. In April 20XX, the system budgeted a volume of 2,000 surgeries but actually performed 1,000. This budget variance of 1,000 fewer surgeries translates into a $150,000 loss of revenue and $10,000 savings on expenses, thus $140,000 less income. Clearly, these results are not good.

Managers' response to the variance differs according to the influencing factor. Some issues are more controllable than others. For example, volume may vary because a physician is on vacation or because advertising is ineffective.

To understand the reasons for variances more thoroughly, managers should analyze influencing factors in more depth. Budget variances can result from changes in volume, price, and efficiency. In exhibit 15.8, the effect of these factors on the variances is not given. To learn how much changes in volume, price, and efficiency influence the budget variances, the analyst divides the variances by their respective volumes (units) and then determines the variance per unit (see exhibit 15.9). The revenues per surgery (per unit) actually increased by $100, but the expenses per unit increased even more, by $165.

EXHIBIT 15.8 Surgical Center Project Budget Variance from Actual Results, April 20XX

	Budget	Actual	Variance
Volume (number of surgeries)	2,000	1,000	1,000
Revenues	$500,000	$350,000	$(150,000)
Expenses	$350,000	$340,000	$ (10,000)
Income (loss)	$150,000	$ 10,000	$(140,000)

EXHIBIT 15.9 Surgical Center Project Actual Variances per Unit, April 20XX

	Budget	Actual	Variance
Volume (surgeries)	2,000	1,000	(1,000)
Revenues/unit	\$500,000 ÷ 2,000 = \$250	\$350,000 ÷ 1,000 = \$350	\$100
Expenses/unit	\$350,000 ÷ 2,000 = \$175	\$340,000 ÷ 1,000 = \$340	\$165
Income (loss)/unit	\$75	\$10	\$(65)

From these data, the dollar amounts of the effects of volume, price, and efficiency can be calculated using the following formulas:

Volume variance = (Actual volume – Budgeted volume)
× Budgeted income/unit.

Price variance = (Actual price/unit – Budgeted price/unit)
× Actual quantity.

Efficiency variance = (Budgeted expenses/unit – Actual expenses/unit)
× Actual quantity.

As shown in exhibit 15.10, volume and efficiency negatively affected the variance from budget, while price had a countering positive effect. This kind of information can help managers better understand and initiate further questions regarding their strategic operations. For example, although the analyst knows that higher prices positively contributed to April's results, the analyst does not know whether prices were higher because rates increased or because more acute surgeries were performed. Likewise, the efficiency variance could have been caused by overstaffing or by a justifiable reason. The manager's job is to ask further questions to identify the underlying cause.

Static budget
A budget that is based on forecasted volumes and does not change when the volume of activity deviates from the forecast.

Static Versus Flexible Budgets

To evaluate compliance to budgets, organizations can use either static or flexible budgets. A **static budget**, as illustrated in the previous example, is less sophisticated because budget projections are based on a single, fixed level of volume and activity. A **flexible budget**, on the other hand, is one that can be adjusted

Flexible budget
A budget that changes according to actual (not forecasted) activity volumes.

EXHIBIT 15.10 Surgical Center Project Volume, Price, and Efficiency Variances, April 20XX

Volume variance	(1,000 – 2,000) × \$250 = \$(250,000)
Price variance	(\$350 – \$250) × 1,000 = \$100,000
Efficiency variance	(\$175 – \$340) × 1,000 = \$(165,000)

according to changes in volume and costs. The flexible budget approach is more useful than the static budget approach because it considers volume changes in the presented budget; actual price and efficiency changes can be more easily examined.

Chapter Summary

The implementation of strategy can be a difficult, time-consuming effort. Many strategic plans and changes fail substantially because of a lack of appropriate implementation and monitoring structures and processes. Successful implementation requires the involvement of an organization's governing body, executives, and key stakeholders as well as integration of the organization's strategic planning, budget, and monitoring processes. Strategy is more than an event—it is an integral part of an organization's ongoing operations.

An organization's CEO is probably not the best person to be in charge of the day-to-day strategic planning process. An executive with requisite planning skills who can facilitate and coordinate divergent opinions is a better choice for this role. This person may be in charge of other duties as well, including business development, marketing, public relations, change management, and project management, depending on the size of the organization and other factors.

The governing board's primary role in strategic planning is to approve the organization's mission, vision, goals, strategic direction, and strategic plan document. The governing board also is responsible for periodically monitoring implemented strategies' status and appointing and coordinating subcommittees (other than the strategic planning committee) as needed to address problems.

Many organizations expand stakeholders' involvement in the planning process by establishing different stakeholder committees, which report to the governing board. Stakeholder committees may have diverse functions but, like other appointed subcommittees, generally monitor progress toward strategic objectives. In clinical organizations, medical staffs are also key stakeholders and must be appropriately involved in the strategic planning process. Many organizations hire consultants to develop at least a portion of their strategic plan.

Organizations should monitor strategic efforts regularly. Specific metrics or key performance indicators (KPIs) should be established for each objective to ensure that the organization is progressing in the right direction, fulfilling its mission, and meeting the needs of key stakeholders. Monitoring is an ongoing learning process that drives positive change to achieve an organization's mission and vision more fully.

One tool many companies use to monitor strategy is the balanced scorecard. The balanced scorecard incorporates multiple measures that can be examined simultaneously and thus provides a more comprehensive view of an organization's progress. Scorecards may include a number of outcome measures, including financial, customer and stakeholder, internal business processes, and learning and growth. Healthcare organizations have adapted these dimensions to include quality and access measures.

Budgets are another key component of strategy. Organizations establish budgets on the basis of their strategies. Strategic projects are prioritized, and resources are allocated accordingly. An organization should monitor a project's progress and direction by analyzing its adherence to its projected budget. Variances from the budget help managers understand the factors affecting achievement of the project's objective.

Strategy is developed and implemented in many different ways, depending on organizations' culture, preferences, bylaws, and mission. However, common to all successful strategic efforts are people, structures, and controls that translate concepts into direction and organizational action.

Chapter Questions

1. How should budgeting reflect strategic planning?
2. What occurs when strategic planning is an event rather than a process?
3. In what role should an organization's CEO serve during the strategic planning process?
4. What might influence the roles and titles of the person in charge of strategic planning?
5. What are the key roles of the governing board in strategic planning?
6. When should an organization create a separate strategic planning committee?
7. What are the advantages of using consultants for strategic planning? What challenges does the use of consultants present?
8. What is a KPI, and how should it be developed?
9. Why is monitoring critical to strategic implementation?
10. What is the difference between a balanced scorecard and traditional goal metrics?
11. How should a capital budget reflect strategic priorities?
12. How can budget variances be used to monitor implementation of strategy?

Chapter Cases

Case Studies

Read "The Struggle of a Safety Net Hospital," "The Battle in Boise," or "Bozeman Health's Competitive Dilemma" in the Case Studies section at the end of this book and answer the questions at the end of the case.

Managing with Budget Variances

Ruth was the chief nursing officer of a midsized hospital in a southwestern community. The hospital had experienced a number of very difficult years and had gradually lost market share to some of the newest market entrants. In its latest strategic plan, achieving competitive efficiencies had become a key priority. To accomplish this aim, the hospital would need to cut 10 percent of its costs. Because she managed the largest portion of hospital personnel, she was asked to defend the recent actual results against the budget, specifically for salary and related costs. She received the following data:

	Budgeted	Actual
Adjusted Patient Days	210,000	178,000
Net Revenues	$52,000,000	$51,285,000
Salary Costs	$22,000,000	$19,435,000
Other	$ 2,350,000	$ 1,650,000
Total Costs	$24,350,000	$21,085,000
Contribution Margin	$27,650,000	$30,200,000

Analyze the data using volume, price, and efficiency variance.

Questions

1. Did Ruth's hospital achieve its 10 percent reduction in salary costs?
2. What effects did volume, price, and efficiency have on the outcomes?
3. What would you present to justify the financial results?

Chapter Assignment

Read the 2003 article by W. Zelman, G. Pink, and C. Mathias titled "Use of the Balanced Scorecard in Health Care" from the *Journal of Health Care Finance*, volume 29, issue 4, pages 1–16. Write a two-page paper on the effective use and misuse of this tool.

CASE STUDIES

1. Move to a Concierge Model or a Direct Primary Care–Medicine Business Model?

Michael Glen runs the General Medical Clinic, a group of 22 primary care physicians in a prosperous suburb of Philadelphia, Pennsylvania. He has held this position for just over ten years and has seen many changes to the healthcare sector. The clinic includes a spectrum of primary care providers, with six general internal medicine, six pediatricians, and ten family practitioners. The clinic has prospered, and almost all the physicians have full or near-full practices. However, in the past five years, expenses have continued to increase, while revenues remained stagnant. Although compared to national standards the physicians appear to make good salaries, their take-home pay has been flat over the past three years, and they are concerned that it may decrease if healthcare reform proceeds. Currently, General Medical Clinic's primary care practitioners make about $190,000 per year, with some variation for age, practice intensity, and other factors.

The clinic has billed insurance and sought to collect the difference from the patient or, if the patient was uninsured, would seek to set up a payment plan. Its patient load consists of 25 percent Medicaid, 40 percent Medicare, 5 percent bad debt, and 30 percent commercial insurance. Currently, it did not have any capitated contracts.

Michael recently attended a conference where he learned about concierge medicine and direct primary care (DPC). The presenter noted that more and more physicians feel overworked, revenues and salaries are flat, and many doctors spend more and more time on nonclinical paperwork. Many primary care physicians, she reported, have begun to look for practice options with alternative financial arrangements. Capitation has been one option, but it has not been very successful for most primary care practices.

Concierge medicine and direct primary care (DPC) are two relatively new options that could solve these problems, the presenter said. In concierge medicine, practices charge their patients a flat fee (monthly or annually) for enhanced services and greater access. These "enhanced" services usually include same-day access to the doctor, which might be done via cellular phone or text messaging. Such practices often also provide online consultations; unlimited office visits with no copayments; and free prescription refills, house calls, and preventive care services. Most concierge medicine services also bill patients' insurance.

The woman also described DPC, which, like concierge medicine, charges a monthly or annual fee to patients for enhanced services and access. DPC differs from concierge medicine, as practices do not bill insurance for medical visits, and generally no third-party involvement occurs. Therefore, all of the work associated with billings, claims, and coding is eliminated (Qamar 2014). DPC services also generally include basic lab tests, vaccinations, and generic drugs at or near cost. Practices using either model derive most of their revenues from membership fees and generally experience an increase in profitability.

The proponents at the conference suggested that both models would work well for patients with complex medical conditions needing careful monitoring and help coordinating multiple specialists. As both are relatively new practice models, only a few studies exist, and they suggest better outcomes. One study showed patients in a DPC model had 27 percent fewer visits to the emergency department and 60 percent fewer hospital days, and their healthcare costs their employers 20 percent less (Beck 2017). A study on concierge medicine showed decreases in preventable hospital use, with 56 percent fewer nonelective admissions and more than 90 percent fewer readmissions (Goodman 2014).

Concierge practices generally charge monthly fees beginning at $175 a month, but they can cost more than $5,000 per year. Most practices that move to concierge medicine retain only 15–35 percent of their existing patients. A concierge physician generally maintains a patient panel of only 300 to 600 patients. DPC practices charge a bit less, however, with monthly fees of about $100. Therefore, DPC practices tend to have larger patient panels of 600–800 per physician (Colwell 2016).

Even though concierge medicine and DPC practices often target upper-middle-class families, some seek higher-income families and maintain an even more restrictive and expensive practice. A few very restrictive practices charge $40,000 to $80,000 per family for an extensive, immediate array of services. These practices may include only 50 families in their patient panels. These high-end practices can increase a primary care physician's annual income to about $600,000 (Schwartz 2017).

General Medical Clinic's primary care physicians each currently serve 2,000–3,000 active patients. The older physicians have enjoyed a relationship with many of their patients for more than 20 years. Moving to either model would mean each physician would lose over 1,000 patients— more than 22,000 individuals for the full clinic.

The insurance market in Pennsylvania has changed and will continue to do so. These changes may encourage families to consider concierge medicine or DPC. One survey shows that over half (51 percent) of workers have a healthcare plan that requires them to pay up to $1,000 of out-of-pocket costs for healthcare before their insurance covers any of the expenses. Patients also complain about the long waits in physician offices and very short physician consultation during visits. Data show that an average primary care physician in a traditional practice spends 13 to 15 minutes seeing a patient, while a physician in a DPC practice would spend 30 to 60 minutes (Ramsey 2017).

Some studies show that patients appear to like concierge medicine and DPC, as the monthly fee provides basic checkups with same-day or next-day appointments and the right to purchase medications and lab tests at or near wholesale prices. These services come with virtually round-the-clock access to a primary care doctor, which might include using FaceTime while a family is on vacation or a meeting in the office for stitches after a bad fall on a Saturday night. Since DPC practices do not accept insurance, patients owe no copayments or other costs beyond the monthly fee for office visits and primary care.

Yet there are a few problems—for example, up-front, prepaid fees in both models do not qualify as medical expenses that can be reimbursed from a flexible spending account or health savings account. The biggest challenge is that patients must have the financial means to pay the fees. In General Medical Clinic's case, most of the less wealthy patients would not participate. A move to either model requires that the clinic target its affluent patients.

Michael also read that a large company from Philadelphia plans to enter concierge medicine and DPC across the East Coast and announced its intent to enroll up to 800,000 workers in the next few years. It plans to offer very high salaries to attract good primary care practitioners for its expansion. Given General Medical Clinic's current business model, Michael fears that he would be unable to match any lucrative salary offers from this company, and his physicians would leave.

Michael also has ethical concerns about both models. Adopting either model forces patients to find a new physician in a market with primary care shortages. Decreasing a physician's patient panel, as both models do, would also intensify the primary care shortage. In addition, currently, primary care physicians refer many patients to specialists. Reducing the primary care panels would directly reduce the number of referrals to specialists, which might affect the clinic's ability to negotiate better commercial insurance contracts.

General Medical Clinic will hold an executive committee meeting in two days. Michael wants to be able to present both options fairly. He needs to develop an overview and make a recommendation.

Questions

1. What are the advantages and disadvantages of the General Medical Clinic moving its primary care physicians to concierge or DPC models?
2. How would General Medical Clinic's business model need to change if it moved to either model? Specifically, how would its value, input, processes, and revenues change?
3. Given the direction of healthcare, what would you recommend if you were Michael?

2. The Virulent Virus

Background

A new disease, aguasangre, was discovered about ten years ago. It is a nonfatal but annoying infirmity that causes the soles of the feet to sweat profusely and emit a terrible smell. It has an infection cycle of about two years. Once it manifests, it takes approximately three months to reach an epidemic stage and then disappears, only to reemerge a couple of years later. Populations can receive immunizations against the disease, but the vaccines must be redeveloped each time it reemerges from its site of origin. This site varies, although it is often somewhere in the Amazon Basin. Each time the virus mutates, the site of origin changes. If someone finds the new site of origin soon enough, a vaccine can be developed and sold, but once the virus reaches an epidemic stage, the value of the vaccine drops precipitously. If the site is found and samples are delivered to the research center in Parana, Argentina, within three months, huge profits could be made.

Situation

An outbreak occurred two and a half months ago. You had information that suggested the origination site was near Iguazu, Brazil. You immediately traveled to Brazil and have been wandering up and down the Paraguay River tributaries for two and a half months. During this dangerous journey, a large spider bit your left hand, and your hand swelled. You also mildly sprained your ankle. At this point, you are low on supplies but determined to persevere.

Amazingly, you finally discover the site and obtain the samples needed to develop the vaccine. You have exactly two weeks to deliver the samples to the research center in Parana. It has been raining off and on for three days. When heavy rains fall in the region, large areas can be flooded for a long time. If you arrive late, the epidemic will have passed and your work will have been in vain. You would like to call in a helicopter to lift you out, but your satellite phone has been damaged and does not work, and there is no other way for you to communicate with the outside world. After careful consideration, you come up with these alternatives:

1. Wait for the rains to end. Your hand and ankle will heal in the meanwhile, and you can enjoy a safe trip home and hope for better luck next year.
2. Cross the Paraguay River basin. This trip can be dangerous. With the heavy rains, parts of it may be impassible. However, you can cross it quickly; the trip takes seven to ten days—if you make it without harm. If you encounter more rain or are injured again before you arrive on the other side of the river, you probably will have to turn back. In either case, you may perish; piranhas, snakes, and other wild animals inhabit the basin, and the water is deep.
3. Go around the head of the river basin. This path is less dangerous and usually passable. It is slow and tiring, however. In good health, you could probably make it in two to three weeks.

   The weather appears only moderately favorable; heavy wet clouds hover over the area. It has been drizzling, but it could clear up or rain intensely. You listen to your radio. Meteorologists are predicting that in 48 hours, they will know if a tropical depression is moving inland or outward to the Atlantic. You think of one more option.
4. Wait two to four days. At that point, choose #2 if the weather permits or #3 if it does not.

What do you do? (Circle your answer.) #1 #2 #3 #4

3. The Case of Humana and Vertical Integration

Humana, Inc., is one of the largest publicly traded managed care companies in the United States. The company has about 6.2 million enrollees in 16 states. It offers primarily HMO and PPO plans, along with Medicare and Medicaid insurance products and other administrative health services. Early in its history, however, Humana pursued and seemingly failed to carry out a vertical integration strategy. The company began in the nursing home industry, developed into a sophisticated integrated healthcare company, and then divested to become a managed care company. This case poses many questions regarding the value and difficulty of becoming a large, vertically integrated company.

Humana is a good subject for analysis and highly relevant to typical corporate healthcare decision making because it has experienced multiple stages of diversification and development, on both a product line and companywide basis. At one time, it was one of the largest hospital companies in the United States, known for its efficiency and centralization. It fervently pursued expansion into health insurance and offered this product first in January 1984.

Humana's History

In 1961, four friends put up $1,000 each to found a nursing home. Subsequently they expanded into more than 40 facilities, and by the late 1960s their company, Extendicare Inc., was one of the largest nursing home companies in the United States. With the passage of Medicare, they branched into the hospital business and by 1970 owned ten hospitals, which became so profitable that they divested their nursing homes in 1972.

They changed the company's name to Humana in 1974. Through intense cost controls, centralization, and high volumes from growth, Humana achieved economies of scale and continued to earn significant profits. By the early 1980s Humana was one of the largest hospital companies in the United States. Humana determined that owning its own insurance products could benefit its hospitals by garnering 70 percent of referrals, and so it began to offer health plans. However, in reality Humana was unable to attract more than 46 percent, and difficulties and conflict erupted among its hospitals, insurance divisions, and medical staff members.

By the late 1980s, Humana's net income plunged, prompting the company to restructure its hospital and insurance businesses. By the early 1990s, its managed care plans were generating more than $2 billion in revenues and had become more profitable than its hospitals. Finally, in 1993, Humana spun off its hospital division of 76 facilities into a company called Galen Health Care Inc., which merged with Columbia Hospital Corporation six months later (see www.fundinguniverse.com/company-histories/humana-inc-history/).

A number of significant problems motivated Humana to divest its hospital business. The first problem was the conflicting economic objectives of the health insurance business and the healthcare-providing business. The purpose of a health insurance company is to sell insurance policies by keeping its premiums low. The best way to control its expenses is to minimize its customers' use of healthcare services. The majority of a health insurance company's savings result from lowering the incidence and length of hospitalization. In contrast, healthcare providers increase their income by increasing utilization. They have an incentive to give their patients the best and most of everything. In this way, they maximize their patients' welfare and their own.

Second, transfer pricing encouraged the use of non-Humana hospitals. Humana, like all integrated companies, used transfer prices (see chapter 4) to account for the sale of its hospital services to its insurance division. Generally, transfer pricing may be set at full charges, at cost of goods, or at a discounted rate. But surprisingly, despite the financial expertise of Humana cofounder

David Jones, Humana set the transfer prices for its own hospitals higher than the market prices for its competitors' hospitals. As a result, Humana's insurance division preferred to refer its patients to non-Humana hospitals. After all, the hospitals that were not owned by Humana charged the insurance division less. Ironically, the vertically integrated firm was paying to put its patients in competitors' hospitals while beds in its own hospitals stayed empty.

Third, Humana's relationships with its physicians were problematic. Predominantly, Humana organized its HMOs around physician practices known as *IPA-model HMOs* instead of employing doctors directly, as did staff-model HMOs. What Humana recognized too late was that the IPAs often did not represent Humana's best interests. Humana's HMOs, like others in the industry, tried to trim costs by cutting the amount of money they paid doctors. Because Humana's doctors were not on the company's staff but under a contractual relationship with Humana as well as other HMOs, the doctors could—and did—retaliate when Humana lowered the amount it paid to the IPA physicians, referring patients away from Humana's hospitals and into competitors' beds.

Another problem concerned doctors not selected to be on Humana's HMO panels. Physicians who had been excluded from the Humana insurance plan were often angry—so angry that they also started referring more of their patients to non-Humana hospitals. Humana welcomed these physicians too late into the insurance plan. When it finally included them, yet another problem surfaced: Humana had diminished its power to influence these physicians' behavior. Humana's health insurance plan was not a significant part of these newly included doctors' practices; it covered only a few of their patients, and Humana therefore had little power over them. This lack of incentive and influence bred indifference among physicians and occasioned an increase in the length of Humana enrollees' hospital stays—and many of these extra hospital days were spent in non-Humana facilities.

The fourth problem was costs. Humana's hospital costs grew because the hospital division's management was distracted by many of the company's new acquisitions and lacked experience in the insurance area. David Jones had started the health insurance division precisely because of the large number of empty beds in Humana's hospitals. The salaried physicians in Humana's primary care centers did little to enhance referrals to Humana's hospitals. Humana's tightly centralized hospital management had no experience in guiding salaried physician practices and could offer little advice to their physician managers. The physicians earned the same salary regardless of the number of patients they saw, and many of them failed to develop a patient following in their communities. As an owner rather than a renter, Humana was forced to pay the full costs of its hospitals and full salaries to its physicians whether they had patients or not.

In the early 1990s, Humana found that owning both HMOs and hospitals put it at a disadvantage when it came time to sign contracts. Jones stated,

> After the strategies began to appear to some extent incompatible, we started having trouble carrying water on both shoulders. It seemed that if we solved a problem for the hospital it would create a problem with the health plan, and [vice versa]. We could see that conflict, but amazingly enough, it did not surface for a number of years. We started in 1983 being an integrated company, and the strategy worked reasonably well for a while. But it got more difficult as we got larger, which surprised me. I would have thought it would have gotten easier as we got larger. (Luke, Walston, and Plummer 2004, 243)

After the hospital divestiture, Humana divested and outsourced other operations. It exited numerous underperforming markets, divested a unit that sold and administered flexible spending accounts, sold its wholly owned health centers, transferred the risk and administration of its long-term disability products to Duncanson & Holt Services, and sold its Medicare supplement and workers' compensation businesses.

These transactions enabled Humana to focus on a core business of health insurance and to invest in technological enhancements. The company sought to position itself as a leader in the "digital health plan industry" and possibly as the first health plan to operate fully through the Internet. During the 1990s, Humana made more than 20 corporate acquisitions and became one of the United States' largest managed healthcare plans. By 2011, Humana's medical benefit plans had grown to about 11.2 million members and its other specialty products to approximately 7.3 million people, with 76 percent of its revenues coming from contracts with the federal government (Humana 2012).

At one time, Humana was one of the most powerful vertically integrated players in the healthcare field. As a result of both environmental pressures and the difficulties of sustaining a vertical organization in healthcare, Humana has become a strong health insurance business.

Questions

1. What can hospitals considering vertical integration learn from Humana's mishaps?
2. Why did Humana integrate and then evolve into a managed care company?
3. Did Humana act most efficiently by divesting its provider assets? What might the company have done to overcome the problems inherent in managing both provider and insurance operations?
4. Did Humana have difficulty transferring managerial knowledge across business lines? Why or why not?
5. Was vertical integration an issue as a result of the four problems mentioned in the case, or is it an issue in all large organizations? How can largeness affect the managerial ability of a company such as Humana?

6. What problems did Humana's choice of transfer pricing present? Why were the transfer prices of Humana's hospitals set higher than market prices? What recommendation would you have given to Humana?
7. What were the specific reasons physician relationships and incentives caused problems? What structural or incentive plans might have helped resolve these problems?

4. An Orthopedic Group Decides to Construct a Specialty Hospital

The "About Us" web page of OrthoIndy, an orthopedic group practice based in Indianapolis, Indiana, states: "With over 80 physicians providing care to central Indiana residents from more than 10 convenient locations, OrthoIndy provides leading-edge bone, joint, spine, and muscle care."

OrthoIndy has adjusted its practice over time. For years its physicians took patient emergency calls for all hospitals in the area and provided services to all types of patients. As the market became more competitive and the physicians' incomes declined slightly, OrthoIndy decided to reduce calls and cover only key facilities (Methodist Hospitals based in Gary, Indiana, and Indianapolis-based St. Vincent Health) and stopped treating Medicaid patients. This decision upset most of the hospitals in the area, as well as orthopedists who were not affiliated with OrthoIndy. Some of OrthoIndy's partners were concerned about the ethical and political ramifications of the decision, but ultimately all parties agreed with it. Although these choices improved the income and lifestyle of the practicing physicians, they wished to augment their salaries further. The group practice already owned a large, profitable surgical center.

The OrthoIndy group had always been supportive of community activities, especially sports. It served more than 15 teams, including professional football, basketball, and racing teams, as well as high school teams. OrthoIndy's patient commitment is stated on its website (Revolvy 2017):

> The physicians and staff at OrthoIndy and IOH are committed to our patients. The following is our commitment to YOU:
>
> At OrthoIndy, our physicians set out to create a patient experience unlike any other in Central Indiana. The result, the Indiana Orthopaedic Hospital [is] one of the highest ranked facilities in the country for patient satisfaction.
>
> Our patients are at the center of everything we do, and their collective experience—both clinically and personally—is the result of every interaction they have with each person in our hospital. And that's why we strive to treat our patients as members of our own family in a like-home environment. At OrthoIndy and IOH, our highly-skilled physicians and staff are committed to our patients' health, safety and the comfort of their individual orthopaedic care.

The opening (or impending opening) of four specialty heart hospitals in the Indianapolis area caused OrthoIndy to analyze the potential for a joint-ventured orthopedic hospital. From many of the physicians' perspectives, the cardiologists working at the new heart hospitals were gaining a new stream of revenue and, along with their partners, would be able to provide new, beautiful facilities and equipment to attract better-paying patients. Following lengthy and somewhat heated arguments, OrthoIndy decided to proceed with a for-profit, partnership-style organization—a state-of-the-art hospital that would specialize in musculoskeletal care. Only members of the group could become partners in the new Indiana Orthopaedic Hospital. Those with ethical or other reservations could distance themselves from the venture.

The plan was to fast-track the opening of Indiana Orthopaedic Hospital by shortening its construction time by six to ten months. OrthoIndy's leaders justified the venture by asserting that their stand-alone, state-of-the-art facility owned and operated by OrthoIndy physicians would provide patients higher-quality care and better treatment options.

By offering various services, OrthoIndy aimed to differentiate the new hospital from the other general hospitals practicing orthopedics in its market area. From admission to discharge, patients would enjoy a "like-home" atmosphere, complete with satellite television and access to e-mail and the Internet. Patient rooms would be spaciously and well appointed and would include a work or reading nook for friends and family members. After discharge, patients would enjoy additional conveniences, such as coordinated postoperative appointments with their physician's office and referrals to the state-of-the-art, on-campus physical therapy center.

With great effort, construction crews completed the hospital on time. The following announcement was published on its opening day (PR Newswire 2005):

> **INDIANAPOLIS, March 1**—OrthoIndy announced today the opening of the Indiana Orthopaedic Hospital, central Ind.'s first and only orthopaedic specialty hospital located at I-465 and West 86th Street. Spanning 130,000 square feet, the hospital represents a $50 million commitment to the city of Indianapolis, its residents and to the patients who will receive care at this state-of-the-art facility. . . .
>
> The Indiana Orthopaedic Hospital was built when OrthoIndy physicians saw an increasing need to deliver specialized orthopaedic care in a patient-focused environment. Approximately 60 physicians from central Ind. will practice at the hospital that will focus on complex surgical procedures, including total joint replacements and spinal cases. Amenities include 10 spacious and technologically advanced operating suites, 37 patient rooms, 39 pre and post-operative rooms, 16 post-anesthesia care unit (PACU) rooms, an imaging center with digital radiography, Magnetic Resonance Imaging (MRI), and CatScan (CT) availability, in and outpatient therapy services, a

pharmacy and cafeteria. Additionally, each patient room features a workspace area for guests and is equipped with the GetWellNetwork™ which provides patients with an Internet connection, satellite television and access to patient educational materials.

Interestingly, about a year later, one of the larger hospitals in the area—St. Vincent Health—spent $9 million to improve its orthopedic services by forming a 61-bed orthopedic center and to create "something that will be the best in the Midwest for orthopedic care." Other area healthcare leaders were expected to respond to St. Vincent's investment in orthopedics and increase the competition in this market (Murphy 2006).

Questions

1. What strategy perspectives did OrthoIndy employ in determining to build its own hospital?
2. Do you believe OrthoIndy's strategic tactics worked? Why or why not?
3. Was the strategy congruent with OrthoIndy's mission? Why or why not?
4. What effect do you think the new construction had on consumers?
5. Do you think that a specialty hospital such as Indiana Orthopaedic Hospital would increase or decrease the costs, quality, and availability of care for consumers?
6. How were the general hospitals near the specialty hospitals affected? Why did St. Vincent Health create its own orthopedic center?
7. How did OrthoIndy's business model differ from those of other competitors?

5. The Struggle of a Safety Net Hospital

The costs of caring for uninsured and underinsured patients are shouldered by both public and private organizations but often fall primarily on older, publicly owned facilities. The cost pressures and demands for care often far exceed the budgets and resources of many public providers.

Wishard Health Services, located in Indianapolis, Indiana, is an example of a public provider that has struggled to position itself strategically to achieve its mission to care for the poor of Marion County. Its mission, vision, and values are as follows (Wishard Health Services 2013):

Our Mission

The mission of Wishard Health Services is to:

- Advocate
- Care

- Teach
- Serve

with special emphasis on the vulnerable populations of Marion County.

Our Vision

Wishard Health Services will enhance continuously our ability to meet the needs of the underserved and all people of Marion County, will be sound economically, and will lead innovatively in clinical care, research, education, and service excellence.

Our Values

- Professionalism
- Respect
- Innovation
- Development
- Excellence

By 2003, Wishard was under tremendous pressure. The hospital was owned and operated by the county and, as noted, had a mission to care for the vulnerable and underserved population of the county. Although there were almost a dozen other hospitals in its service area that provided some care to the indigent, the county hospital was seen as the main provider for this segment of the population. Although the other hospitals did not refuse to provide emergency care for the poor, most elective Medicaid and indigent patients were routinely sent to Wishard's facilities. Almost 90 percent of its patients were covered by a government program or had no insurance coverage. As a result, revenues were always short, operating losses had to be subsidized by tax revenues, and capital projects were constantly deferred. With no funds to expand or refurbish its facilities, Wishard Hospital and Wishard's clinics were extremely crowded and looked old and worn. The facilities' condition, coupled with their location in a poor part of Indianapolis, Indiana, discouraged the patronage of insured patients.

In 2003, the situation seemed to be worsening further. Wishard was in deep financial trouble, and its executives discussed ways to reduce the system's losses. Wishard's CEO publicly stated a deep concern about the 144-year-old institution's future. Wishard Health Services included its 492-bed hospital, six community health clinics, and Midtown Community Mental Health Center, which together served about 800,000 patients per year. According to Dr. Robert B. Jones, the hospital's medical director, 50 percent of those patients were insured by Medicaid or Medicare, and 40 percent had no insurance.

City officials also were worried about the financial health of Wishard and talked about a potential shortfall of between \$20 million and \$80 million out of a \$385 million budget. The best estimate was that Wishard was on track to end the year with spending at $35 million, but it could turn out to be much worse. The hospital did have cash reserves that could cover this deficit in 2003, according to Wishard's president Matthew Gutwein. But if the deficit continued and worsened in 2004 as expected, this reserve would be completely empty, and Wishard essentially would be broke by the end of 2004 with even worse years to come.

Wishard's ability to survive and fulfill its mission was seriously challenged. The primary factors contributing to the deep losses included the following:

- Declining reimbursements from the Medicare and Medicaid programs for the elderly and poor (For every $1 in hospital bills submitted to the two federal programs, Medicare paid just 82 cents, compared to 89 cents four years earlier. Medicaid paid 70 cents for every dollar of service, down from 90 cents.)
- Increasing numbers of patients without insurance to pay their bills (Nationwide, the number of uninsured had reached 43 million residents, 700,000 of whom were in Indiana.)
- Continual hikes in the prices of drugs and new equipment and in wages for nurses and specialists, who were always in short supply
- Stiff competition from specialty hospitals and surgery centers that appealed to well-off, paying patients, whom mainline hospitals depended on to earn their profits
- A weak stock market that sent hospital endowment investment income plummeting

Something had to be done, and Wishard was seriously considering almost all of its options, including these:

- Closing Wishard's heavily used and highly respected emergency department
- Merging with Clarian Health, which operates Indiana University, Riley Children's, and Methodist hospitals, or entering joint ventures, potentially involving construction projects
- Building a hospital to replace Wishard facilities, some of which had been built in 1914
- Increasing copayments for outpatients to reduce unnecessary outpatient visits

Wishard's CEO stressed that construction of a new hospital would not be likely for another 5, 10, or even 15 years, depending on the pace at which fundraising set aside sufficient monies for construction or on the ability to pass a county bond to fund the construction. The construction would be very expensive; replacement of the whole facility could cost up to $750 million.

While Wishard was struggling to decide what to do, a construction boom occurred and competition increased among area hospitals. Hospitals around Indianapolis were spending lavishly, investing more than $700 million in new or updated facilities, most with interior decor and lobbies fit for luxury hotels. These elaborate new facilities made Wishard appear even worse off.

This new focus on consumerism and profligate spending in the hospital business gave rise to what Daniel Evans, president of Clarian Health, called "mindless competition." For example, the $60 million Heart Center of Indiana in Carmel, which opened in December 2002, offered cooked-to-order meals. City-focused Clarian, the largest healthcare system in the area, expanded its market to the suburbs by building a $150 million hospital in Hendricks County and a $235 million hospital in Carmel. The Hendricks County Medical Center was situated in a parklike setting that included a half-mile of walking trails in a serene environment intended to reduce the stress of a visit or stay in the hospital. To keep patients and attract new ones, both St. Vincent and Community Hospital took on physician groups as equity partners in their heart hospital projects, while Clarian sought to partner with physicians at its two for-profit suburban hospitals. St. Vincent opened a $24 million children's hospital in 2003, becoming the first facility to compete head to head with Clarian's Riley Hospital for Children, previously the only children's hospital in central Indiana. St. Vincent also opened a $15 million cancer center, complete with a serenity garden and an indoor waterfall, while Clarian planned to counter with an even larger cancer center near IU Hospital.

Area hospitals' struggle to compete was compounded by the market entry of national for-profit providers. For example, almost all local hospitals offering cancer care lost business to an aggressive for-profit operator, U.S. Oncology, which opened four cancer treatment centers in the Indianapolis area in the previous six years under the name Central Indiana Cancer Centers. These freestanding centers were projected to treat more than 43,000 patients in 2003. The cancer centers could handle patients at a lower cost because they lacked large hospitals' overhead stemming from their big maintenance staffs, parking garages, and building needs.

The hospitals also faced competition from OrthoIndy, a large orthopedics practice that was building a $30 million orthopedic hospital, and the 60-room Heart Center of Indiana, which featured a highly trained staff, one of the first all-computerized patient record systems, and furnishings befitting a *Fortune* 500 firm. Other hospital sites also demonstrated opulence. Clarian's futuristic $40 million People Mover was designed to ferry doctors and staff over city streets to its scattered hospitals, and the lobby of Clarian's two-year-old, $30 million cardiovascular center featured a terrazzo stone floor.

Amid all of this change, most hospitals were receiving lower reimbursements from insurers than they had previously, and the growing demand for charity care decreased the profitability of three of Indianapolis's four largest hospital networks. The following table shows these three networks' revenue, earnings, and full-time equivalents in 2002 and the percentage change in revenue and earnings from 2001. The figures for St. Vincent, the fourth network, are from the first eight months of the 2002–2003 fiscal year and include its hospital in Carmel.

Hospital Network	Revenue	Earnings	Full-Time Equivalent Employees
Clarian Health Partners	$1.66 billion (up 15%)	$51 million (down 27%)	9,344, reduced by 100 in 2002
Community Health Network	$755 million (up 12.5%)	$26.6 million (down 15.5%)	8,700
St. Francis Hospital & Health Centers	$362 million (up 10%)	$11.4 million (no change)	3,215, reduced by 337 in 2002–2003
St. Vincent Indianapolis Hospital	$498 million (up 0.7% over budget)	$32 million (up 8.3% over budget)	5,455, reduced in 2002

Although their reimbursements and profits decreased, all of the healthcare systems except Wishard still made money in 2002.

What Should Wishard Do?

Some believed that the days of a stand-alone Wishard were over. Dr. Brater, dean of the IU Medical School, believed that there were strong reasons to consider bringing Wishard into the Clarian network in a formal way. Few (if any) inner-city, tertiary hospitals providing high-level, specialized care could survive within a one-mile radius of each other. In 1995 Methodist Hospital merged with IU's hospitals, which were located less than one mile from Wishard. A merger would potentially eliminate duplication of services and create economies of scale.

Would Clarian agree to take on Wishard's massive community burden of indigent care? What effect would this liability have on the competitiveness of Clarian Health Partners, especially after the construction and financial commitments it had recently made?

Short of a merger—which was not a foregone conclusion—Clarian and Wishard discussed ways to collaborate and save money. They considered options that would be invisible to patients and the public, such as joint billing and purchasing. Collaboration on medical initiatives, even joint ventures involving construction, also was a possibility. Some collaboration already existed between the two. Wishard did not provide open-heart surgery, so it sent its open-heart surgery patients to Clarian. Wishard operated a burn unit, whereas Clarian's local Methodist Hospital did not, so Clarian sent its burn patients to Wishard.

Wishard was recognized as an important part of the area's healthcare system. The other area hospitals and community knew that closing Wishard would have a devastating impact on area healthcare providers in that they would have to absorb the indigent care. Indigent patients would also have a much more difficult time finding care.

Mark Mueller, a patient whose perspective on Wishard had changed with his own fortunes and health problems, exemplified the struggle of indigent people to obtain care. He counted on Wishard for almost all of his healthcare—in fact, his life depended on it. He had been diagnosed with diabetes, and his kidneys had failed. He had been unemployed for six years and lived on disability. He had lost his insurance coverage, so Wishard was the only place he could go for care. "I wouldn't have any options," said Mueller, a widower. "I just don't see how the poor . . . well, a lot of them won't survive if Wishard goes down the tubes" (Penner 2003a).

An Interim Solution

Wishard had to do something to stem its losses. Frustrated, Wishard's board realized that most of the options it had considered were too long-term or impractical. However, it seriously discussed yet another option—increasing and enforcing copayments. While the overall purpose of Wishard was to care for the poor, the more poor patients it served, the greater the hospital's losses. In an effort to reduce the number of visits by poor patients, Wishard implemented a new copayment policy on October 1, 2003, that dramatically increased copayments for patients visiting physician clinics and using emergency department services. Although revisions of this policy in 2004 decreased the amount of up-front (time of service) copayment required of self-pay patients, copayments still ranged from $35 to $120, a significant amount for most indigent patients.

Collection of copayments also became vigorously enforced. In the past, the clinics and the emergency department often overlooked it, understanding that many of their patients had little or no money. Beginning in late 2003, each clinic, hospital, and emergency department was required to collect copayments from all nonemergency patients up front.

Some board members and physicians were concerned that this policy would discourage vulnerable patients from seeking care. They speculated that pregnant women might skip physician visits and wind up rushing to the emergency department at the time of delivery. They also feared that patients with diabetes and hypertension might self-treat and seek care only in emergencies, which could increase hospital stays and the overall cost of care.

Wishard continued to struggle to find its strategic direction. The only certainty was that the future would become only more difficult for all healthcare providers, especially those like Wishard that primarily served poor and vulnerable populations.

Sources: Penner (2003a, 2003b); Swiatek (2003).

Questions

1. What was Wishard's competitive situation?
2. Did Wishard have direct competitors? If so, in what areas did it compete?
3. What strategic leverage did Wishard have over the other area hospitals?
4. From a societal perspective, what problems occur by having a stand-alone public hospital with a primary mission of serving the indigent population?
5. What strategic steps would you recommend for Wishard?

6. St. John's Reengineering

St. John's Hospital, a medium-sized hospital located in Seattle, Washington, was established in 1894 with a primary mission of caring for the sick and downtrodden. The hospital had grown and developed as a solo facility until 2000, when it merged with a suburban hospital, St. Agnes. This merger caused many changes in the organizational structure of both hospitals. A corporate office was established and located approximately halfway between the facilities. The president of St. John's, Abhishek Ghosh, was promoted to the position of corporate president, and the president of St. Agnes became the senior vice president.

The early 2000s was a busy time for the corporate office. By 2002, it had 45 employees. The hospitals diversified their organization by purchasing a number of urgent care centers, physician office practices, and skilled nursing facilities. Ghosh was certain that integration would create stability and financial success. However, the urgent care centers and the skilled nursing facilities barely broke even, and the physician office practices lost almost half a million dollars per year. As the years progressed, it became increasingly critical for the hospitals to generate enough cash flow and profit to subsidize the other parts of the corporation.

Both hospitals did reasonably well in the early 2000s, but with reductions in Medicaid and Medicare reimbursements, their margins narrowed. By 2003, both hospitals were earning less than a 2 percent net profit margin, and the prospects for 2004 seemed worse. In 2003, patient revenues did not cover expenses for the first time. After seeing these figures, Ghosh called an emergency executive session. Those in attendance included the presidents of both hospitals, Ghosh, and corporate legal counsel. The only item on the agenda was to figure out what to do to get back into the black.

The first to speak was Joe Alexander, who at that point had served as corporate counsel for four years. He had been a staunch promoter of total quality management (TQM) since it had been introduced in 1993. However, because the system had not prospered recently, he and many others had become discouraged with the principles of TQM. Something stronger was needed to reenergize the hospitals and corporation. A few weeks prior to the meeting, Alexander was pondering this dilemma as he opened the afternoon mail. Among his many letters, a bright mailer caught his eye. It was an invitation to a local seminar on hospital reengineering. He had read material about reengineering in *Fortune* and other popular magazines and knew that prominent companies like Taco Bell and AT&T claimed they had experienced huge improvements as a result of their reengineering efforts. The local seminar cost only $250, so he decided to attend. He finished the seminar the day before the emergency executive session.

"I just came back from a seminar that may be the ticket to saving our hides," said Alexander. "Reengineering has been widely used in many industries to radically improve firms' costs, quality, and speed. I wish we had learned more about this opportunity earlier; we might not have wasted so much time on TQM."

"Tell us more about it," said Ghosh.

"Well, it's a way to improve processes. Everything we do in an organization involves processes. Reengineering involves designing and implementing the most efficient, needed processes. It dramatically lowers costs—some say as much as 30 percent—and improves quality."

Additional discussion ensued, during which the decision was reached to put Alexander in charge of an effort to reengineer both hospitals.

With great enthusiasm, Alexander took the corporate chief financial officer (CFO), Yoon Tae Chong, to another conference to learn how to implement this great process innovation. They wanted to be thorough, so they worked with an external consulting firm and developed a series of principles on which to focus. Alexander presented them to Ghosh for approval.

Alexander stated, "Thank you for the opportunity to develop this process. I think with our team and these guiding principles we can really reduce our costs and strategically position ourselves for competitive advantage."

Ghosh said, "Tell me again the seven principles you developed."

Alexander responded, "First, process-oriented organization, benchmarks set as achievement goals, and blank sheets (biases are too strong among established people). After those three, standardization between the hospitals and employee-led teams (which are the most efficient structure because they reduce the need for middle managers). Then we shift to three key areas of focus: access, materials, and delivery of care. And finally, dealing with union issues de facto. I just need your approval to get moving and to get Yoon to help us start saving money."

"Joe, I think you've done a wonderful job," replied Ghosh. "Get to work and let's get this hospital system in shape."

Alexander quickly began to organize an implementation team. He brought in Second Chance Consulting Inc., and with the CFO, selected 36 employees from each of the two hospitals to design changes. These employees were divided into three groups. One group was put in charge of access, one in charge of materials, and one in charge of delivery of care. The consultants set benchmarks of 20 percent reductions in costs in each area. Alexander was concerned that staff in the key areas might be resistant to changing their processes, and he wanted a fresh perspective. He therefore asked that all of the people invited to participate be assigned to areas outside their own. He also decided not to include any of the hospital managers and department heads, believing they would not represent the best for the hospital as a whole.

The teams spent a total of six weeks intensively designing new standardized processes that could be implemented across the two hospitals. At hospital roadshows, corporate personnel talked about the great changes that the teams were designing. Staff were told that the changes would save the hospitals from ruin and reverse their fortunes.

However, some expressed skepticism. As the date of implementation neared, the hospitals' administrators—perturbed by what they considered a show of disloyalty—told managers that those who did not support the effort should look for other work. Dissent immediately went underground, and the administrators believed they finally had all managers on board.

At the end of the six weeks, leadership drafted a detailed "battle plan" to reengineer the organization. Four from each team were retained to implement the designed solutions. The rest of the team members disbanded. Each employee involved in designing the changes was given a laptop computer as thanks for her work.

The first action was to eliminate two-thirds of the nursing middle managers. This change was projected to yield savings of $2 million per year. It was instituted to promote team-based authority among the nursing units, although many nurses feared that quality and communication would suffer. Other changes soon followed. The cafeteria was eliminated; patient food menus were minimized; a new position combining food service, housekeeping, and transportation was created; and the admissions staff was cut by half, among other major changes.

Hospital executives required that employees implement changes, but managers and rank and file found that many were impractical. Some issues caused by the changes were not addressed, such as admitting Medicaid patients after half of the admissions staff had been eliminated. Access to the hospital slowed to a crawl because many Medicaid patients had to wait for verification of benefits. The elimination of the cafeteria forced employees to bring in food or leave for meals, reducing employees' work time. The minimization of patient food menus was a disaster. The three same menus were rotated over and over, and dinner on Wednesdays was always the same: corned beef and cabbage. Patient complaints about food skyrocketed.

The hospital unions also complained and refused to cooperate. The new position required a lot of cross-training, and the union demanded wage increases for each new skill employees had to acquire. Most new positions increased existing personnel's wages by about $1.00/hour. Materials management was decentralized, and 18 new people had to be hired as a result; this change seemed to increase, not decrease, costs.

Although the changes clearly were not producing positive results, managers were reluctant to express their concerns to hospital administrators. The executives remained positive and were certain that the changes would save their hospitals. Alexander continued to be a big supporter of reengineering and cited sabotage and bad attitudes as reasons for the lack of success. His focus was to stay the course and fully implement the plan. He reminded managers that loyalty and commitment were required to move forward.

After a tumultuous year of implementing the changes, the hospitals' financial losses accelerated. Costs did not decline significantly, but the number of patients declined. Employee and patient satisfaction were at an all-time low. St. John's board of trustees became concerned and began to question the organization's direction.

Questions

1. What problems arose during the reengineering at St. John's?
2. How could the executives have improved the process of change at St. John's?
3. What next steps would you have recommended to the corporation's board?

7. The Battle in Boise

One would not expect Idaho, a state with fewer than 2 million residents, to be highlighted nationally as an example of heightened conflict among physicians and hospitals. Nevertheless, competitive pressures and the trend of physician employment have profoundly changed the state's healthcare market. In 2012, the dominant St. Luke's Health System and its smaller competitor, Saint Alphonsus Health System, employed about half of the 1,400 doctors in southwestern Idaho.

St. Luke's is a regional health system consisting of seven medical centers in southwestern Idaho. Its largest facility is a 399-bed hospital in Boise. The system has expanded in the recent past and controls hospitals in Twin Falls (228 beds), Jerome (25 beds), Ketchum (25 beds), and McCall (15 beds) (St. Luke's 2013). The system also aggressively prepared itself for the changes that will be instituted by the Affordable Care Act.

Saint Alphonsus, on the other hand, belonged to Trinity Health, a large national system of approximately 30 hospitals. Saint Alphonsus had two facilities in southwestern Idaho: the 381-bed Saint Alphonsus Regional Medical Center in Boise and a 152-bed hospital in Nampa (Trinity Health 2017).

By 2012, according to an article in the *New York Times*, many independent doctors were complaining that both hospitals in Boise, especially St. Luke's, had too much power and control over their medical practices (Creswell and Abelson 2012b). The doctors accused St. Luke's of dictating which tests and procedures to perform, how much to charge, and which patients to admit. Independent specialists claimed that their referrals from the physicians employed by St. Luke's had dropped sharply and that patients frequently paid more for treatment at the hospital than they would pay at an independent physician's office.

At the same time, employed physicians voiced growing pressure to meet the financial goals the hospitals had set for them, which in the physicians' opinions often entailed unnecessary tests, procedures, and hospital admissions.

Although the two hospitals have competed for decades, their rivalry intensified in the years just prior to 2013. Saint Alphonsus, trying to slow St. Luke's perceived domination, even sought a court injunction to stop St. Luke's from buying physician practices. This legal maneuver claimed that St. Luke's market dominance allowed them to raise prices and to demand exclusive or preferential agreements with insurance companies. As an example, Saint Alphonsus claimed that the price of a colonoscopy had quadrupled, and that St. Luke's charges for laboratory work were nearly three times the fees charged by others in the market. Saint Alphonsus argued that St. Luke's dominance was hurting Saint Alphonsus's business and creating steep declines in hospital admissions and referrals from physicians employed by St. Luke's.

St. Luke's justified its actions, saying it was positioning itself to better compete and improve its ability to coordinate patient care when it was to become an accountable care organization (ACO). ACOs require close coordination between hospitals and physicians and are predicted to cut healthcare costs by eliminating unneeded procedures and tests and keeping patients out of the hospital.

As a result, the Federal Trade Commission (FTC) and the Idaho attorney general began to investigate St. Luke's. Jeffrey Perry, an assistant director in the FTC's Bureau of Competition, was quoted in the *New York Times*: "We're seeing a lot more consolidation than we did 10 years ago. Historically, what we've seen with the consolidation in the health care industry is that prices go up, but quality does not improve" (Creswell and Abelson 2012a).

The number of independent physicians in the United States is rapidly decreasing. In 2000, 1 in every 20 physician specialists was a hospital employee. By 2012, 1 in 4 was employed and 40 percent of primary care physicians were hospital employees. By one estimate, Medicare is paying upward of a billion dollars more annually for the same services because hospitals can charge more when their doctors are employees. For instance, laser eye surgery can cost $738 when performed by a hospital-employed doctor, compared to $389 when done by an independent doctor. Likewise, an echocardiogram can cost $319 if done in a hospital versus $143 if performed in an independent doctor's office.

Employed physicians in Boise also stated that they were strongly encouraged to refer to other doctors working for their employer, even if those doctors were not the best choice of provider for their patients. (Hospitals employing physicians have financial incentives to retain referrals and admissions.) In Boise, doctors employed by St. Luke's were pressured to refer only within the St. Luke's system, according to Saint Alphonsus's complaint. Saint Alphonsus claimed a 90 percent drop in admissions to its hospitals by physicians employed by St. Luke's. The complaint also contended that independent doctors in a nearby community often sent patients 40 miles away for CT scans because of the much higher prices at St. Luke's.

Mr. Pate, St. Luke's CEO, stated in the *New York Times* that prices for some of their services had increased, but he justified the increase by suggesting that the services had been exceptionally underpriced. He believed that overall costs would decline at St. Luke's as a result of physician employment because it would be better able to coordinate care, prevent expensive emergency department visits, and eliminate redundant tests. Nevertheless, many area physicians remained skeptical that patients would be better served, especially after the price increases.

Sources: Creswell and Abelson (2012b); Jameson (2012).

Questions

1. The Affordable Care Act encouraged vertical integration and consolidation to improve the coordination of care. However, too much consolidation can give one organization too much market power. What could be done to balance the need to coordinate care and maintain some level of competition?
2. What are the advantages to directing physician referrals within one system of care? Disadvantages?

3. Why could costs (or charges) increase if services are performed within a hospital setting versus in an independent physician's office?
4. How could virtual integration be used to coordinate care without raising fixed costs?

8. Response to St. Kilda's ACO Offer

In January 2013, St. Kilda's, a healthcare system located on the West Coast, was selected by the US Department of Health & Human Services (HHS) to form a new accountable care organization (ACO) to encourage greater physician and healthcare provider coordination and higher-quality care. At that time, HHS had assisted in setting up 250 ACOs for Medicare beneficiaries that set standards for quality and furnished shared savings for providers. Quality measures were guided by the 33 indicators that the Centers for Medicare & Medicaid Services (CMS) had established.

St. Kilda's reasons for creating the ACO included the following:

- Taking a leadership role in providing effective, evidence-based care that truly serves the needs of today's patients, families, caregivers, and communities
- Building a strong network of primary care—a medical home where patients build a real relationship with their healthcare team
- Focusing on prevention to keep patients healthy and out of the hospital
- Moving toward a system that rewards providers for quality care, successful outcomes, and cost-efficiency—not just for the number of procedures they perform
- Eliminating waste in resources, time spent waiting, and duplication of tests

By 2015, St. Kilda's reported having over 24,000 patients participate in its ACO and having saved nearly $5 million, but, even with this, it did not reach the necessary 2.4 percent minimum savings to achieve the government's shared-savings payment. However, St. Kilda's leaders thought participating in this program was worthwhile, as it allowed the organization to harness new and innovative ways to improve health. Its leadership believed that "as we move away from the fee-for-service model and get closer to a fee-for-value approach, we must master the concept of population management. To make that happen, we must step up our efforts in prevention and health maintenance."

In 2016, St. Kilda's Health Partners (SKHP), a wholly owned subsidiary of the St. Kilda's Health System, had an integrated network of approximately

1,400 employed and affiliated healthcare providers in its ACO. It was anticipated that by January 2017, SKHP would be in value-based arrangements with multiple payers to provide care for approximately 170,000 members. The anticipated patients spanned the health–illness continuum from healthy to high-risk disease conditions.

As most of the value-based business, existing and anticipated, would be paid by capitation, SKHP sought ways to reduce its costs. For example, in November 2016, a request for proposals (RFP) identified high-cost services unavailable in its system and sought to establish preferred providers and centers of excellence that would be willing to meet both quality and cost criteria. It requested responses in the following specialty areas:

- Transplantation, including single organ, multiple organ, and bone marrow
- Women's health
- Gastroenterology
- Bariatrics
- Oncology
- Neurosciences and spine services
- Musculoskeletal and orthopedics
- Cardiology
- Urology
- Rehabilitation
- Behavioral and mental health
- Endocrinology and diabetes
- Pediatrics

Successful bidders would have to improve access to quality care and ensure seamless care and communication with primary and specialty care providers. The bid listed the following "value propositions" that successful bidders would have to address:

- Improved quality
- Improved value
- Reduced barriers to access
- Enhanced patient and caregiver comfort and convenience
- Standardization
- Efficiencies
- Patient satisfaction
- Physician satisfaction

- Improved processes
- Improved communication

Respondents to the bid were asked to provide a long list of specific data pertinent to their area of expertise and specialty related to the above criteria, including

- Length of stay
- Risk-adjusted mortality index
- Procedural infection rate
- Operating room time
- Procedure volume
- Patient compliance to treatment plan
- Disease-specific improvement rates (e.g. diabetes control, weight loss)
- Transplant wait time
- Transplant graft survival rate
- Experience with CMS or payer and employer bundled payments
- Readmission rate
- Cost per case
- Ability to demonstrate affordability and convenience to patient and caregiver while seeking care away from home (e.g., access to low-cost or complimentary lodging, utilities, meals, transportation)
- Patient perception of ease of access and timeliness of appointments
- Clinical Group Hospital Consumer Assessment of Healthcare Providers and Systems and the Hospital Consumer Assessment of Healthcare Providers and Systems
- Patient communication with healthcare team
- Accreditation information
- Ability to demonstrate accessibility and timeliness of care
- Ability to demonstrate a plan to manage the care of SKHP population
- Proof of a multidisciplinary, patient-centered approach to care delivery

Respondents were also requested to submit a cost proposal that would delineate the method and amount the respondent would charge St. Kilda's for agreed-on services, including, but not limited to, medical expenses, necessary travel, overhead, supplies, and miscellaneous costs. The cost proposal had to be valid for at least one year. Contracts were to be for three years, beginning April 1, 2017.

In December 2016, Elizabeth Narvaez-Luna, director of strategy at a large, nationally known pediatric medical center, was contemplating the bid with her staff. In the past, its medical staff and administration had enjoyed a positive relationship with St. Kilda's and certainly wanted to maintain this rapport. They did not want other facilities to siphon away the pediatric volumes currently coming from St. Kilda's primary market area. However, a number of significant issues, both positive and negative, caught the staff members' attention. These included the following:

1. St. Kilda's Hospital (not its ACO) had been incrementally adding pediatric capabilities for years. Some of these services were appropriate for their population, but recently some were venturing into areas believed potentially unsafe, as well as inefficient for the larger region (such as a pediatric blood and marrow transplantation program for a handful of patients or a pediatric cardiac surgery program). Partnering with Narvaez-Luna's pediatric medical center would allow St. Kilda's to eliminate or diminish these marginal programs and get high-quality services to its community through the contract.
2. The bid did not guarantee or even address channeling patients. It contained no provision for directing patients into pediatric specialty care. Prior experience suggested that responding to such bids takes a lot of work and data sharing on the medical center's part, but the pediatric medical center gains little in return, because the bids allow patients to go any hospital they wish. Currently, St. Kilda's pediatric oncologists refer to a large number of pediatric oncology programs across the west. Without a steering mechanism, the staff was concerned that the medical center would receive no additional volumes. On the other hand, working through this bid might help better position individual providers at St. Kilda's, to expand their referral networks.
3. The bid asked broadly for cost information, but the type of requested proposal was unclear. The medical center had a very powerful cost accounting system and could price services quite accurately—therefore, the pediatric medical center has experience providing care under capitation and bundled payments. There are advantages and disadvantages to each payment system.
4. The RFP called for bids in three weeks. It was not reasonable to develop bundled payment proposals in that period. In addition, the staff felt some fundamental opposition to bundled payments, seen as a "race to the bottom," in which much energy is expended to set a price that is soon to be undercut by a competitor, triggering yet another cut. The hospital had experienced this cycle in the past in other opportunities to set bundled payments. One option is to share the hospital's overall cost position compared to competitors (which is very good) but not to commit to specific prices.

Discussion continued. Ultimately, the director and staff knew they had to develop a recommendation to their CEO. Some of the points they would have to cover in the recommendation included the following:

1. What is the value in responding to the proposal?
2. How should the medical center address the lack of patient-steering mechanisms in the proposal?
3. What type of cost proposal or cost information should be included in the bid?
4. What could be the anticipated response from competitors?

9. Deciding on a Population Health Referral Contract Approach

Jackie, the director of strategic planning at Healthy Hospital, was working with her CEO to determine what strategy their organization should take for specialist providers to whom they refer their capitated business. Currently, 15 percent of their business was paid on a population health or capitated basis, but when specialists were required, patients were referred to outside doctors and paid out of the capitated pool of money. This amount has become significant, with most payments made at full cost. Jackie's boss believes there must be a way to lower costs and, at the same time, improve quality by creating a smaller specialist panel.

She realizes that the continued move to population health, in effect, restricts more of Healthy Hospital's market's patients by contract to specific providers and, as it accepts more fully capitated arrangements, it needs to expand its network from employed providers to a group of specialists, which would effectively lock down the referral patterns.

Rather than only looking at the financials, Jackie has written the assumptions it has used to date. These include the following:

1. Although capitated payments have been slow to materialize, the number of patients covered by such payments will double in the next two years and quadruple in the next four years.
2. Payers would prefer to have fully capitated population contracts.
3. High-quality specialist providers are willing to contract to promote population health.
4. Healthy Hospital has the ability to screen potential providers for efficiency, quality, and effectiveness.
5. Better quality of care can be delivered by a population health focus.
6. Large provider systems are required to provide population health.

She has also listed the hospital's possible choices:

- Do nothing and continue to pay billed charges for referrals.
- Establish a pay-for-performance contract. Contract with specialists for improvements in overall cost and quality.
- Move to bundled payments. This system works best for high-volume, elective procedures with some predictability in costs. It could lead to a race to the bottom.
- Enter into traditional capitation for all patients. More patients would be present to moderate variability, but it would be challenging because of the breadth of contracting.
- Enter into specialty capitation for the highest cost patients. A smaller number of patients creates higher variation in patient costs.
- Enter into a specialty capitation for a broad group of conditions across multiple specialties. This arrangement would require contracting with a large group of multispecialty providers.

Jackie plans to present the assumptions and possible choices to her CEO to determine which options are realistic to pursue.

Questions

1. Are all of Jackie's assumptions credible? Have any of these changed or are changing?
2. How could Jackie strengthen her presentation by incorporating her organization's mission, vision, and values?
3. What additional problems may arise with each of the choices she presents?

10. Build a New Service Because of a Large Donation?

You are the regional vice president of a midsize healthcare system in West Hadley. A wealthy philanthropist has served with you for years on the system's board. Recently, his youngest brother in Little Barrington developed kidney problems and required dialysis. However, the community, with only 40,000 residents, lacks dialysis services. This shortfall necessitated a 50-mile drive, three times a week, to the nearest dialysis center. As the travel time and four hours of treatment at the center took up three full days a week, this scarcity was a significant burden on this family.

The philanthropist wanted to improve the care and met with Little Barrington's mayor and the CEO of a hospital in your system. During the meeting, he announced that he was willing to give $8 million to establish a dialysis center in the community. The mayor was ecstatic, while the CEO was publicly appreciative but privately a bit apprehensive. After the meeting, the mayor issued a press release praising the forthcoming donation and the CEO immediately called you to discuss the matter.

The healthcare system had struggled with this issue in the past. Donors had offered to give a large financial gift for a service (an intensive care unit, pediatric wing, or other expensive item). These individuals were generally highly aligned with the health system and frequently prominent in the community. In addition, the donor was almost always highly committed to her pet cause. Frequently, however, community volumes made the service unsustainable. On top of this, the volumes at the new services would sometimes cannibalize the volumes at a larger site within the system, making the new service even less efficient systemwide. Quality of care could also be affected by the halved volumes after the loss of critical mass and support services needed round the clock and the difficulty of hiring people into specialty roles without adequate volume to keep them busy.

You discuss the situation with the CEO, recognizing the aforementioned issues and acknowledging that the $8 million that was offered was enough capital to begin the service but would not provide funds for continuing operation costs. The state currently has one dialysis center for every 76,000 residents, few being profitable. Given this, it is probable that the proposed dialysis center could run at a loss. The CEO would like direction from you.

Questions

1. Who are the key stakeholders in this case? Who would be the most influential and engaged?
2. If you were the VP, what type of analysis would you ask the CEO (or his/your staff) to complete prior to making a decision? What are the key decision factors?
3. How could/should the mission of the health system and individual hospital be tied to your decision?
4. What alternatives to a fixed dialysis center might you suggest to the philanthropist?

11. Dissolving a Long-Standing Affiliation and Moving On

By Khanhuyen Vinh

Partnerships and affiliations may last a long time. However, when they dissolve, animosity and increased competitiveness may result. A renowned medical school had a productive working relationship for decades with a hospital. However, increasing clashes and perceived competitive moves caused the school to sever the decades-old affiliation. As a result, the hospital is urgently seeking to initiate immediate changes through the development of several initiatives. The changes will help attract superstar surgeons and researchers to partner with the hospital in its quest to become a world-class academic healthcare provider, while seriously damaging its former partner.

L Hospital (LH) is an 800-operating bed teaching hospital in an extraordinarily financially strong healthcare system that includes three community hospitals and a home health agency. LH, as the flagship hospital, was affiliated with J School of Medicine (JSM), a local medical school ranked among the top 15 in the country by *US News and World Report*. LH was accustomed to winning annual accolades for several of its service lines.

However, when the medical school terminated its affiliation with the hospital, LH's leadership was angry and almost immediately began aggressively pursuing multiple initiatives to combat the loss of the former affiliation and fulfill its goal of becoming a top-tier academic healthcare institution. The new initiatives consisted of employing primary care physicians and establishing a graduate medical education (GME) program, building a research institute, and building a new outpatient clinic—all of which would be located near the hospital and owned primarily by the hospital. LH also sought an affiliation with another medical school. Although perhaps strategically sound, these developments tested the relationships and loyalty of key physicians, required immense financial resources, and taxed administrative and clinical leaders.

LH had experience in employing primary care physicians. In previous years, the hospital simultaneously pursued both foundation and equity models to acquire primary care physician practices throughout the city. The foundation model later dissolved, while a modified framework of the equity model remained. Following the termination of the partnership, LH chose to directly employ primary care physicians and place their office practices physically adjacent to the hospital, thereby establishing its own general medicine service and, to a lesser degree, contribute to the pipeline of patients admitted into LH. Direct employment, as opposed to relocating an acquired practice into the hospital facility, would expedite assimilation into the LH culture, as LH was attempting to build its medical service swiftly.

To be a teaching hospital requires a pipeline of medical residents. LH realized that it either must depend on another medical school to provide this pipeline or build its own source of medical residents. Typical of its "going solo" mentality, LH decided to build its own GME program to be accredited by the American Council for Graduate Medical Education (ACGME). Medical students would apply directly to LH for residency, thereby bypassing the hospital's dependency on a medical school.

The new research institute served the purpose of attracting researchers at the forefront of their fields by providing a venue for well-funded, cutting-edge research. The combination of preeminent researchers conducting novel investigations that may redirect the course of medicine would elevate the hospital's image and secure its position as a top-tier academic medical center.

Medical advances have allowed for more procedures to take place in an outpatient setting without requiring an inpatient hospital stay. The hospital's current outpatient building, located across the street, had reached capacity. A new outpatient building would accommodate additional volume to capture downstream patient revenue, especially as managed care increasingly directed payments to outpatient procedures.

A merger with another medical school would be critical to the hospital's vision of being a premier teaching hospital and formed the basis for developing these new initiatives. This medical school needed to be reputable, so that LH could attract prominent physicians and researchers.

The dissolution of the hospital and medical school affiliation represented a novel phenomenon. LH and JSM built their 50-year relationship on a foundation of power and prestige. JSM boasted nationally recognized physicians and research programs. LH brought its extensive financial resources to fund the medical school's academic services and research, a state-of-the art institution, and patients for medical residents to study. The hospital treated celebrities, a former US president, international royalty, and established patients across the city and nation. A world-renowned cardiovascular surgeon claimed affiliation with both institutions. Together, both entities aimed to claim a position on the national and international stage. Because of their top physicians and research programs, JSM believed it contributed increasingly to LH's profitability. However, LH believed its financial success resulted from its own strategic initiatives and not from its relationship with JSM.

The increasingly tumultuous affiliation between the institutions ultimately crumbled because of the desire for control, as well as the personalities involved. LH had been providing approximately $50 million annually to JSM's academic services and announced it wanted an accounting of these expenditures. On the other hand, JSM wanted to build its own outpatient clinic to generate revenue. Furthermore, JSM wanted only its academic physicians to make decisions, thereby usurping all authority held by private physicians. LH vehemently refused a JSM-controlled outpatient clinic, fearing competition with its hospital. The affiliation agreement required both parties to concur on such construction. LH insisted that its private physicians be included because they brought in more than 60 percent of hospital revenues.

The personalities of senior leadership from the entities also seemed to constantly clash. Board members from both facilities consisted of individuals with strong roots in the community. The JSM chairperson came from a prominent family with multigenerational philanthropic contributions to the arts and sciences throughout the city. The newly recruited JSM president was touted as an experienced negotiator. The LH chairperson was the former leader of a

Fortune 500 company, while the LH system CEO held deep-rooted ties to the hospital and local community for more than 20 years. All four people failed to understand the opposite party's needs and seemed willing to battle to the end.

Distrust by both parties led to stalled discussions. Aggravating the situation, numerous internal leaks to the press revealed that the sides had labeled each other "antagonistic," "dishonest," and "not forthright." The breaking point was reached when JSM publicly announced it had entered into negotiations to affiliate with St. X Hospital, a competitor of LH, which would offer JSM more autonomy but less financial support. LH took this announcement to be a de facto termination of its affiliation with JSM and, subsequently, LH responded by announcing its change initiatives.

LH's and JSM's primary stakeholders consisted of academic physicians and private physicians, both of whom counted superstar surgeons among their ranks. The chiefs of service at LH also traditionally assumed department chair positions at the medical school. The severed affiliation between JSM and LH forced the academic physicians to choose sides. They had to assess their roles at each entity and weigh the future of their research programs, which were supported by LH's deep pockets and stellar facilities and equipment. The private physicians were incensed that JSM wanted to exclude them from negotiations, thereby severely limiting their influence on hospital decisions.

Other primary stakeholders included the boards of both the medical school and hospital. The JSM board wanted more financial autonomy, control, and decision-making authority but stood to lose substantial funding, as few hospitals in the country possessed LH's financial capability. The LH hospital board desired an affiliation with a brand-name medical school to attract top physicians and lead cutting-edge research to elevate the hospital's reputation and prominence.

The secondary group of stakeholders consisted of patients, who traveled from across the city, country, and world to receive care. These patients were well insured or cash-paying. Their social prominence augmented the hospital's reputation.

The system- and hospital-level CEOs at LH, along with the renowned chief of neurosurgery, maintained routine communications with both the large physician practice groups and the individual academic and private physicians. Those communication efforts served to open the flow of information between the leadership and the physicians. The board and senior hospital executives aggressively sought to attract academic and private superstar surgeons, while inviting all physicians who would join forces with LH. To this end, they announced an initial commitment of approximately $100 million for the research institute and $70 million for the outpatient center.

The LH CEO established committees for each initiative change (physician employment, GME, research institute, and outpatient center), which were cochaired by a hospital vice president and a chief of service (or an influential physician designee, in cases where the service chief had remained loyal to JSM). Other physicians participated in the committee work groups by providing input to create a successful implementation plan. Each work group met weekly or biweekly to flesh out details, provide updates, and identify next steps. The chair of the board, system and hospital CEOs, consultants, and legal experts handled approaching another medical school with which to pursue an affiliation.

At the same time, LH implemented policy changes. A new policy required its chiefs of service to admit the majority of their patients to LH. As a result, chiefs of service could not concurrently maintain their department chair positions at the medical school and admit the majority of their patients to a competing hospital. This measure forced the academicians to identify their affiliation with either entity explicitly. In addition, office leases for academic physicians in the LH buildings were to soon expire. LH hinted at either eviction or a rate increase for its nonaffiliate physicians. The hospital justified rate increases to meet fair market value, as rates had not been comparably adjusted for about a decade.

Established academicians with deep ties to both entities sought for reconciliation through letters to both boards and multiple meetings. Once it was clear no reconciliation would result, physicians who supported LH welcomed the new direction. The private physicians, in particular, rejoiced in the absence of JSM. However, many academic physicians were both concerned and upset about the division.

LH proceeded with its changes, ultimately resulting in completion of all the planned initiatives. A hospital physician organization was created to employ general medicine doctors, thereby establishing a medicine service at LH. The GME program was established for medical and surgical services. Approximately a decade after the dissolution, LH offers 36 GME programs accredited by ACGME. The hospital purchased land within walking distance, demolished the existing building, and built a research institute. As of 2015, the research institute supports 277 principal investigators and scientists performing more than 840 ongoing clinical studies conducted in 540,000 square feet of space, and has received $70 million in grant funding.

To build an outpatient center connected to its existing buildings, the hospital purchased an adjacent lot from a local university, constructed a building for the university at another location, demolished the former university building on the lot, and then constructed the outpatient center. These land purchases represented a significant feat because the hospital was landlocked, and real estate in that vicinity commanded premium prices as a result of high demand. As of 2015, the outpatient center consists of 14 operating rooms, 36 pre-op beds, and 30 postanesthesia care unit beds located in a 1.6-million-square-foot building. While a few prominent chiefs of service remained with the medical school, a greater number of chiefs of service pledged their loyalty to the hospital. Finally, LH announced a $100 million merger with an Ivy League medical school as its primary academic affiliate; at that time, *US News and World Report* ranked this medical school higher than its former partner. Physicians from LH were to be granted academic privileges at the Ivy League medical school. Over the years, the LH System added community hospitals and physician practices. The 2013 consolidated financial statement for the LH System reported gross revenue of $2.6 billion and net revenue of $683 million.

Questions

1. What caused the long-standing affiliation between LH and JSM to dissolve? What could or should have been done to rectify the problems that led to the dissolution?
2. Was LH ultimately better off without JSM? Why or why not?
3. What factors do you think contributed to the success of LH's change initiatives?
4. How did LH involve primary stakeholders in its decision-making processes?
5. How did participation by physicians in the various work groups affect the outcome?
6. What elements in this scenario were beyond the control of hospital management? How could or should these be mitigated?

12. Value in Capitation for Hospitalists?

By Khanhuyen Vinh

A business opportunity arose for a hospitalist physician practice (MCHA) to partner with an insurance payer (Healthsprings) to manage the insurance company's dual-eligible patients admitted to the hospital where it currently treats patients. Healthsprings currently has a contract with a competing hospitalist physician group but is dissatisfied with its performance. This partnership would position MCHA to manage this patient group at the hospital exclusively. Although an exciting option, partners have questioned whether this capitation contract with Healthsprings will add value for the group of hospitalists.

MCHA is a 20-physician hospitalist group practicing at a large, prestigious, teaching hospital in the Southwest with just under 900 beds. The hospital recently transitioned to a closed panel for hospital medicine physicians, which gave hospitalist groups exclusive care for all medicine patients. Currently, the hospital has contracted with six hospitalist groups that manage approximately 1,300 patient cases monthly.

MCHA is the largest group and manages the highest volume of patient cases. It performs competitively on hospital key performance indicators consisting of length of stay (LOS) index, mortality index, 30-day all-cause readmission, patient satisfaction, and core measures. In particular, MCHA usually leads on the LOS index measure and reported the lowest LOS index of all groups from January through May 2015. MCHA operates on a fee-for-service model with no capitation contracts. Its payer mix consists of 44 percent Medicare or Medicaid, 54 percent private insurance, and 2 percent self-pay.

Referrals by specialists and other primary care physicians (PCPs) provide the primary source of patient volume for all six hospitalist groups, thereby increasing competition. Referrals from these two sources are largely based on professional relationships and physician preference for practice styles. Although MCHA manages twice as many patient cases on average as the second-largest hospitalist group, it continues to compete for patient volume.

The group's goal is to continue to increase patient volume from various sources. The group is also one of two groups that have expanded their practice to cover emergency department (ED) services. MCHA physicians also manage patients at Long-Term Acute Care Hospital (LTACH), which serves as another source of patient volume for the group. MCHA believes that expansion opportunities include caring for patients at LTACH and taking on capitation contracts.

To understand more thoroughly where the hospitalists groups compete, MCHA's director created the following figure, which displays sources of patient volume as compared to level of competition among the six hospitalist groups. The strategy canvas illustrates three hospitalist physician groupings. Four hospitalist practices (groups 1–4) together represent one category because they demonstrate the same patient volume characteristics. Group 5 constitutes the second category because it currently has the dual-eligible capitation contract with Healthsprings, and MCHA is the third category. Only group 5 and MCHA manage the ED's "no-doctor" admissions. Admitted to the hospital from the ED, these patients either do not have a PCP who has hospital privileges, have a doctor who does not want to make rounds at the hospital, or simply do not have a PCP.

The hospital exclusively approached MCHA to provide patient care at the LTACH located on the west side of the city. This exclusive partnership has benefited both parties with more efficient care for the hospital and greater billings for MCHA.

Although managed care and capitation payments have not yet taken hold in its metropolitan area, MCHA wants to look beyond the traditional referral sources to augment its patient volume. Because few other providers currently have managed care contracts, the business opportunity with Healthsprings

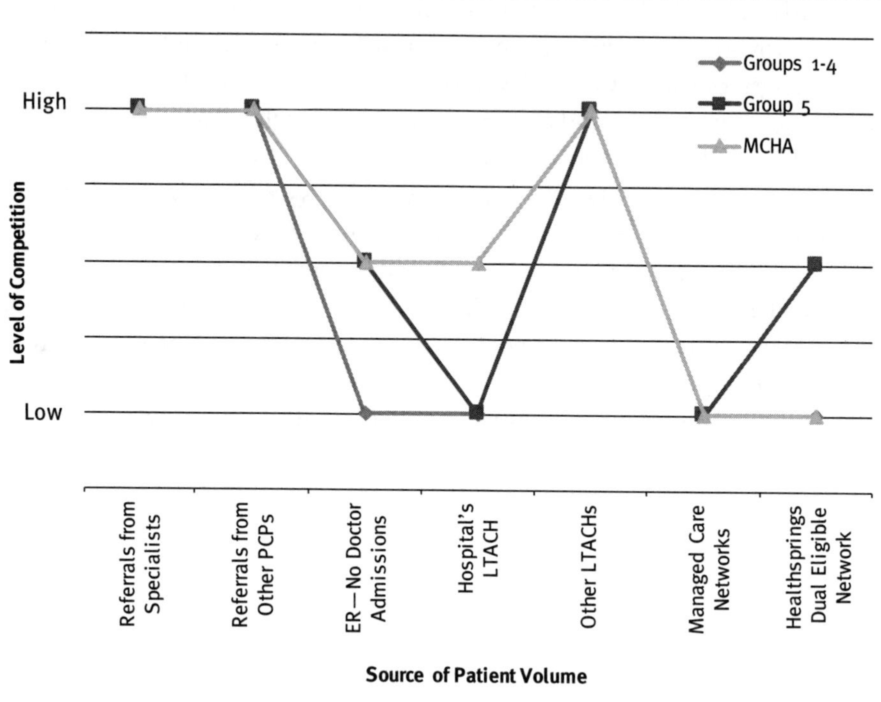

provides MCHA an entry to a potential first-mover advantage. MCHA believes that with this contract it could capture another immediate source of patient volume and position itself for a future in which capitation becomes the norm. The capitation contract with Healthsprings would also allow MCHA to manage the dual-eligible patient population exclusively. Given the group's ability to provide quality patient care while managing LOS, the contract could yield a net profit depending on the negotiated reimbursement amount per patient case and number of patients expected from this specific payer. The additional costs could be marginal unless Healthsprings were to increase its high patient volume dramatically—given MCHA's current physicians and existing capacity, it would not need to add physicians initially.

While MCHA feels it needs new sources of patient volume, the profitability from this new patient base remains uncertain. Medicare patients, on average, have more comorbidities and require a higher level of medical care, and they form the majority of Healthsprings patients. Healthsprings also tends to transfer its patients from community hospitals to the teaching hospital at which MCHA practices. These patient transfers translate to Healthsprings' enrollment of sicker patients who require more specialized medical services and often prolonged treatment in the intensive care unit. As a result, Healthsprings patients have longer LOS. Initially, the insurance company offered a capitation contract of $550 per patient per admission for an anticipated 15 patients per month. Healthsprings also would require MCHA physicians to meet with the Healthsprings' case managers twice a week. This patient volume would constitute only a small percentage of MCHA's total volume, but the longer LOS and additional meetings would result in more work per patient for MCHA physicians.

The group was discussing the positives and negatives of this possible arrangement. The members did not know whether Healthsprings would provide a larger patient volume or an increase in their capitated amount.

Questions

1. What are the advantages and disadvantages of this offer?
2. What are the specific risks MCHA will take under capitation?
3. What could it do or negotiate to modify the risks?
4. What would be MCHA's marginal cost and opportunity costs of this proposal?
5. What other information would you want from Healthsprings?
6. Given the information you have, what would you recommend to the group?

13. Bozeman Health's Competitive Dilemma

By Eric Connell

Bozeman Health is a not-for-profit health system that operates in southwest Montana. The main hospital in Bozeman has 86 beds, a Level 3 trauma center designation, and a medical staff of over 200. It has patient revenue of approximately $350 million. Bozeman is home to Montana State University (approximately 15,000 students) and is a haven for outdoor recreation because of its proximity to mountains, rivers, and Yellowstone National Park. The population of Bozeman is 40,000. Bozeman Health is the primary healthcare provider for Gallatin County, which has a population of 100,000. The community continues to be one of the fastest growing micropolitan areas in the United States.

You are the new CEO of Bozeman Health (BH) and have inherited an organization that has its share of challenges. Following a long-tenured CEO, at BH for over 20 years, the last two CEOs have been unable to stay long. One CEO resigned after nine months, stating differences with the board of directors. Rumor was that the CEO was pushing for productivity increases and staff reductions, upsetting certain doctors, who used their personal relationships with the board to force the CEO out.

The next executive was fired for ethical issues. He had failed to disclose a criminal conviction during the hiring process. Although the offense occurred over 30 years before his hiring, the board's public explanation was the CEO had failed to be completely honest and lied on his application that he had never had a felony criminal conviction. Although this was the board's public position, rumors spread that the ethical consideration was only an excuse. Stories surfaced that the CEO was actively engaged in trying to merge the hospital with Sanford Health, a large health system in the Dakotas—and being paid under the table by Sanford. In a short time, the CEO pushed the organization to implement an electronic health record system hosted by Sanford, despite contrary recommendations from BH's information technology department. The implementation was a failure. The CEO also made a unilateral decision to join Sanford's group purchasing organization (GPO) and change the name of the organization from Bozeman Deaconess Health Services to Bozeman Health, which was too similar for many to Sanford Health.

You know that the BH culture is very stable, and its leaders are deeply entrenched in the way the organization operates. You are worried that it could be a serious threat to BH's long-term viability. During the interview process, you recognized that most of the senior leaders at Bozeman Health are closer to the end of their careers than the beginning and estimate that most will be retiring within the next five years.

The main hospital in Bozeman is neither loved nor hated in the community, and this lukewarm response is also troublesome. You know that your biggest advantage is that Bozeman Health is the only hospital in the county, essentially giving the organization a monopoly. But Bozeman has a relatively high percentage of commercial payers and a growing population. You recognize that eventually there may be another hospital in your primary market.

Billings Clinic, which operates a women's health clinic, has an interest in the market. It had previously expressed plans to build a hospital in the resort town of Big Sky, 45 miles from Bozeman. Bozeman Health viewed this as a threat and fast-tracked its own plans to build a hospital in the town. Because BH already owned the land, it was easy to turn the first shovel of dirt and keep the Billings Clinic from entering the market. The four-bed hospital opened in December 2015 and was largely a defensive move. The Big Sky Medical Center is unlikely to break even for the next eight years.

The main campus in Bozeman is a sprawling web of various construction projects intended to meet the services demands in the growing community. The original hospital building was constructed in 1986. A $10 million addition to the emergency department was completed in 2012; an additional office tower was completed in 2015; and in 2016, BH opened a $10 million, 37,000-square-foot outpatient clinic in a bedroom community nine miles from Bozeman.

It seems as though every department is asking for additional space. Your family birth center, for example, had 1,300 births in the last year and was frequently required to divert patients to other hospitals because of a lack of space. Nurses struggle to operate in tiny ICU rooms that were designed in the 1980s and are now filled with life-sustaining equipment. Operating in spaces that are not optimized for workflows creates additional work and stress for providers and staff members. Patients rightly complain of limited parking. Fortunately, the organization owns hundreds of acres of land adjacent to the campus that were doanted to the organization and has yet to determine how to use the space.

After speaking with key physicians, board members, and department heads, you wonder what you have gotten yourself into. You face a multitude of challenges and a very uncertain future. If you are unable to implement an effective strategy, it is highly likely that the organization will struggle and you will lose your job. Estimate that you have two to three years to get Bozeman Health on a path to success, but you want to take a few months to get to know the organization better before you lay out a detailed plan.

However, time is not your friend. Four months before you started, the Billings Clinic announced the following in the Bozeman Daily Chronicle.

Billings Clinic Buys 54 acres in Bozeman

By Lewis Kendall, Staff Writer,

Jan 6, 2016

Billings Clinic announced Wednesday that it has purchased 54 acres of land as it prepares to expand its medical services in Bozeman.

The lot, purchased for an undisclosed amount, is located west of Costco near the North 19th Avenue interchange. Clinic officials will now meet to decide what type of facility to develop, said Julie Burton, the clinic's director of communications.

"We will have that conversation and make decisions when the time is right," said Burton. "It will have to run its course."

For comparison, the lot size of the adjacent Costco is about 13 acres, while Bozeman Health Deaconess Hospital sits on approximately 34 acres, according to state tax records.

The clinic has long been looking to grow its offerings in Bozeman, Burton added.

"This was an opportunity that came up and the location of the land was ideal," she said. "We thought this was the perfect place to look forward."

The clinic already operates an OB-GYN facility on Highland Boulevard, which has been around for more than a decade.

Founded in 1911, the nonprofit employs around 4,000 people in Montana, Wyoming and North and South Dakota.

The Billings Clinic is a formidable foe. It has been aggressive in the region but had done relatively little in Bozeman. You have spoken with Billings Clinic providers, and they suggest that the Billings Clinic might move slowly, but this pace cannot be guaranteed. You are concerned that the clinic might seek a capital partner should it decide to move quickly in Bozeman.

Today you arrive at BH at 7 am for a brainstorming session to outline key issues with your vice presidents. You know that you just do not have the necessary time to construct a thorough and vetted strategic planning process. In fact, you may only have months to develop a strategic direction. You need to formulate an agenda and desired outcomes for your upcoming meeting now.

Questions

1. Given the challenges, how would you structure a strategic planning process?
2. In your competition with Billings Clinic, who are the key stakeholders?
3. What alliances and partnerships could you consider to improve BH's competitive position?
4. What should your public position be regarding the possible entry of the Billings Clinic into Bozeman? What would your internal, strategic positioning toward Billings be?

APPENDIX

This appendix is a reprint of a project charter template from the Centers for Disease Control and Prevention. The modifiable electronic version is available at www2.cdc.gov/cdcup/library/templates/CDC_UP_Project_Charter_Template.doc.

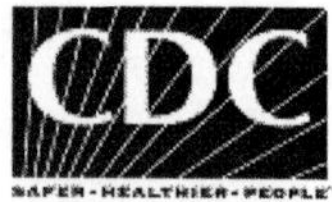

<PROJECT NAME>

PROJECT CHARTER

Version *<1.0>*

<mm/dd/yyyy>

[Insert appropriate Disclaimer(s)]

VERSION HISTORY

[Provide information on how the development and distribution of the Project Charter up to the final point of approval was controlled and tracked. Use the table below to provide the version number, the author implementing the version, the date of the version, the name of the person approving the version, the date that particular version was approved, and a brief description of the reason for creating the revised version.]

Version #	Implemented By	Revision Date	Approved By	Approval Date	Reason
1.0	*<Author name>*	*<mm/dd/yy>*	*<name>*	*<mm/dd/yy>*	*<reason>*

UP Template Version: 11/30/06

Note to the Author

[This document is a template of a Project Charter document for a project. The template includes instructions to the author, boilerplate text, and fields that should be replaced with the values specific to the project.

- *Blue italicized text enclosed in square brackets ([text]) provides instructions to the document author, or describes the intent, assumptions and context for content included in this document.*
- *Blue italicized text enclosed in angle brackets (<text>) indicates a field that should be replaced with information specific to a particular project.*
- *Text and tables in black are provided as boilerplate examples of wording and formats that may be used or modified as appropriate to a specific project. These are offered only as suggestions to assist in developing project documents; they are not mandatory formats.*

When using this template for your project document, it is recommended that you follow these steps:

1. *Replace all text enclosed in angle brackets (i.e., <Project Name>) with the correct field values. These angle brackets appear in both the body of the document and in headers and footers. To customize fields in Microsoft Word (which display a gray background when selected):*
   a. *Select File>Properties>Summary and fill in the Title field with the Document Name and the Subject field with the Project Name.*
   b. *Select File>Properties>Custom and fill in the Last Modified, Status, and Version fields with the appropriate information for this document.*
   c. *After you click OK to close the dialog box, update the fields throughout the document with these values by selecting Edit>Select All (or Ctrl-A) and pressing F9. Or you can update an individual field by clicking on it and pressing F9. This must be done separately for Headers and Footers.*
2. *Modify boilerplate text as appropriate to the specific project.*
3. *To add any new sections to the document, ensure that the appropriate header and body text styles are maintained. Styles used for the Section Headings are Heading 1, Heading 2 and Heading 3. Style used for boilerplate text is Body Text.*
4. *To update the Table of Contents, right-click and select "Update field" and choose the option- "Update entire table"*
5. *Before submission of the first draft of this document, delete this "Notes to the Author" page and all instructions to the author, which appear throughout the document as blue italicized text enclosed in square brackets.]*

[Insert appropriate disclaimer(s)]

TABLE OF CONTENTS

1 INTRODUCTION

1.1 PURPOSE OF PROJECT CHARTER

[Provide the purpose of the project charter.]

The *<Project Name>* project charter documents and tracks the necessary information required by decision maker(s) to approve the project for funding. The project charter should include the needs, scope, justification, and resource commitment as well as the project's sponsor(s) decision to proceed or not to proceed with the project. It is created during the Initiating Phase of the project.

The intended audience of the *<Project Name>* project charter is the project sponsor and senior leadership.

2 PROJECT AND PRODUCT OVERVIEW

[Typically, the description should answer who, what, when and where, in a concise manner. It should also state the estimated project duration (e.g., 18 months) and the estimated project budget (e.g., $1.5M).

3 JUSTIFICATION

3.1 BUSINESS NEED

[Example: A data collection system is necessary to conduct a national program of surveillance and research to monitor and characterize the x epidemic, including its determinants and the epidemiologic dynamics such as prevalence, incidence, and antiretroviral resistance, and to guide public health action at the federal, state and local levels. Data collection activities will assist with monitoring the incidence and prevalence of x infection, and x-related morbidity and mortality in the population, estimate incidence of x infection, identify changes in trends of x transmission, and identify populations at risk.)]

3.2 PUBLIC HEALTH AND BUSINESS IMPACT

[Example: System x collects information about x infection as the jurisdictional, regional, and national levels and will assist in monitoring trends in x transmission rates, incidence rates and x morbidity and mortality trends to help determine public health impact.]

3.3 STRATEGIC ALIGNMENT

Goal	Project Response Rank	Comments
Scale: **H** – High, **M**- Medium, **L** – Low, **N/A** – Not Applicable		
NC / Division / Branch Strategic Goals:		
combo		
CDC Strategic Goals:		
<Reference Appendix C for goals>		
Department of Health and Human Services (DHHS) Strategic Goals:		

Goal	Project Response Rank	Comments
<Reference Appendix C for goals>		
DHHS IT Goals:		
<Reference Appendix C for goals>		
President's Management Agenda (PMA) Strategic Goals:		
<Reference Appendix C for goals>		

4 SCOPE

4.1 OBJECTIVES

[Example: Improving epidemiologic analyses by provisioning consistent data or to making progress towards a 2010 goal]

The objectives of the *<Project Name>* are as follows:

- *[Insert Objective 1]*
- *[Insert Objective 2]*
- *[Add additional bullets as necessary]*

4.2 HIGH-LEVEL REQUIREMENTS

The following table presents the requirements that the project's product, service or result must meet in order for the project objectives to be satisfied.

Req. #	Requirement Description

4.3 MAJOR DELIVERABLES

The following table presents the major deliverables that the project's product, service or result must meet in order for the project objectives to be satisfied.

Major Deliverable	Deliverable Description

4.4 BOUNDARIES

[Describe the inclusive and exclusive boundaries of the project. Specifically address items that are out of scope.]

5 DURATION

5.1 TIMELINE

[An example of a high-level timeline is provided below.]

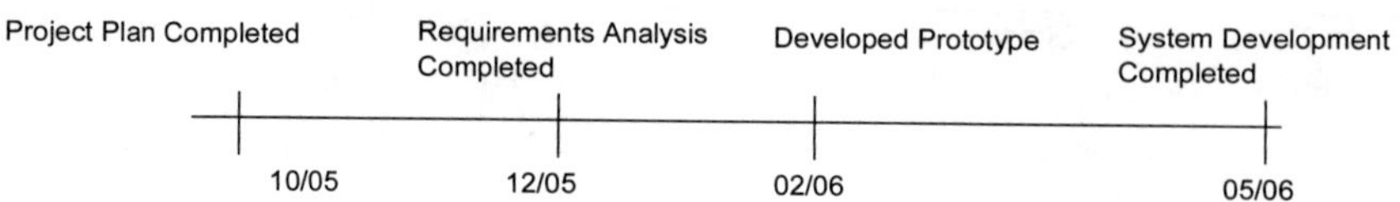

5.2 EXECUTIVE MILESTONES

[Example: For CPIC major/tactical projects, these milestones could be used to complete the Funding Plan/Cost and Schedule section of the OMB Exhibit 300.]

The table below lists the high-level Executive Milestones of the project and their estimated completion timeframe.

Executive Milestones	Estimated Completion Timeframe
[Insert milestone information (e.g., Project planned and authorized to proceed)]	*[Insert completion timeframe (e.g., Two weeks after project concept is approved)]*
[Insert milestone information (e.g., Version 1 completed)]	*[Insert completion timeframe (e.g., Twenty-five weeks after requirements analysis is completed)]*
[Add additional rows as necessary]	

6 BUDGET ESTIMATE

6.1 FUNDING SOURCE

[Example: grant, terrorism budget, or operational budget.]

6.2 ESTIMATE

This section provides a summary of estimated spending to meet the objectives of the *<Project Name>* project as described in this project charter. This summary of spending is preliminary, and should reflect costs for the entire investment lifecycle. It is intended to present probable funding requirements and to assist in obtaining budgeting support.

[For CPIC major/tactical projects complete and attach the required sections of the OMB Exhibit 300 located at http://intranet.cdc.gov/cpic/. For all other projects, provide a summary of the project's expected spending below.]

Object Code	Budget Item	Qtr1	Qtr2	Qtr3	Qtr4	Total
11/12	Personnel.......	$ -	$ -	$ -	$ -	$0.00
20	Contractual Services......	$ -	$ -	$ -	$ -	$0.00
21	Travel......	$ -	$ -	$ -	$ -	$0.00
22	Transportation of things.....	$ -	$ -	$ -	$ -	$0.00
23	Rent, Telecom, Other Comm & Utilities.....	$ -	$ -	$ -	$ -	$0.00
24	Printing & Reproduction......	$ -	$ -	$ -	$ -	$0.00
26	Supplies......	$ -	$ -	$ -	$ -	$0.00
31	Equipment......	$ -	$ -	$ -	$ -	$0.00
41	Grants/Cooperative Agreements......	$ -	$ -	$ -	$ -	$0.00
	Total	$ -	$ -	$ -	$ -	$ -

7 HIGH-LEVEL ALTERNATIVES ANALYSIS

[Example: Alternatives to developing a custom system may have included looking at existing COTS products or reusing an existing system.]

1. *[Provide a statement summarizing the factors considered.]*
2. *[Provide a statement summarizing the factors considered.]*

8 ASSUMPTIONS, CONSTRAINTS AND RISKS

8.1 ASSUMPTIONS

[Example: The system is being developed to capture data from public health partners. One assumption is that data is entered electronically into the system.]

This section identifies the statements believed to be true and from which a conclusion was drawn to define this project charter.

1. *[Insert description of the first assumption.]*
2. *[Insert description of the second assumption.]*

8.2 CONSTRAINTS

[Example: There might be time constraints on developing a system that is used to track data of highly infectious diseases like SARS.]

This section identifies any limitation that must be taken into consideration prior to the initiation of the project.

1. *[Insert description of the first constraint.]*
2. *[Insert description of the second constraint.]*

8.3 RISKS

[Example: The risk of accessibility or unavailability of public health partners for obtaining requirements to develop a data collection system may delay project deliverables. A possible mitigation strategy might be to schedule requirement sessions with the partners as early as possible. List the risks that the project sponsor should be aware of before making a decision on funding the project, including risks of not funding the project.]

Risk	Mitigation

9 PROJECT ORGANIZATION

9.1 ROLES AND RESPONSIBILITIES

[Depending on your project organization, you may modify the roles and responsibilities listed in the table below.]

This section describes the key roles supporting the project.

Name & Organization	Project Role	Project Responsibilities
<Name> <Org>	Project Sponsor	Person responsible for acting as the project's champion and providing direction and support to the team. In the context of this document, this person approves the request for funding, approves the project scope represented in this document, and sets the priority of the project relative to other projects in his/her area of responsibility.
<Name> <Org>	Government Monitor	Government employee who provides the interface between the project team and the project sponsor. Additionally, they will serve as the single focal point of contact for the Project Manager to manage CDC's day-to-day interests. This person must have adequate business and project knowledge in order to make informed decisions. In the case where a contract is involved, the role of a Government Monitor will often be fulfilled by a Contracting Officer and a Project Officer.
<Name> <Org>	Contracting Officer	Person who has the authority to enter into, terminate, or change a contractual agreement on behalf of the Government. This person bears the legal responsibility for the contract.
<Name> <Org>	Project Officer	A program representative responsible for coordinating with acquisition officials on projects for which contract support is contemplated. This representative is responsible for technical monitoring and evaluation of the contractor's performance after award.

Name & Organization	Project Role	Project Responsibilities
<Name> <Org>	Project Manager (This could include a Contractor Project Manager or an FTE Project Manager)	Person who performs the day-to-day management of the project and has specific accountability for managing the project within the approved constraints of scope, quality, time and cost, to deliver the specified requirements, deliverables and customer satisfaction.
<Name> <Org>	Business Steward	Person in management, often the Branch Chief or Division Director, who is responsible for the project in its entirety.
<Name> <Org>	Technical Steward	Person who is responsible for the technical day-to-day aspects of the system including the details of system development. The Technical Steward is responsible for providing technical direction to the project.
<Name> <Org>	Security Steward	Person who is responsible for playing the lead role for maintaining the project's information security.

9.2 STAKEHOLDERS (INTERNAL AND EXTERNAL)

[Examples of stakeholders include an epidemiologist performing a behavioral research project and people in the field collecting data using a software application (the proposed project) to collect the data required for a behavioral research project.]

10 PROJECT CHARTER APPROVAL

The undersigned acknowledge they have reviewed the project charter and authorize and fund the *<Project Name>* project. Changes to this project charter will be coordinated with and approved by the undersigned or their designated representatives.

[List the individuals whose signatures are desired. Examples of such individuals are Business Steward, Project Manager or Project Sponsor. Add additional lines for signature as necessary. Although signatures are desired, they are not always required to move forward with the practices outlined within this document.]

Signature: ______________________ Date: __________

Print Name: ______________________

Title: ______________________

Role: ______________________

Signature: ______________________ Date: __________

Print Name: ______________________

Title: ______________________

Role: ______________________

Signature: ______________________ Date: __________

Print Name: ______________________

Title: ______________________

Role: ______________________

APPENDIX A: REFERENCES

[Insert the name, version number, description, and physical location of any documents referenced in this document. Add rows to the table as necessary.]

The following table summarizes the documents referenced in this document.

Document Name and Version	Description	Location
<Document Name and Version Number>	*[Provide description of the document]*	*<URL or Network path where document is located>*

APPENDIX B: KEY TERMS

[Insert terms and definitions used in this document. Add rows to the table as necessary. Follow the link below for definitions of project management terms and acronyms used in this and other documents.

http://www2.cdc.gov/cdcup/library/other/help.htm

The following table provides definitions for terms relevant to this document.

Term	Definition
[Insert Term]	*[Provide definition of the term used in this document.]*
[Insert Term]	*[Provide definition of the term used in this document.]*
[Insert Term]	*[Provide definition of the term used in this document.]*

APPENDIX C: GOALS

- **CDC Strategic Goals**
  URL: **http://www.cdc.gov/about/goals/**
  - **Goal 1** - Healthy People in Every Stage of Life
  - **Goal 2** - Healthy People in Healthy Places
  - **Goal 3** - People Prepared for Emerging Health Threats
  - **Goal 4** - Healthy People in a Healthy World

- **Department of Health and Human Services (DHHS) Strategic Goals**
  URL: **http://aspe.hhs.gov/hhsplan/2004/goals.shtml** (Search for "HHS IT Strategic Plan")
  - **Goal 1** - Reduce the major threats to the health and well-being of Americans
  - **Goal 2** - Enhance the ability of the Nation's health care system to effectively respond to bioterrorism and other public health challenges
  - **Goal 3** - Increase the percentage of the Nation's children and adults who have access to health care services, and expand consumer choices
  - **Goal 4** - Enhance the capacity and productivity of the Nation's health science research enterprise
  - **Goal 5** - Improve the quality of health care services
  - **Goal 6** - Improve the economic and social well-being of individuals, families, and communities, especially those most in need
  - **Goal 7** - Improve the stability and healthy development of our Nation's children and youth
  - **Goal 8** - Achieve excellence in management practices

- **Department of Health and Human Services (DHHS) IT Goals**
  URL: **http://aspe.hhs.gov/hhsplan/2004/goals.shtml**
  - **Goal 1** - Provide a secure and trusted IT environment
  - **Goal 2** - Enhance the quality, availability, and delivery of HHS information and services to citizens, employees, businesses, and governments
  - **Goal 3** - Implement an enterprise approach to IT infrastructure and common administrative systems that will foster innovation and collaboration
  - **Goal 4** - Enable and improve the integration of health and human services information
  - **Goal 5** - Achieve excellence in IT management practices, including a governance process that complements program management, supports e-government initiatives, and ensures effective data privacy and information security controls

- **President's Management Agenda (PMA) Strategic Goals**
  URL: **http://www.whitehouse.gov/omb/budintegration/pma_index.html**
  Government-wide Initiatives
  - **Goal 1** - Strategic Management of Human Capital
  - **Goal 2** - Competitive Sourcing
  - **Goal 3** - Improved Financial Performance
  - **Goal 4** - Expanded Electronic Government
  - **Goal 5** - Budget and Performance Integration

Program Initiatives

- **Goal 1** - Faith-Based and Community Initiative
- **Goal 2** - Privatization of Military Housing
- **Goal 3** - Better Research and Development Investment Criteria
- **Goal 4** - Elimination of Fraud and Error in Student Aid Programs and Deficiencies in Financial Management
- **Goal 5** - Housing and Urban Development Management and Performance
- **Goal 6** - Broadened Health Insurance Coverage through State Initiatives
- **Goal 7** - A "Right-Sized" Overseas Presence
- **Goal 8** - Reform of Food Aid Programs
- **Goal 9** - Coordination of Veterans Affairs and Defense Programs and Systems

GLOSSARY

Accountable care organization (ACO): A payment and healthcare delivery model in which a group of healthcare providers work together to coordinate a patient's care, improve quality, and reduce costs.

Accounts receivable: The monies customers owe to a business for goods and services they have received.

Acid (or quick) ratio: The combined amount of an organization's cash and marketable securities divided by its current liabilities. This ratio examines an organization's ability to pay its current liabilities from cash and cash equivalents.

Acquisition: The purchase (or merger) of an existing organization. Through this method of growth, the acquiring organization gains an established product in the market and may also reduce competition by eliminating one of its competitors.

Activity (or efficiency) ratios: Measures of how efficiently an organization uses its resources.

Affordable Care Act (ACA): A law passed by the federal government in 2010 that sought to decrease the number of uninsured to improve health outcomes and streamline the delivery of healthcare.

Annual budget process: Yearly generation of action plans and budgets to drive implementation of strategies and subsequent control of problems and evaluation of progress.

Asset turnover: An organization's operating revenues divided by its total assets. This ratio identifies the amount of money each dollar of assets creates over a defined period.

Average payment period: An organization's accounts payable divided by its annual purchases divided by 365. This ratio presents the number of days an organization takes to pay its credit purchases.

Balance sheet: A financial statement of an organization's assets, liabilities, and capital at a given point in time.

Balanced scorecard: A monitoring system used to simultaneously evaluate multiple metrics and gather feedback on strategic progress.

Barriers to entry: Obstacles that impede an organization as it seeks to enter a market.

Behavioral segmentation: Major category of consumer market segmentation that divides consumers by their perception and use of a product or service, including their familiarity with it, attitude toward it, and response to it.

Benchmarking: Comparison of internal data to those of outside organizations for purposes of evaluating an organization's performance.

Broad differentiation strategies: Strategies aimed at offering products that consumers perceive to be distinct from competitors' products and that appeal to a wide segment of a market.

Broad low-cost strategy: A type of strategy aimed at providing low-cost products to a broad customer segment.

Budget variance: The difference between a budgeted amount and actual expenditures.

Business model: The underlying structure of an organization; the means through which an organization creates and delivers value to its customers and earns revenues.

Business-level strategy: The strategic scope and direction of strategic business units (SBUs). SBUs focus on specific product/service lines while under the umbrella of corporate direction.

Business plan: A written document that defines, analyzes, and promotes a specific proposal, a line of business, or an innovative concept.

Capital budget: The estimated dollar amount to be expended on projects in a given fiscal period.

Certificate of need (CON): State laws in the United States that require organizations to obtain approval from a state planning agency before beginning a major capital project.

Chain of command: The formal channel that defines the line of authority, as well as reporting relationships up and down an organization's hierarchy.

Coalition: An alliance of individuals and groups that support a cause or an effort.

Competencies: Activities "that a company has learned to perform with proficiency." (Thompson et al. 2016, 93)

Concierge medicine: Also known as retainer medicine, a relationship between a patient and a primary care physician in which the patient pays an annual fee or a retainer for enhanced services.

Core competencies: Activities "that a company performs proficiently that [are] also central to its strategy and competitive success." (Thompson et al. 2016, 93)

Corporate-level strategy: The overall strategic scope and direction of a corporation. The primary function of corporate-level strategy is to allocate capital funds to SBUs and decide which businesses to enter or exit.

Corporate structure: An overarching management configuration that controls and supervises divisions or strategic business units. A corporation is a legal structure that can be instituted to limit owners' personal liability and centralize management under a governing board.

Current ratio: An organization's current assets divided by its current liabilities. This calculation determines the degree to which an organization can pay its current liabilities with liquid assets.

Customer value: The perceived benefits of a product or service. Consumers may find value in many aspects of products and services, including range and type, degree of customization, ease of availability and access, and the trade-off between quality and cost.

Dashboard: A data visualization tool that displays the statuses of key metrics and performance indicators.

Days cash on hand: The combined amount of an organization's cash and marketable securities divided by its operating expenses less depreciation, all divided by 365. This liquidity indicator evaluates how many days an organization could pay its daily operating expenses without additional cash inflows.

Days in accounts receivable: An organization's accounts receivable divided by its average daily revenue. This ratio shows how many days of billings are owed to the organization and the average time it takes a bill to be paid.

Debt (or capital structure) ratios: Measures indicating how an organization's assets are financed and its capacity for additional debt.

Demographic segmentation: Major category of consumer market segmentation that divides customers into markets on the basis of such factors as age, gender, disease or diagnosis, payer type, and income.

Differentiation: Dividing and separating activities, functions, and products to make them distinct from others.

Disruptive innovations: Innovations that create new markets by discovering new categories of customers. They do this partly by harnessing new technologies but also by developing new business models and exploiting old technologies in new ways. (A. W. 2015)

Diversification: Strategic expansion into different businesses.

Division of labor: Specialization of work that breaks down tasks within a production process so that personnel become highly proficient in components of the process.

Driving forces: The major factors causing change in an industry.

Economies of scale: Reductions in unit cost as a result of an increase in number of products or services produced.

Emergent strategy: A pattern of actions that develop over time and become an organization's strategy de facto. This type of strategy is identified by examining decisions that were made and the patterns that occurred as a result. Also called *realized strategy*.

Exit barriers: The costs an organization will incur if it exits a market.

First movers: Organizations that are the earliest to enter a market or an industry.

Five Forces model: A framework devised by Michael Porter that identifies five factors affecting the degree of competition in a market and the ability of established organizations to influence prices: (1) the potential for new entrants, (2) the threat of substitute products, (3) the power of suppliers, (4) the power of buyers, and (5) rivalry among competing sellers.

Flexible budget: A budget that changes according to actual (not forecasted) activity volumes.

Focused differentiation strategy: A type of strategy aimed at offering products that consumers perceive to be distinct from competitors' products and that appeal to a limited industry niche or customer segment.

Focused factories: A manufacturing strategy that concentrates on core (often single) products and a defined set of technologies and customers.

Focused low-cost strategy: A type of strategy aimed at providing low-cost products to a limited subset of the broad mass market.

Force field analysis: A technique used to evaluate whether environmental influences support or undermine an organization's decisions or plans.

Four-firm concentration ratio: A measure of market concentration calculated by summing the market shares of the four largest firms in a market.

Four Ps: Four attributes that have traditionally been used to establish an organization's market position: (1) product, (2) price, (3) promotion, and (4) place.

Functional-level strategy: Strategic scope and direction at the operating division, department, or project level. This type of strategy is driven by product or service line.

Functional organization: An organizational structure that is divided into subunits based on specialized functional areas such as finance, marketing, and so on.

Gantt charts: Bar charts that lay out the schedules, steps, and time frames of a project or projects.

Gap analysis: A method of identifying the distance between the organization's current position and its desired position with regard to its mission, vision, and values.

Generic strategies: Commonly used strategies that combine a target market (e.g., a small segment of a population) and a type of differentiation (e.g., low cost).

Geographic segmentation: Major category of consumer market segmentation that divides customers by political and physical land units.

Goals: Broad results that an organization seeks to achieve.

Governing board: An overarching entity whose principal responsibility is to oversee and direct an organization.

Group purchasing organizations (GPOs): Alliances formed to give member organizations greater negotiating power and concessions on price, delivery times, and quality when purchasing products or services.

Herfindahl-Hirschman Index (HHI): A measure of market concentration calculated by squaring the market share percentage of each organization in a market and then summing the numbers.

Horizontal expansion: The acquisition or merger of two or more organizations that produce similar products or services.

Hubris: Excessive pride and arrogance.

Industry: A particular category of business or economic activity; an aggregation of sellers whose products are close substitutes.

Inputs: The combination, type, and mix of resources an organization uses to provide a product or service, such as personnel; materials; and strategic assets such as facilities, equipment, location, patents, networks, and partnerships.

Intangible resources: Nonphysical resources, including reputation, brand name, skills, and knowledge.

Integration: Combining, coordinating, and collaborating duties and tasks to facilitate communication and efficiency.

Internal environmental analysis: Evaluation of an organization's products, assets, operations, and other factors to determine whether the organization is carrying out its mission effectively and efficiently.

Internal expansion: A method of business growth that builds on an organization's capabilities and resources and may include developing new products and services, launching marketing efforts to increase market share, or introducing existing products into new markets.

Inventory turnover: The cost of supplies (cost of goods sold) divided by an organization's average inventory. This ratio measures the number of times inventory is used or sold during a specific period.

Isomorphic: The tendency of organizations in a market to become similar in form and structure, offer similar products, and adopt similar practices over time.

Joint-venture alliance: A partnership between a small number of organizations in which each member has a direct ownership position in a shared investment and directional authority over the investment.

Key performance indicators (KPIs): Critical milestones that can be used to measure progress toward an objective or a goal.

Leaders' and participants' readiness: The degree of experience leaders and participants have leading change, their skill level, their motivation, and their values.

Liquidity: An organization's ability to convert assets into cash.

Market analysis: A study that examines competitors and relevant markets, including the market position in which an organization will be placed, relative to other industry competitors.

Marketing: The activities involved in promoting products and services, including creating, communicating, and delivering offerings that customers value.

Marketing and sales management: An organization's approach to promoting and selling its products or services—the type of marketing to be used (e.g., salespersons, direct mail, media advertising), as well as potential distribution channels and their related advantages (e.g., Internet, distributors, retailers).

Marketing plan: A written document that details an organization's marketing strategies.

Markets: Places, systems, and processes through which buyers and sellers exchange goods and services.

Market structure: The organizational characteristics of a market that exert a strategic influence on the intensity and form of competition.

Matrix organization: An organizational structure that has dual reporting relationships, generally to a functional manager and a product manager.

Medical staff: An organized body of licensed professionals who are approved and given privileges to practice medicine at hospitals and other healthcare facilities.

Medical technology: The procedures, equipment, and processes used to deliver medical care.

Middle strategy: A strategy that seeks to deliver low cost and differentiation simultaneously.

Mission: A statement of an organization's purpose, aims, and values.

Mobility barriers: Intraindustry obstacles that impede organizations in a strategic group from joining and competing in another group. Examples of mobility barriers include advertising, expenditures on research and development, distribution channels, breadth of product lines, and patents.

Monopolistic competition: One of the four basic types of market structure. Monopolistic competition exists in markets composed of many organizations offering differentiated products.

Monopoly: One of the four basic types of market structure. Monopolies exist in markets that are dominated by a single organization.

Most-favored-nation clause: A clause in a contract between a provider and an insurance company that guarantees that the provider will charge the insurance company prices that are lower than the prices the provider charges all other insurance companies it does business with.

Net assets to total assets: An organization's net assets divided by its total assets. In the case of a not-for-profit organization, this ratio indicates the proportion of assets that is financed by retained earnings and donations; in the case of a for-profit organization, this ratio indicates the proportion of assets that is financed by equity from profits and private contributions (the sale of stock and private investments). The higher the ratio, the lesser the debt and the greater an organization's capacity to borrow and to pay back existing debt.

Net margin: An organization's net income divided by its total revenues. This ratio demonstrates the actual flow of all revenues, including nonoperating revenues, into an organization.

Net present value: A measure that extends the concept of time value of money to evaluate the cumulative present value of an investment, which is the difference between the present value of cash inflows and the present value of cash outflows.

Network outsource alliance: An arrangement in which a core organization outsources functions to contract organizations. For example, some pharmaceutical companies use this type of alliance for drug discovery and clinical trials.

Networks: Joint ventures and alliances between established organizations for growth purposes. By forming networks, organizations can enter a market more quickly and with minimal risk.

Objectives: Objectives are narrow "stepping stones" that quantifiably support and elaborate on goals.

Oligopoly: One of the four basic types of market structure. Oligopolies exist in markets dominated by a few large organizations that offer similar or identical products.

Operating margin: An organization's net operating income divided by its net operating revenues. This ratio measures the percentage of revenues from operations (the organization's primary businesses) that accumulates as profits and exceeds expenses.

Operating statement: A financial statement containing operating results for a specific period; includes revenues (monies taken in), expenses (monies paid out), and the difference between the two (profit or loss). Also referred to as a *profit and loss (P&L) statement*, *revenue statement*, *statement of financial performance*, *earning statement*, and *statement of operations.*

Organizational capabilities: Internal resources, such as physical assets, human resources, reputation, culture, and processes and routines, that enable an organization to accomplish its mission.

Organizational preparedness: The degree to which an organization understands planned changes and the rationales behind them, the alignment of an organization's culture with the planned changes, and leaders' and participants' readiness (preparedness) for change.

Organization and management: The structure, management team, ownership, and governance of an organization.

Patient origin study: Data that describe the proportion and number of an organization's customers (patients) who come from different geographic locations. These data can be arrayed and graphed to display the provider's primary and secondary service areas.

Perfect competition: One of the four basic types of market structure. Perfect competition exists in markets composed of many small organizations that produce an undifferentiated, homogeneous product.

PEST analysis: An analytical method of deriving forces that are driving change in an industry. Categories of forces explored include political, economic, social, and technological.

Physician–hospital organization (PHO): A strategic alliance between a hospital and its medical staff established to develop new services and compete effectively for managed care business.

Planning structure: The person(s) or unit with responsibility for strategic planning.

Pooled interdependence: An arrangement in which organizational subunits group their resources but mostly have their own separate processes and require little coordination.

Pooled-service alliance: An arrangement in which the resources of a large number of organizations are grouped to produce value for member organizations. Group purchasing organizations are an example of this type of alliance.

Positioning: Designing and promoting an organization's products and services so that they occupy a distinctive place in the market.

Present value: The value of future earnings in today's terms, calculated by multiplying future earnings by $[1/(1 + i)^n]$, where i equals the interest or discount rate and n equals the number of years in the future.

Process: A series of steps that transforms inputs into products or services (outputs). Processes usually are established to organize functions and interface with external entities.

Profitability: The degree to which the revenues generated by a product or service exceed the costs of producing that product or service.

Profitability ratios: Measures that examine an organization's ability to produce earnings or profits.

Project charter: A tool commonly used in project management that clarifies a project's key components, including scope, desired outcomes, participants, resources, time frames, and responsible parties, and ensures that the project's definition and desired outcomes coincide with the organization's strategic priorities and goals.

Prospective strategy: A planning function that forecasts an organization's future situation and designs means to guide an organization's future decisions.

Psychographic segmentation: Major category of consumer market segmentation that categorizes consumers by lifestyle, personality, or values.

Ratio analysis: A quantitative analysis that uses financial data from an organization's financial statements to highlight its financial strengths and weaknesses.

Reciprocal interdependence: An arrangement in which organizational subunits have multiple interactions and make multiple exchanges of outputs or products among organizational subunits prior to producing a final outcome. Complex products that necessitate constant learning and communication are developed through reciprocal interdependence.

Related diversification: Expansion into a different business that uses similar technologies (also called *concentric diversification*) or adds new products or services to an organization's existing offerings (also called *horizontal diversification*).

Resource interdependence: The relationships, dependencies, and interactions among organizational resources.

Return on assets: A ratio calculated by dividing net profits by total assets showing the amount of earnings or profits gained for each dollar of invested assets.

Scenario analysis: A technique of proposing alternative futures that could come to pass if a specified environmental change occurs. This type of analysis is used by leaders to better understand and plan for future contingencies.

Segmentation: The division of a market into subsets of consumers with similar needs and wants; enables marketers to focus their marketing efforts on consumers most likely to buy a product or use a service.

Sequential interdependence: An arrangement in which resources or tasks are handed off from one organization or organizational subunit to another. Information, materials, products, and resources must be highly coordinated among organizational subunits because these exchanges occur in a particular order.

Service or product line: The particular kind or type of services or products offered by an organization.

Societal environment: The public and socioeconomic factors surrounding and influencing an organization, such as general economic conditions, population demographics, cultural values, governmental regulations, and technology.

Span of control: The number of subordinates reporting to a supervisor.

Stakeholders: Persons who have a claim to or obtain some benefit from an organization.

Static budget: A budget that is based on forecasted volumes and does not change when the volume of activity deviates from the forecast.

Statistical budget: Merger of an organization's capital budget forecasts with estimated statistical projections for an organization's services or products for a given fiscal period.

Strategic action cycle: The four stages of the strategic action cycle are (1) strategic planning, (2) budgeting, (3) implementing strategy, and (4) controlling problems or monitoring progress.

Strategic alliance: A mutually beneficial, long-term, formal relationship formed between two or more parties to pursue a set of common goals or to meet a critical business need while remaining independent organizations. Also called *quasi-firm* and *hybrid arrangement.*

Strategic business units: Profit centers in an organization that focus on a product line or market segment.

Strategic groups: Clusters of organizations that use the same or similar strategies in an industry. By classifying organizations into strategic groups, leaders can better analyze the structure of an industry.

Strategic intent: Statements, including mission, vision, and values, that describe an organization's perception of its purpose, its direction, and acceptable conduct.

Strategic management: Overseeing and directing daily activities in an organization to ensure they support achievement of the organization's mission and vision. Responsibilities may include designing organizational structures, policies, and procedures; evaluating budgets and progress toward goals; and coordinating staff training.

Strategic plan: A formal, written document that guides an organization's actions and informs stakeholders about the organization's direction and future activities.

Strategic planning committee: A standing or ad hoc committee that is responsible for organizing and leading an organization's strategic planning process.

Strategic priorities: The most important areas addressed by a strategic plan.

Strategic thinking: The generation and application of unique business insights and opportunities intended to create competitive advantage for a firm or an organization.

Switching costs: The costs associated with changing a product, brand, marketplace, or supplier.

SWOT analysis: An analytical tool used to develop an overview of an organization's strategic situation and better understand its environment. This type of analysis examines four important aspects of an organization: its strengths and weaknesses (i.e., the internal environment) and its opportunities and threats (i.e., the external environment).

Tangible resources: An organization's physical assets, including land, buildings and plant, equipment, cash, and personnel.

Times interest earned ratio: A ratio that shows an organization's ability to produce the earnings or profit necessary to pay the interest costs on its loans. For-profit organizations calculate it by dividing an organization's profits (EBIT or EBITDA) by its interest expense. For not-for-profit organizations, it is calculated by dividing an organization's net revenues less expenses plus interest expense by its interest expense.

Time value of money: The concept that money available at the present time is worth more than the same amount in the future because the value of money diminishes over time as a result of inflation, risk, and uncertainty of returns from investments.

Total debt to total assets ratio: An organization's long-term debt divided by its net assets. This ratio measures the proportion of an organization's assets that is funded by debt.

TOWS analysis: A variant of SWOT analysis that helps leaders make better strategic decisions. Leaders compare external opportunities and threats to internal strengths and weaknesses to determine whether their organization's strengths can leverage its opportunities, minimize its threats, and so forth.

Transaction cost economics: A theory that suggests that organizational boundaries influence organizations' efforts to mitigate the costs of the transactions and contractual hazards incurred by buying and selling assets and services.

Transfer pricing: The price charged for intraorganization trade (i.e., the sale or transfer of goods and services within an organization).

Trend data: Data that portray changes over time (generally from one year to the next).

Unrelated (conglomerate or lateral) diversification: The addition of new products or services that have little or no overlap with an organization's current products or services and assets.

Valuable resources: Resources that lack substitutes and are critical, rare, and difficult to imitate.

Value chain: The key internal processes or activities that an organization performs to create value for its stakeholders. The value chain provides a framework for analyzing an organization's strengths and weaknesses across the flow of product or service development and delivery.

Values: Statements expressing the ethics that guide an organization's actions and processes and standards for behavior among its staff.

Vertical expansion: Acquisition of a business that is a source of supplies for the acquiring organization (backward expansion) or that purchases from the acquiring organization (forward expansion).

Vertical integration: Assimilation of the vertical components of an organization through greater internal control and coordination.

Virtual integration: Coordination of intraorganization processes, flows, and outcomes through contractual, nonowned mechanisms.

Vision: A statement of the desired future state of an organization.

White paper: An authoritative paper or analysis of an issue or a problem.

REFERENCES

AARP. 2017. *Chronic Conditions Among Older Americans: Chronic Illness on the Rise.* Accessed May 26. https://assets.aarp.org/rgcenter/health/beyond_50_hcr_conditions.pdf.

Abelson, R. 2016. "Retail Health Clinics Result in Higher Spending, Survey Finds." *New York Times.* Published March 7. www.nytimes.com/2016/03/08/business/retail-health-clinics-result-in-higher-spending-survey-finds.html.

Adams, S. 2017. "Mission Statements." *Dilbert.* Accessed May 26. http://dilbert.com/search_results?terms=Mission+Statement.

Adamy, J. 2016. "Changing US Demographics Favor Democrats in Election, Report Says." *Wall Street Journal.* Published February 25. www.wsj.com/articles/changing-u-s-demographics-favor-democrats-in-election-report-says-1456376460.

Adler, R., J. Dunagan, B. Kreit, M. Liebhold, J. Tester, and A. Townsend. 2009. *HC2020 Perspectives.* Institute for the Future. Accessed July 5, 2017. www.iftf.org/uploads/media/IFTF_SR-1276_HC2020_Perspectives.pdf.

Administration on Aging. 2015. "A Profile of Older Americans: 2015." Accessed August 24, 2017. https://www.acl.gov/sites/default/files/Aging%20and%20Disability%20in%20America/2015-Profile.pdf.

Advisory Board. 2014. "From 32 to 19: Three More ACOs Drop Out of Pioneer Program." Published September 26. www.advisory.com/daily-briefing/2014/09/26/from-32-to-19-three-more-acos-drop-out-of-pioneer-program.

Aetna. 2015. "Aetna to Acquire Humana, Combined Entity to Drive Consumer-Focused, High-Value Health Care." Accessed May 31, 2017. https://news.aetna.com/2015/08/aetna-to-acquire-humana/.

Agency for Healthcare Research and Quality. 2014. *The Effective Health Care Program Stakeholder Guide.* Reviewed February. www.ahrq.gov/research/findings/evidence-based-reports/stakeholderguide/chapter3.html.

Ahlquist, G. 2013. "New Approaches for Community Hospitals and Health Systems." *H&HN.* Published June 6. www.hhnmag.com/articles/6134-new-approaches-for-community-hospitals-and-health-systems.

Albrecht, K., and R. Zemke. 2008. *Service America! Doing Business in the New Economy.* San Diego: Karl Albrecht International.

ALDI. 2013. "Market Force." Accessed August 24, 2017. www.marketforce.com/case-study-grocery-aldi-case-study.

Alexander, R., and R. Gunderman. 2010. "EMI and the First CT Scanner." *Journal of the American College of Radiology* 7 (10): 778–81.

American College of Healthcare Executives. 2017. "Strategic Plan, 2017–2019." Accessed June 19. www.ache.org/abt_ache/planning.cfm.

———. 2016. "ACHE Healthcare Executive 2017 Competencies Assessment Tool." Accessed August 29, 2017. www.ache.org/pdf/nonsecure/careers/competencies_booklet.pdf.

American Hospital Association (AHA). 2017. "AHA Fast Facts on US Hospitals." Updated January. www.aha.org/research/rc/stat-studies/fast-facts.shtml.

———. 2014. "Trendwatch: The Value of Provider Integration." Published March. www.aha.org/content/14/14mar-provintegration.pdf.

American Hospital Directory. 2017. Database. Accessed August 8. www.ahd.com.

American Marketing Association. 2016. "Definition of Marketing." Accessed June 2. www.ama.org/AboutAMA/Pages/Definition-of-Marketing.aspx.

American Red Cross. 2017. "Mission and Values." Accessed June 2. www.redcross.org/about-us/mission.

Andersen, E. 2013. "It Seemed Like a Good Idea at the Time: 7 of the Worst Business Decisions Ever Made." *Forbes.* Published October 4. www.forbes.com/sites/erikaandersen/2013/10/04/it-seemed-like-a-good-idea-at-the-time-7-of-the-worst-business-decisions-ever-made/.

Anderson, L. 2014. "Patent Expirations Through 2016 Predicted to Lower Brand Spending by $127 Billion." Drugs.com. www.drugs.com/article/patent-expirations.html.

Andrews, J. 2000. "Failed Ties." *H&HN* 74 (10): 52–56.

Anthem. 2017. "Company History." Accessed August 28. www.antheminc.com/aboutantheminc/companyhistory/index.htm.

———. 2013. "WellPoint Reports Fourth Quarter and Full Year 2012 Results and Provides 2013 Outlook." Published January 23. http://phx.corporate-ir.net/phoenix.zhtml?c=130104&p=irol-newsArticle&ID=1776927.

Aquirre, D., and M. Alpern. 2014. "10 Principles of Leading Change Management." *Strategy + Business.* Published June 6. www.strategy-business.com/article/00255?gko=9d35b.

Assistant Secretary for Planning and Evaluation. 2016. "Strategic Goal 1: Strengthen Health Care." Reviewed February 9. www.hhs.gov/about/strategic-plan/strategic-goal-1/.

Associated Press. 2016. "Some Nonprofit Hospitals Are Among the Most Profitable." Published May 2. www.cbsnews.com/news/some-nonprofit-hospitals-are-among-the-most-profitable/.

A. W. 2015. "What Disruptive Innovation Means." *Economist.* Published January 25. www.economist.com/blogs/economist-explains/2015/01/economist-explains-15.

Bader, B., E. Kazemek, P. Knecht, and R. Witalis. 2007. "Strategic Planning: Work for the Full Board or a Committee?" BoardRoom Press. Published April. https://

static1.squarespace.com/static/5487509fe4b0672ae6c16f81/t/54a42712e4b0d05e1a9f0816/1420044050114/Strategic_Planning-Work_for_the_Full_Board_or_a_Committee.pdf.

Bailey, D. 1994. "Forces in Customer Service." *Training and Management Development Methods* 8 (5): 701.

Baker, L., M. Bundorf, and D. Kessler. 2014. "Vertical Integration: Hospital Ownership of Physician Practices Is Associated with Higher Prices and Spending." *Health Affairs* 33 (5): 756–63.

Barkholz, D. 2016. "HCA's Growth Plan Is to Drop Anchor, Not Shop Around." *Modern Healthcare*. Published January 28. www.modernhealthcare.com/article/20160128/NEWS/160129851.

Barnard, C. 1968. *The Functions of the Executive*. Cambridge, MA: Harvard University Press.

Barnes, D., R. Palmer, D. Kresevic, R. Fortinsky, J. Kowal, M. Chren, and S. Landefeld. 2012. "Acute Care for Elders Units Produced Shorter Hospital Stays at Lower Cost While Maintaining Patients' Functional Status." *Health Affairs* 31 (6): 1227–36.

Barney, J. 1991. "Firm Resources and Sustained Competitive Advantage." *Journal of Management* 17: 99–120.

Barney, J., and W. Hesterly. 2014. *Strategic Management and Competitive Advantage: Concepts*, 5th ed. Boston: Pearson.

Baroto, M., M. Madi Bin Abdullah, and H. Wan. 2012. "Hybrid Strategy: A New Strategy for Competitive Advantage." *International Journal of Business and Management* 7 (20): 120–33.

Bazigos, M., and J. Harter. 2016. "Revisiting the Matrix Organization." *McKinsey Quarterly*. Published January. www.mckinsey.com/business-functions/organization/our-insights/revisiting-the-matrix-organization.

Bazzoli, F. 2016. "Trump Election Puts Future of Value-Based Care in Doubt." Health-Data Management. Published November 9. www.healthdatamanagement.com/news/trump-administration-offers-unknown-future-for-value-based-care.

Beatty, K. 2010. "The Three Strengths of a True Strategic Leader." *Forbes*. Published October 27. www.forbes.com/2010/10/27/three-strengths-strategy-leadership-managing-ccl.html.

Beck, M. 2017. "With Direct Primary Care, It's Just Doctor and Patient." *Wall Street Journal*. Published February 27. www.wsj.com/articles/with-direct-primary-care-its-just-doctor-and-patient-1488164702.

Becker, A. 2011. "Hospitals and Insurers Unite Against Anthem on Contract Provision." *CT Mirror*. Published March 22. https://ctmirror.org/2011/03/22/hospitals-and-insurers-unite-against-anthem-contract-provision/.

Beckham, D. 2016a. "How to Make Strategic Planning Work for Your Health Care Organization." *H&HN*. Published June 20. www.hhnmag.com/articles/7361-how-to-make-strategic-planning-work-for-your-health-care-organization.

———. 2016b. "10 Surprising Keys to Strategic Thinking for Health Care CEOs." *H&HN*. Published April 18. www.hhnmag.com/articles/7096-surprising-keys-to-strategic-thinking-for-health-care-ceos.

Belicove, M. 2013. "Understanding Goals, Strategy, Objectives, and Tactics in the Age of Social." *Forbes*. Published September 27. www.forbes.com/sites/mikalbelicove/2013/09/27/understanding-goals-strategies-objectives-and-tactics-in-the-age-of-social/#6f9441e7658e.

Benko, L. 2007. "Quiet Giant." *Modern Healthcare* 37 (8): 28–30.

Bennett, A. 2012. "Accountable Care Organizations: Principles and Implications for Hospital Administrators." *Journal of Healthcare Management* 57 (4): 244–54.

Berdan, B. 2016. "Climbing the Healthcare Summit." Association for Talent Development. Published February 8. www.td.org/Publications/Magazines/TD/TD-Archive/2016/02/Climbing-the-Healthcare-Summit.

Berenson, R., P. Ginsburg, J. Christianson, and T. Yee. 2012. "The Growing Power of Some Providers to Win Steep Payment Increases from Insurers Suggests Policy Remedies May Be Needed." *Health Affairs* 31 (5): 973–81.

Berenson, R., P. Ginsburg, and N. Kemper. 2010. "Unchecked Provider Clout in California Foreshadows Challenges to Health Reform." *Health Affairs* 29 (4): 699–705.

Berrett, B. R. 2012. Personal correspondence with the author. No date.

Berry, E. 2011. "Pace of Mergers, Acquisitions Revs Up for Physician Practices." *American Medical News*. Published August 1. www.amednews.com/article/20110801/business/308019963/4/.

Bertakis, K., A. Azari, L. Helms, E. Callahan, and J. Robbins. 2000. "Gender Differences in the Utilization of Health Care Services." *Journal of Family Practice* 49 (2): 147–52.

Bhasin, H. 2016. "Role of Strategic Planning in an Organization." *Marketing 91*. Published November 30. www.marketing91.com/role-strategic-planning-organization/.

Bilchik, G. S. 1997. "Can Rivals Play Nice?" *H&HN* 71 (8): 24–26, 28.

Biography. 2014. "Frederick W. Taylor." Updated April 2. www.biography.com/people/frederick-w-taylor-9503065.

Bolch, M. 2012. "States Move Forward with Unique ACO Models for Medicaid." *Managed Healthcare Executive* 22 (9): 31–32.

Boukus, E., A. Cassil, and A. O'Malley. 2009. "A Snapshot of US Physicians: Key Findings from the 2008 Health Tracking Physician Survey." Center for Studying Health System Change. Published September. http://hschange.org/CONTENT/1078/.

Bourgeois, L. J., I. M. Duhaime, and J. L. Stimpert. 1999. *Strategic Management: A Managerial Perspective*. Fort Worth, TX: Dryden Press.

Bradt, G. 2015. "The Root Cause of Every Merger's Success or Failure: Culture." *Forbes*. Published June 29. www.forbes.com/sites/georgebradt/2015/06/29/the-root-cause-of-every-mergers-success-or-failure-culture/#191894fbd305.

Brown, D., J. Bersin, W. Gosling, and N. Sloan. 2016. "Engagement: Always On." Deloitte University Press. Published February 29. https://dupress.deloitte.

com/dup-us-en/focus/human-capital-trends/2016/employee-engagement-and-retention.html.

Bryant, A. 1995. "Continental Is Dropping 'Lite' Service." *New York Times*. Published April 14. www.nytimes.com/1995/04/14/business/company-reports-continental-is-dropping-lite-service.html.

Bryson, J. 2004. "What to Do When Stakeholders Matter: Stakeholder Identification and Analysis Techniques." *Public Management Review* 6 (1): 21–53.

Buchmueller, T. C. 2006. "Consumer Demand for Health Insurance." Bureau of Economic Research. Published Summer. www.nber.org/reporter/summer06/buchmueller.html.

Budetti, P. P., S. M. Shortell, T. M. Waters, J. A. Alexander, L. R. Burns, R. R. Gillies, and H. Zuckerman. 2002. "Physician and Health System Integration." *Health Affairs* 21 (1): 203–10.

Buell, J. 2017. "The Care Continuum Universe: Delivering on the Promise." *Healthcare Executive*, January/February, 10–18.

Burns, J. 2015. "Study: Little Evidence That Integrating Hospital, Physician Care Improves Quality or Reduces Costs." Association of Health Care Journalists. Published March 13. http://healthjournalism.org/blog/2015/03/study-little-evidence-that-integrating-hospital-physician-care-improves-quality-or-reduces-costs/.

Burns, L. R. 2002. "Competitive Strategy." In *A Physician's Guide to Health Care Management*, edited by D. M. Albert, 46–56. Malden, MA: Blackwell Science.

———. 2000. "Physician Responses to the Marketplace: Group Practices and Hospital Alliances." *LDI Issue Brief*. Published May. www.upenn.edu/ldi/issuebrief5_8.pdf.

Burns, L. R., J. Cacciamani, J. Clement, and W. Aquino. 2000. "The Fall of the House of AHERF: The Allegheny Bankruptcy." *Health Affairs* 19 (1): 7–41.

Burns, L. R., and M. V. Pauly. 2012. "Accountable Care Organizations May Have Difficulty Avoiding the Failures of Integrated Delivery Networks of the 1990s." *Health Affairs* 31 (11): 2407–16.

———. 2002. "Integrated Delivery Networks: A Detour on the Road to Integrated Care?" *Health Affairs* 21 (4): 128–43.

Burns, L. R., and Wharton School colleagues. 2002. *The Health Care Value Chain: Producers, Purchasers, and Providers*. San Francisco: Jossey-Bass.

Burns, L. R., and D. R. Wholey. 1993. "Adoption and Abandonment of Matrix Management Programs: Effects of Organizational Characteristics and Inter-organizational Networks." *Academy of Management Journal* 36 (1): 106–38.

Business Dictionary. 2017. "Transfer Price." Accessed June 8. www.businessdictionary.com/definition/transfer-price.html.

Business Wire. 2012a. "Clinigen Announces Keats Healthcare Integration and Outlines Ambitious Growth Plans." Published February 14. www.businesswire.com/news/home/20120214005755/en.

———. 2012b. "UnitedHealthcare, North Shore-LIJ Health System to Offer New Tiered Benefit Plan Options Based on Accountable Care Concepts." Published

October 23. www.businesswire.com/news/home/20121023006639/en/UnitedHealthcare-North-Shore-LIJ-Health-System-Offer-Tiered.

Butcher, L. 2016. "Consumer Segmentation Has Hit Health Care. Here's How It Works." *H&HN*. Published March 8. www.hhnmag.com/articles/6932-consumer-segmentation-just-hit-health-care-heres-how-it-works.

———. 2014. "More Than a Building." *H&HN*. Published April 8. www.hhnmag.com/articles/4612-more-than-a-building.

Capps, C., and D. Dranove. 2004. "Hospital Consolidation and Negotiated PPO Prices." *Health Affairs* 23 (2): 175–81.

Carlson, J. 2012. "Midwest Health Organizations Form 'Virtual' Network." *Modern Healthcare*. Published March 8. www.modernhealthcare.com/article/20120308/NEWS /303089976.

Casalino, L. P., H. Pham, and G. Bazzoli. 2004. "Growth of Single-Specialty Medical Groups." *Health Affairs* 23 (2): 82–90.

Catton, B. 1971. *The Civil War*. New York: American Heritage Press.

Cayton, J., T. Kennedy, B. O'Dell, M. Stine, and D. Lee. 2012. "Current Market Trends of Cardiac Stents." *Journal of Medical Marketing* 12 (1): 5–12.

CB Insights. 2016. "Fools Rush In: 27 of the Worst Corporate M&A Flops." Published October 6. www.cbinsights.com/blog/merger-acquisition-corporate-fails/.

Centers for Disease Control and Prevention (CDC). 2017a. "Introduction to Program Evaluation for Public Health Programs: A Self-Study Guide." Accessed July 3. www.cdc.gov/eval/guide/step1/.

———. 2017b. "Public Health Genomics." Updated August 24. www.cdc.gov/genomics/public/index.htm.

———. 2016a. "Chronic Diseases and Health Promotion." Updated February 23. www.cdc.gov/chronicdisease/overview/index.htm.

———. 2016b. "Going Abroad for Medical Care." Updated December 5. www.cdc.gov/features/medicaltourism/.

———. 2016c. "Nursing Home Care." Updated July 6. www.cdc.gov/nchs/fastats/nursing-home-care.htm.

———. 2006. Project chapter template. Posted November 30. www2a.cdc.gov/cdcup/library/templates/CDC_UP_Project_Charter_Template.doc.

Centers for Medicare & Medicaid Services (CMS). 2017a. "Accountable Care Organizations." Updated May 12. www.cms.gov/ACO.

———. 2017b. "NHE Fact Sheet." Modified March 21. www.cms.gov/research-statistics-data-and-systems/statistics-trends-and-reports/nationalhealthexpenddata/nhe-fact-sheet.html.

———. 2016. "CMS Quality Strategy." Accessed June 9, 2017. www.cms.gov/Medicare/Quality-Initiatives-Patient-Assessment-Instruments/QualityInitiativesGenInfo/Downloads/CMS-Quality-Strategy.pdf.

———. 2015. *Hospital Value-Based Purchasing*. Published September. www.cms.gov/Outreach-and-Education/Medicare-Learning-Network-MLN/MLNProducts/downloads/Hospital_VBPurchasing_Fact_Sheet_ICN907664.pdf.

Centura Health. 2016. "Centura Health Facts." Accessed June 12, 2017. www.centura.org/About-Us/Centura-Health-Fast-Facts/.

Chandler, A. D. 1962. *Strategy and Structure: Chapters in the History of the Industrial Enterprise*. Cambridge, MA: MIT Press.

Chandler, C. 2010. "St. Dominic Partners with Walmart to Enter Retail Health Market." *Mississippi Business Journal* 32 (44): 4.

Chase, D. 2013. "The Hot Spotters Sequel: Population Health Heroes." *Forbes*. Published April 30. www.forbes.com/sites/davechase/2013/04/30/the-hot-spotters-sequel-population-health-heroes/.

Chen, P. W. 2010. "Can Concierge Medicine for the Few Benefit the Many?" *New York Times*. Published August 26. www.nytimes.com/2010/08/26/health/26pauline-chen.html.

Chesbrough, H. 2007. "Business Model Innovation: It's Not Just About Technology Anymore." *Strategy and Leadership* 35 (6): 12–17.

Chorus. 2017. "About Us." Accessed June 9. www.choruspharma.com/about-us.html.

———. 2009. "The Chorus Story." Accessed August 24, 2017. www.choruspharma.com/Chorus.Brochure.02June2009.pdf.

Christensen, C. 1997. *The Innovator's Dilemma: When Technologies Cause Great Firms to Fail*. Boston: Harvard Business School Press.

Christensen, C., H. Baumann, R. Ruggles, and T. Sadtler. 2006. "Disruptive Innovation for Social Change." *Harvard Business Review* 84 (12): 94–101.

Christensen, C. M., and M. E. Mangelsdorf. 2009. "Good Days for Disruptors." *MIT Sloan Management Review* 50 (3): 67–70.

Churchill, W. 1931. *The World Crisis, 1911–1918*. London: Four Square Books.

Clarke, R. 2009. "A Mission of Value." *Healthcare Financial Management* 63 (4): 144–45.

Coca-Cola Company. 2013. "Mission, Vision, and Values." Accessed June 12, 2017. www.coca-colacompany.com/our-company/mission-vision-values.

Colorado Springs Gazette. 2011. "What Next for Twitter? Company Faces Key Challenges." Published August 19. www.gazette.com/articles/jose-123518-keycalif.html.

Colwell, J. 2016. "Concierge Medicine Becomes an Option in Reform Era." *Medical Economics*. Published August 10. http://medicaleconomics.modernmedicine.com/medical-economics/news/concierge-medicine-becomes-option-reform-era.

Coman, A., and B. Ronen. 2009. "Focused SWOT: Diagnosing Critical Strengths and Weaknesses." *International Journal of Production Research* 47 (20): 5677–89.

Cook, D. 1995. *The Long Fuse: How England Lost the American Colonies, 1760–1785*. New York: Atlantic Monthly Press.

Cook, D., J. Thompson, E. Habermann, S. Visscher, J. Dearani, V. Roger, and B. Borah. 2014. "From 'Solution Shop' to 'Focused Factory' in Hospital Surgery: Increasing Care Value and Predictability." *Health Affairs* 33 (5): 746–55.

Cook, J., G. Hunter, and J. A. Vernon. 2009. "The Future Costs, Risks and Rewards of Drug Development: The Economics of Pharmacogenomics." *Pharmaco-Economics* 27 (5): 355–63.

Crans, F. W. 2009. "How Costly Is the Consignment Convenience?" *Healthcare Purchasing News*. Published November 1. www.hpnonline.com/inside/2008-11/0811-Iggy-Fred.html.

Crean, K. W. 2010. "Accelerating Innovation in Information and Communication Technology for Health." *Health Affairs* 29 (2): 278–83.

Creswell, J., and R. Abelson. 2012a. "A Giant Hospital Chain Is Blazing a Profit Trail." *New York Times*. Published August 14. www.nytimes.com/2012/08/15/business/hca-giant-hospital-chain-creates-a-windfall-for-private-equity.html.

———. 2012b. "A Hospital War Reflects a Bind for Doctors in the U.S." *New York Times*. Published November 30. www.nytimes.com/2012/12/01/business/a-hospital-war-reflects-a-tightening-bind-for-doctors-nationwide.html.

CSIMarket.com. 2017. "Healthcare Sector Financial Strength Information." Accessed August 9. https://csimarket.com/Industry/industry_Financial_Strength_Ratios.php?s=800.

Curry, L., E. Spatz, E. Cherlin, H. Krumholz, and E. Bradley. 2011. "What Distinguishes Top-Performing Hospitals in Acute Myocardial Infarction Rates?" *Annals of Internal Medicine* 154 (6): 384–90.

Curtright, J., S. Stolp-Smith, and E. Edell. 2000. "Strategic Performance Management: Development of a Performance Measurement System at the Mayo Clinic." *Journal of Healthcare Management* 45 (1): 58–68.

Cutler, D., and F. Morton. 2013. "Hospitals, Market Share and Consolidation." *Journal of the American Medical Association* 310 (18): 1964–70.

Cylus, J., M. Hartman, B. Washington, K. Andrews, and A. Catlin. 2010. "Pronounced Gender and Age Differences Are Evident in Personal Health Care Spending Per Person." *Health Affairs*. Published December. http://content.healthaffairs.org/content/early/2010/12/07/hlthaff.2010.0216.full.

Dans, E. 2016. "The Delicate Balance Between Competition and Monopoly." *Forbes*. Published January 6. www.forbes.com/sites/enriquedans/2016/01/06/the-delicate-balance-between-competition-and-monopoly/.

Darbi, W. 2012. "Of Mission and Vision Statements and Their Potential Impact on Employee Behavior and Attitudes." *International Journal of Business and Social Science* 3 (14): 95–109.

Das, R. 2016. "Five Technologies That Will Disrupt Healthcare by 2020." *Forbes*. Published March 30. www.forbes.com/sites/reenitadas/2016/03/30/top-5-technologies-disrupting-healthcare-by-2020/2/.

Dave, D., and H. Saffer. 2012. "Impact of Direct-to-Consumer Advertising on Pharmaceutical Prices and Demand." *Southern Economic Journal* 79 (1): 97–126.

D'Aveni, R., and D. Ravenscraft. 1994. "Economies of Integration Versus Bureaucracy Costs: Does Vertical Integration Improve Performance?" *Academy of Management Journal* 35 (3): 596–625.

Davis, K., C. Schoen, and K. Stremikis. 2010. "Mirror, Mirror on the Wall: How the Performance of the U.S. Health Care System Compares Internationally, 2010 Update." Commonwealth Fund. Published June 23. www.commonwealthfund.org/publications/fund-reports/2010/jun/mirror-mirror-update.

Davison, B. 2003. "Management Span of Control: How Much Is Too Wide?" *Journal of Business Strategy* 24 (4): 22–29.

Day, G. 1981. "The Product Life Cycle: Analysis and Application Issues." *Journal of Marketing* 45 (4): 60–67.

DeBord, M. 2016. "That New Tesla Probably Won't Be as Cheap as You Think." *Business Insider*. Published February 11. www.businessinsider.com/teslas-model-3-strategy-will-keep-price-high-2016-2.

Definitive Healthcare. 2016. "Top 10 GPOs by Member Hospital Beds." Published August 16. www.definitivehc.com/top-10-lists/top-10-gpos-by-member-hospital-beds.

Deloitte. 2016. "Global Life Sciences Outlook: Moving Forward with Cautious Optimism." Accessed June 15, 2017. www2.deloitte.com/content/dam/Deloitte/global/Documents/Life-Sciences-Health-Care/gx-lshc-2016-life-sciences-outlook.pdf.

Deloitte Center for Health Solutions. 2008. *Medical Tourism: Consumers in Search of Value*. Accessed June 15, 2017. www.deloitte.com/assets/Dcom-UnitedStates/Local%20Assets/Documents/us_chs_MedicalTourismStudy(3).pdf.

Denning, S. 2013. "It's Official! The End of Competitive Advantage." *Forbes*. Published June 2. www.forbes.com/sites/stevedenning/2013/06/02/its-official-the-end-of-competitive-advantage/.

DePamphilis, D. 2014. *Mergers, Acquisitions, and Other Restructuring Activities*, 7th ed. New York: Elsevier.

Dezzani, L. 2016. "Top 10 Pharmaceutical Companies 2016." IgeaHub. Published May 6. https://igeahub.com/2016/05/06/top-10-pharmaceutical-companies-2016/.

Diamond, D. 2014. "Hospital Mergers Are Out. 'Strategic Alliances Are In.' Is Obamacare Responsible?" *California Healthline*. Published July 30. http://californiahealthline.org/news/hospital-mergers-are-out-strategic-alliances-are-in-is-obamacare-responsible/.

Dietsche, E. 2015. "6 of the Largest GPOs." *Becker's Hospital Review*. Published July 2. www.beckershospitalreview.com/finance/6-of-the-largest-gpos-2015.html.

Dignity Health. 2017. "Our History: Rooted in Kindness." Accessed August 24. www.dignityhealth.org/about-us/our-organization/mission-vision-and-values.

———. 2013. "Sustaining Our Healing Ministry: Fiscal Year 2013 Social Responsibility Report." Accessed August 24, 2017. www.dignityhealth.org/stellent/groups/public/@xinternet_con_sys/documents/webcontent/stgss045842.pdf.

———. 2008. "Mission Integration: Standards and Indicators." Accessed June 15, 2017. www.dignityhealth.org/stellent/groups/public/@xinternet_con_sys/documents/webcontent/stgss044503.pdf.

DiMaggio, P. J., and W. W. Powell. 1983. "The Iron Cage Revisited: Institutional Isomorphism and Collective Rationality in Organizational Fields." *American Sociological Review* 48 (2): 147–60.

Dougherty, C. 2016. "They Promised Us Jet Packs. They Promised the Bosses Profits." *New York Times*. Published July 23. www.nytimes.com/2016/07/24/technology/they-promised-us-jet-packs-they-promised-the-bosses-profit.html.

Drucker, P. F. 1959. "Long-Range Planning—Challenge to Management Science." *Management Science* 5 (3): 238–49.

Drummond-Hay, R., and D. Bamford. 2009. "A Case Study into Planning and Change Management Within the UK National Health Service." *International Journal of Public Sector Management* 22 (4): 324–37.

Duffy, J. 1991. *Hitler Slept Late and Other Blunders That Cost Him the War*. Westport, CT: Praeger Publishers.

Dunn, M. 2016. "Here Are 20 of the Worst Predictions Ever Made About the Future of Tech." News.com.au. Published March 8. www.news.com.au/technology/gadgets/here-are-20-of-the-worst-predictions-ever-made-about-the-future-of-tech/news-story/2300ac1ffb8a3ba18ce3219636700937.

Dye, R., and O. Sibony. 2007. "How to Improve Strategic Planning." *McKinsey Quarterly*. Published August. www.mckinsey.com/business-functions/strategy-and-corporate-finance/our-insights/how-to-improve-strategic-planning.

Dyer, J., P. Kale, and H. Singh. 2004. "When to Ally and When to Acquire." *Harvard Business Review* 82 (7/8): 109–15.

Eager, K. 2010. "Alliance Management and Project Management: Working Together as a Team." *Pharmaceutical Outsourcing*. Published July 1. www.pharmoutsourcing.com/Featured-Articles/120783-Alliance-Management-and-Project-Management-Working-Together-as-a-Team/.

Eastaugh, S. R. 2014. "Hospital Diversification Strategy." *Journal of Health Care Finance* 40 (3): 1–13.

Edelstein, B. 2011. "Examining Whether Dental Therapists Constitute a Disruptive Innovation in US Dentistry." *American Journal of Public Health* 101 (10): 1831–35.

Ellison, A. 2016. "7 Hospital Bankruptcies So Far in 2016." *Becker's Hospital Review*. Published July 27. www.beckershospitalreview.com/finance/7-hospital-bankruptcies-so-far-in-2016-july27.html.

E*TRADE. 2017. "Humana Inc. Com." Accessed June 22. www.etrade.wallst.com/v1/stocks/snapshot/snapshot.asp?symbol=HUM.

Evans, M. 2016. "Merger Indigestion: Big Hospital Mergers Failing to Deliver Promised Results." *Modern Healthcare*. Published April 23. www.modernhealthcare.com/article/20160423/MAGAZINE/304239980.

———. 2015. "Two More Pioneer ACOs Exit as New CMS Model Emerges." *Modern Healthcare*. Published November 4. www.modernhealthcare.com/article/20151104/NEWS/151109941.

———. 2013. "Highmark Completes West Penn Deal, Announces New System." *Modern Healthcare*. Published April 29. www.modernhealthcare.com/article/20130429/NEWS/304299948.

Farfan, B. 2016. "Why Trader Joe's Has No Grocery Competition: How to Beat, Not Compete." The Balance. Updated November 11, 2017. www.thebalance.com/why-trader-joes-has-no-competition-2892549.

Fausz, A. 2014. "Ideal Span of Control for Lean Organizations." *Lean Healthcare*. Published June 19. www.leanhealthcareexchange.com/?p=4489.

Federal Highway Administration. 2016. "Supporting Performance-Based Planning and Programming Through Scenario Planning." US Department of Transportation. Published June. www.fhwa.dot.gov/planning/scenario_and_visualization/scenario_planning/scenario_planning_guidebook/fhwahep16068.pdf.

Field, R. I. 2007. *Health Care Regulation in America: Complexity, Confrontation, and Compromise*. New York: Oxford University Press.

Finkler, S. A., and D. M. Ward. 2006. *Accounting Fundamentals for Health Care Management*. Sudbury, MA: Jones and Bartlett Publishers.

———. 1999. *Essentials of Cost Accounting for Health Care Organizations*, 2nd ed. Gaithersburg, MD: Aspen Publishers.

Firger, J. 2015. "Prescription Drugs on the Rise: Estimates Suggest 60 Percent of Americans Take at Least One Medication." *Newsweek*. Published November 11. www.newsweek.com/prescription-drugs-rise-new-estimates-suggest-60-americans-take-least-one-390354.

Flanagan, N. 2016. "Reputation Is Everything: How 2 Hospitals Are Weathering PR Firestorms." HealthcareDIVE. Published January 31. www.healthcaredive.com/news/reputation-is-everything-how-2-hospitals-are-weathering-pr-firestorms/412982/.

Ford, E., T. Huerta, R. Schilhavy, N. Menachemi, and V. Walls. 2012. "Effective US Health System Websites: Establishing Benchmarks and Standards for Effective Consumer Engagement." *Journal of Healthcare Management* 57 (1): 47–64.

Friedman, A., J. Howard, E. Shaw, D. Cohen, L. Shahidi, and J. Ferrante. 2016. "Facilitators and Barriers to Care Coordination in Patient-Centered Medical Homes from Coordinators' Perspectives." *Journal of the American Board of Family Medicine* 29 (1): 90–101.

Furnas, B., and R. Buckwalter-Poza. 2010. "Health Care Competition: Insurance Market Domination Leads to Fewer Choices." Center for American Progress. Published June. www.americanprogress.org/issues/economy/reports/2010/06/25/7986/making-health-care-competition-work/.

Galbraith, J. 2012. "The Evolution of Enterprise Organization Designs." *Journal of Organizational Design* 1 (2): 1–13.

Galbraith, J. R., and G. Quelle. 2009. "Matrix Is the Ladder to Success." *Bloomberg Businessweek*. Published August 9. www.businessweek.com/debateroom/archives/2009/08/matrix_is_the_l.html.

Gapenski, L., and K. Reiter. 2015. *Healthcare Finance: An Introduction to Accounting and Financial Management*, 5th ed. Chicago: Health Administration Press.

Garcia, A. 2016. "US Sues to Block 2 Major Healthcare Mergers." CNN Money. Published July 21. http://money.cnn.com/2016/07/21/news/companies/doj-anthem-cigna-humana-aetna/.

Garguilo, L. 2016. "The Creation of Shire's Outsourcing Model." Outsourced Pharma. Published May 20. www.outsourcedpharma.com/doc/the-creation-of-shire-s-outsourcing-model-0001.

Garrido, T., B. Raymond, and B. Wheatley. 2016. "Lessons from More Than a Decade in Patient Portals. *Health Affairs.* Published April 7. http://healthaffairs.org/blog/2016/04/07/lessons-from-more-than-a-decade-in-patient-portals/.

Gelineau, S. 2015. "Preventing a Merger Fail." *H&HN.* Published January 8. www.hhnmag.com/articles/3769-preventing-a-merger-fail.

George, W. W. 2001. "Medtronic's Chairman William George on How Mission-Driven Companies Create Long-Term Shareholder Value." *Academy of Management Executive* 15 (4): 39–47.

Gerhard, U., and B. Hahn. 2005. "Wal-Mart and Aldi: Two Retail Giants in Germany." *GeoJournal* 62 (1-2): 15–26.

Ghoshal, S., and C. A. Bartlett. 1995. "Building the Entrepreneurial Corporation: New Organisational Processes, New Managerial Tasks." *European Management Journal* 13 (2): 139–55.

Ghoshal, S., and L. Gratton. 2002. "Integrating the Enterprise." *MIT Sloan Management Review* 44 (1): 30–38.

Gimbert, X. 2011. *Think Strategically.* New York: Palgrave Macmillan.

Glanton, D., and L. Boweau. 2015. "In About-Face, U of C Medicine to Build Adult Trauma Center on Hyde Park Campus." *Chicago Tribune.* Published December 17. www.chicagotribune.com/news/ct-university-of-chicago-trauma-center-hyde-park-campus-20151217-story.html.

Gluck, A. 2016. "Symposium: The New Health Care Industry—Consolidation, Integration, Competition, in the Wake of the ACA." *Health Affairs.* Published February 24. www.healthaffairs.org.org/do/10.1377/hblog20160224.053315/full/.

Goktan, A. B., and G. Miles. 2011. "Innovation Speed and Radicalness: Are They Inversely Related?" *Management Decision* 49 (4): 533–47.

Goldman, E. 2007. "Strategic Thinking at the Top." *MIT Sloan Management Review* 48 (4): 75–81.

Goldman, E., T. Cahill, R. Filho, and L. Merlis. 2009. "Experiences That Develop the Ability to Think Strategically." *Journal of Healthcare Management* 54 (6): 403–16.

Goldsmith, J., L. Burns, A. Sen, and T. Goldsmith. 2015. *Integrated Delivery Networks: In Search of Benefits and Market Effects.* National Academy of Social Insurance. Published February. www.nasi.org/sites/default/files/research/Integrated_Delivery_Networks_In_Search_of_Benefits_and_Market_Effects.pdf.

Gonzalez, A., M. Mahesh, K. Kim, M. Bhargavan, R. Lewis, F. Mettler, and C. Land. 2009. "Projected Cancer Risks from Computed Tomographic Scans Performed in the United States in 2007." *Archives of Internal Medicine* 169 (22): 2071–77.

Goodman, J. 2014. "Everyone Should Have a Concierge Doctor." *Forbes.* Published August 28. www.forbes.com/sites/johngoodman/2014/08/28/everyone-should-have-a-concierge-doctor/.

Gov 2020. 2017. "Health Care." Deloitte. Accessed August 7. http://government-2020.dupress.com/category/healthcare/.

Gratton, L., and A. Scott. 2016. "Our Assumptions About Old and Young Workers Are Wrong." *Harvard Business Review.* Published November 15. https://hbr.org/2016/11/our-assumptions-about-old-and-young-workers-are-wrong.

Gray, B. 1986. *For-Profit Enterprise in Health Care.* Institute of Medicine. Washington DC: National Academies Press.

Greising, C. H. "How Hospitals Should Approach Financial Planning in Changing Times." *Trustee.* Published October 13. www.trusteemag.com/articles/772-how-hospitals-should-approach-financial-planning-in-changing-times.

Grenny, J., D. Maxwell, and A. Shimberg. 2007. "How Project Leaders Can Overcome the Crisis of Silence." *MIT Sloan Management Review* 48 (4): 46–52.

Griffioen, J. 2016. "Why You Should Hire a Strategic Planning Consultant." Griffioen Consulting Group. Published September 1. http://griffioenconsulting.com/blog/2016/09/why-hire-a-strategic-planning-consultant/.

Grobart, S., and I. Austen. 2012. "The Blackberry: Trying to Avoid the Hall of Fallen Giants." *New York Times.* Published January 28. www.nytimes.com/2012/01/29/business/blackberry-aiming-to-avoid-the-hall-of-fallen-giants.html.

Grogan, K. 2011. "Lilly Hails Success of Its New R&D Models." *PharmaTimes Online.* Published February 17. www.pharmatimes.com/news/lilly_hails_success_of_its_new_r_and_d_models_979582.

Gurd, B. and T. Gao. 2007. "Lives in the Balance: An Analysis of the Balanced Scorecard (BSC) in Healthcare Organizations." *International Journal of Productivity and Performance Management* 57 (1): 6–21.

Halle, M., C. B. Lewis, and M. Seshamani. 2009. "Health Disparities: A Case for Closing the Gap." Healthcare.gov. Accessed October 2, 2017. https://smhs.gwu.edu/rodhaminstitute/sites/rodhaminstitute/files/HCReform%20-%20Disparities%20Report.pdf.

Hambrick, D., I. MacMilan, and D. Day. 1982. "Strategic Attributes and Performance in the BCG Matrix—A PIMS-Based Analysis of Industrial Product Business." *Academy of Management Journal* 25 (3): 510–31.

Harris, G. 2011. "U.S. Scrambling to Ease Shortage of Vital Medicine." *New York Times.* Published August 19. http://www.nytimes.com/2011/08/20/health/policy/20drug.html.

Hartman, M., A. Martin, O. Nuccio, A. Catlin, and National Expenditure Accounts Team. 2010. "Health Spending Growth at a Historic Low in 2008." *Health Affairs* 29 (1): 147–55.

Hatten, K., and M. Hatten. 1987. "Strategic Groups, Asymmetrical Mobility Barriers and Contestability." *Strategic Management Journal* 8 (4): 329–42.

Hawk, B. 2010. *Annual Proceedings of the Fordham Competition Law Institute*. Fordham Competitive Law Institute. Huntington, NY: Juris Publishing.

HCA. 2017. "Our Mission and Values." Accessed June 20. http:// hcahealthcare.com/about/our-mission-and-values.dot.

———. 2016. *Advancing the Patient Care Experience: 2015 Annual Report to Shareholders*. Accessed August 23. http://investor.hcahealthcare.com/sites/hcahealthcare.investorhq.businesswire.com/files/report/file/HCA_2015_Annual_Report_Web_Version.pdf.

He, W., D. Goodkind, and P. Kowal. 2016. *An Aging World: 2015*. United States Census Bureau. Published March 28. www.census.gov/library/publications/2016/demo/P95-16-1.html.

Health Care Service Corporation (HCSC). 2016. "Who We Are." Accessed August 24. www.hcsc.com/who-we-are.

Health Research & Educational Trust. 2014. *Building a Leadership Team for the Health Care Organization of the Future*. Published April. www.hpoe.org/Reports-HPOE/leadership-team-future-2014.pdf.

Healthcare Financial Management Association. 2017. "Health Care 2020." Accessed June 28. www.hfma.org/healthcare2020/.

Healthcare.gov. 2017. "Health Insurance Plan and Network Types: HMOs, PPOs, and More." Accessed June 28. www.healthcare.gov/choose-a-plan/plan-types/.

Healthcarereform.gov. 2017. "Healthcare Disparities: A Case for Closing the Gap." Accessed August 24. https://smhs.gwu.edu/rodhaminstitute/sites/rodhaminstitute/files/HCReform%20-%20Disparities%20Report.pdf.

Healthcare Supply Chain Association. 2014. "Healthcare Group Purchasing Organizations Generate Up to $55 Billion in Annual Cost Savings for Hospitals, Medicare, and Medicaid, According to New Empirical Analysis of US Data." Published July 9. http://c.ymcdn.com/sites/www.supplychainassociation.org/resource/resmgr/press_releases_2014/hsca_press_release_on_dobson.pdf.

Hennessy, M. 2016. "Will More Retail Clinic Ownership Shift to Health Systems?" *Contemporary Clinic*. Published February 1. http://contemporaryclinic.pharmacytimes.com/journals/issue/2016/february2016/from-the-chairman-will-more-retail-clinic-ownership-shift-to-health-systems.

Hensel Jr., B. 2004. "Airline Experts Can Agree on Need for Change." *Houston Chronicle*. Published September 19. www.highbeam.com/doc/1G1-122273905.html.

Herbert, K. 2012. *Hospital Reimbursement: Concepts and Principles*. New York: CRP Press.

Herman, B. 2015. "Lost Appetite: The Expected Surge in Insurers Buying Physician Practices Never Materialized." *Modern Healthcare*. Published October 10. www.modernhealthcare.com/article/20151010/MAGAZINE/310109979.

———. 2014. "Six Wisconsin Systems Create Pact, Aim for ACO." *Modern Healthcare*. Published August 6. www.modernhealthcare.com/article/20140806/NEWS/308069947.

———. 2013. "Highmark to Buy West Penn Debt, Salvages Merger Proposal." *Becker's Hospital Review*. Published January 17. www.beckershospitalreview.com/finance/highmark-to-buy-west-penn-debt-salvages-merger-proposal.html.

Hersher, R. 2017. "Aetna and Humana Call Off Merger After Court Decision." NPR. Published February 14. www.npr.org/sections/thetwo-way/2017/02/14/515167491/aetna-and-humana-call-off-merger-after-court-decision.

Herzlinger, R. 2000. "Market-Driven, Focused Healthcare: The Role of Managers." *Frontiers of Health Services Management* 16 (3): 3–12.

———. 1997. *Market-Driven Health Care*. Reading, MA: Addison-Wesley.

Hiiemaa, K. 2016. "Retail Store Differentiation in 2016." ERPLY. Published February 25. https://erply.com/retail-store-differentiation-in-2016/.

Hill, C., and G. Jones. 1998. *Strategic Management: An Integrated Approach*. New York: Houghton Mifflin.

Hitt, M., R. D. Ireland, R. Hoskisson. 2016. *Strategic Management: Competitiveness an Globalization*, 12th ed. Boston: Cengage Learning.

Hoffman, J. 2014. "Eight Reasons Hospital Partnerships Fail." *H&HN*. Published September 30. www.hhnmag.com/articles/3962-eight-reasons-hospital-partnerships-fail.

Hogg, P. 2015. "Who Are the Top 10 Pharmaceutical Companies in the World?" Proclinical Life Sciences Blog. Published June 15. http://blog.proclinical.com/who-are-the-top-10-pharmaceutical-companies-in-the-world.

Holland, K. 2007. "In Mission Statements, Bizspeak and Bromides." *New York Times*. Published September 23. http://www.nytimes.com/2007/09/23/jobs/23mgmt.html.

Hoye, S. 2016. "BCBSTX Could Drop Texas Health from Network." WFAA. Published December 7. www.wfaa.com/news/bcbstx-could-drop-texas-health-from-network/364436630.

Hruska, J. 2016. "Windows Drops Below 90% Market Share for the First Time in Years: Windows 7 Falls Below 50%." ExtremeTech. Published May 3. www.extremetech.com/computing/227693-windows-drops-below-90-market-share-for-the-first-time-in-years-windows-7-falls-below-50.

Hull, P. 2013. "5 Tips for a Great Business Plan." *Forbes*. Published February 28. www.forbes.com/sites/patrickhull/2013/02/28/5-tips-for-a-great-business-plan/#47cc76f47b1e.

Humana. 2012. *2011 Annual Report*. Published February 28. http://phx.corporate-ir.net/phoenix.zhtml?c=92913&p=irol-reportsannual.

Huotari, P., and Z. Havrdova. 2016. "Stakeholders, Roles and Responsibilities Regarding Quality of Care." *International Journal of Health Care Quality Assurance* 29 (8): 864–76.

Hwang, J., and C. M. Christensen. 2008. "Disruptive Innovation in Health Care Delivery: A Framework for Business-Model Innovation." *Health Affairs* 27 (5): 1329–35.

Ice, J. 2007. "Strategic Intent: A Key to Business Strategy Development and Culture Change." *Organization Development Journal* 25 (4): 169–76.

Institute for Healthcare Improvement. 2017. "Ensuring Healthcare Improvements Stick." *Healthcare Executive* 32 (1): 66–69.

Internal Revenue Service (IRS). 2011. "Notice 2011-52: Notice and Request for Comments Regarding the Community Health Needs Assessment Requirements for Tax-Exempt Hospitals." Accessed August 23, 2017. www.irs.gov/pub/irs-drop/n-11-52.pdf.

———. 2010. "Notice 2010-39: Request for Comments Regarding Additional Requirements for Tax-Exempt Hospitals." Published June 14. www.irs.gov/irb/2010-24_IRB/ar08.html#d0e766.

Ireland, R., M. Hitt, and D. Vaidyanath. 2002. "Alliance Management as a Source of Competitive Advantage." *Journal of Management* 28 (3): 413–46.

Irving Levin Associates, Inc. 2010. "Key Deals and Multiples for Managed Care Mergers and Acquisitions Announced from 2000 to 2009, Revealed by DealSearchOnline.com." *Business Wire*. Published April 6. www.businesswire.com/news/home/20100406006901/en/Key-Deals-Multiples-Managed-Care-Mergers-Acquisitions.

Jacobs, L. 2016. "Looking Ahead in 2016: Top 10 Trends in Health Care." *H&HN*. Published January 5. www.hhnmag.com/articles/6800-looking-ahead-in---top---trends-in-health-care.

Jacobsen, D. 2012. "6 Big Mergers That Were Killed by Culture (and How to Stop It from Killing Yours)." Globoforce. Published September 26. www.globoforce.com/gfblog/2012/6-big-mergers-that-were-killed-by-culture/.

James, B., and G. Poulsen. 2016. "The Case for Capitation." *Harvard Business Review* 94 (7–8): 102–11.

Jameson, M. 2012. "As Hospitals Take Over Doctors' Practices, Fees Rise." *Orlando Sentinel*. Published September 15. http://articles.orlandosentinel.com/2012-09-15/health/os-hospitals-buy-physicians-20120915_1_hospital-executives-hospital-employee-physician-practices.

Johnson, L. 2015. "Here Are the 6 Reasons Why Prescription Drugs Are So Expensive." *Business Insider*. Published September 25. www.businessinsider.com/ap-multiple-factors-cause-high-prescription-drug-prices-in-us-2015-9.

Johnson, S. 2014. "Dialysis Demand Strong as Kidney Disease Grows." *Modern Healthcare*. Published October 11. www.modernhealthcare.com/article/20141011/NEWS/141019999.

Johnson & Johnson. 2017. "Products." Accessed August 16. www.jnj.com/healthcare-products.

———. 2016. "Annual Report: 2015." Published March. http://files.shareholder.com/downloads/JNJ/2431646896x0x881109/474857DD-8E67-43B1-BB38-0A9712D93545/2015_annual_report_.pdf.

Jones, L. 1999. "Plan to Convert Hospital to Mixed-Use Project Gets RDA OK." *Enterprise* 28 (47): 1.

Joseph, J., and R. Klingebiel. 2016. "Centralized Decision Making Helps Kill Bad Products." *Harvard Business Review*. Published October 18. https://hbr.org/2016/10/centralized-decision-making-helps-kill-bad-products.

Joskow, P. 2010. "Vertical Integration." *Antitrust Bulletin* 55 (3): 545–86.

Journal Record. 2001. "OU Regents Approve Licensing Agreement." Published May 16. www.questia.com/library/1P2-5749024/ou-regents-approve-licensingagreement.

Judge, W., and J. Ryman. 2001. "The Shared Leadership Challenge in Strategic Alliances: Lessons from the U.S. Healthcare Industry." *Academy of Management Executive* 15 (2): 71–79.

Kaiser Family Foundation. 2015. "2015 Employer Benefits Survey." Published September 22. http://kff.org/report-section/ehbs-2015-summary-of-findings/.

———. 2014a. "Distribution of Certified Nursing Facilities by Ownership Type." Accessed July 31, 2017. http://kff.org/other/state-indicator/nursing-facilities-by-ownership-type/.

———. 2014b. "Market Share and Enrollment of Largest Three Insurers." Accessed July 31, 2017. http://kff.org/other/state-indicator/market-share-and-enrollment-of-largest-three-insurers-individual-market/.

Kaiser Permanente. 2017. "Senior Consultant: Strategic Planning and Learning (Community Benefit)." Published June 27. www.kaiserpermanentejobs.org/job/pasadena/senior-consultant-strategic-planning-and-learning-community-benefit/641/4988350.

Kale, P., and H. Singh. 2009. "Managing Strategic Alliances: What Do We Know Now and Where Do We Go from Here?" *Academy of Management Perspectives* 23 (3): 45–62.

Kaluzny, A., H. Zuckerman, and T. Ricketts. 2002. *Partners: Forming Strategic Alliances in Health Care*. Washington, DC: Beard Books.

Kaplan, R. 2012. "Have You Checked Your Assumptions Lately?" *Inc*. Published February 14. www.inc.com/robert-kaplan/have-you-challenged-your-assumptions-lately.html.

Kaplan, R. S., and D. P. Norton. 2006. *Alignment: Using the Balanced Scorecard to Create Corporate Synergies*. Boston: Harvard Business School Publishing Corporation.

Kaplan, R., and M. Porter. 2011. "The Big Idea: How to Solve the Cost Crisis in Health Care." *Harvard Business Review*. Published September. https://hbr.org/2011/09/how-to-solve-the-cost-crisis-in-health-care.

Kapur, S. 2016. "GOP's Delayed-Repeal Obamacare Plan Faces Major Obstacles." *Bloomberg Business*. Published December 1. www.bloomberg.com/politics/articles/2016-12-01/gop-s-delayed-repeal-obamacare-strategy-faces-major-obstacles.

Kash, B., and D. Tan. 2016. "Physician Group Practice Trends: A Comprehensive Review." *Journal of Hospital and Medical Management* 2 (1): 1–8.

Kelley, B. 2016. *Charting Change: A Visual Toolkit for Making Change Stick*. New York: Palgrave Macmillan.

Kendall, B., and A. Mathews. 2016. "Justice Department to Challenge Two Health-Insurance Mergers." *Wall Street Journal.* Published July 19. www.wsj.com/articles/justice-department-to-challenge-two-health-insurance-mergers-1468947479.

Kesselheim, A., J. Avorn, and A. Sarpatwari. 2016. "The High Cost of Prescription Drugs in the United States." *Journal of the American Medical Association* 316 (8): 858–71.

Kharpal, A. 2016. "Nokia Phones Are Back After Microsoft Sells Mobile Assets for $350M to Foxonn, HMD." CNBC. Published May 18. www.cnbc.com/2016/05/18/nokia-phones-are-back-after-microsoft-sells-mobile-assets-for-350-million-to-foxconn-hmd.html.

Kilpatrick, A., and L. Silverman. 2005. "The Power of Vision." *Strategy & Leadership* 33 (2): 24–26.

King Faisal Specialist Hospital. 2017. "About Us." Accessed July 26. www.kfshrc.edu.sa/en/home/aboutus.

Koenig, M. 2016. "Nonprofit Mission Statements: Good and Bad Examples." Nonprofit Hub. Accessed July 26, 2017. http://nonprofithub.org/starting-a-nonprofit/nonprofit-mission-statements-good-and-bad-examples/.

Kohli, S. 2014. "When Weird Al Yankovic Sings About Business Jargon, He's Mocking These Companies." *Quartz.* Published July 17. http://qz.com/236031/when-weird-al-yankovic-mocks-csny-flavored-business-jargon-hes-singing-about-these-companies/.

Koort, K. 2014. "The 10 Biggest Killers of Employee Motivation." Talent Management and HR. Published December 1. www.eremedia.com/tlnt/the-10-biggest-killers-of-employee-motivation/.

Koppenheffer, M. 2015. "Want to Please Patients? Maybe You Should Start a Specialty Hospital." Advisory Board. Published April 1. www.advisory.com/research/health-care-advisory-board/blogs/at-the-helm/2015/04/patient-experience-and-specialty-hospitals.

Koronowski, R. 2017. "68 Times Trump Promised to Repeal Obamacare." ThinkProgress. Published March 24. https://thinkprogress.org/trump-promised-to-repeal-obamacare-many-times-ab9500dad31e.

Kotler, P., J. Shalowitz, and R. Stevens. 2008. *Strategic Marketing for Health Care Organizations.* San Francisco: Jossey-Bass.

Kowitt, B. 2010. "Inside the Secret World of Trader Joe's." *Fortune.* Published August 23. http://archive.fortune.com/2010/08/20/news/companies/inside_trader_joes_full_version.fortune/index.htm.

Krentz, S., and R. Gish. 2000. "Using Scenario Analysis to Determine Managed Care Strategy." *Healthcare Financial Management* 54 (9): 41–43.

Krivich, M. 2016. "How Does One Make Provider Marketing Meaningful?" Healthcare Marketing Matters. Published October 30. http://healthcaremarketingmatters.blogspot.com/2016_10_01_archive.html.

Kuttner, R. 1996. "Columbia/HCA and the Resurgence of the For-Profit Hospital Business." *New England Journal of Medicine* 335 (6): 446–51.

Lackmeyer, S. 2001. "3 Hospitals May Take OU Name Regents OK Deal; HCA Nod Needed." *NewsOK*. Published May 12. http://newsok.com/3-hospitals-may-take-ou-name-regents-ok-deal-hca-nod-needed/article/2741049.

Langley, K., B. Toland, S. Twedt, and R. Lord. 2012. "Highmark, UPMC Reach Agreement Until 2015." *Pittsburgh Post-Gazette*. Published May 2. www.post-gazette.com/local/region/2012/05/02/Highmark-UPMC-reach-agreement-until-2015/stories/201205020314.

Lasser, A. 2016. "How to Make Population Health a Strategic Priority in Your Hospital." *H&HN*. Published July 28. www.hhnmag.com/articles/7490-how-to-make-population-health-a-strategic-priority-in-your-hospital.

Laszewski, R. 2015. "Health Insurer Merger Mania: Muscle-Bound Competitors and a New Cold War in Health Care." *Forbes*. Published July 27. www.forbes.com/sites/robertlaszewski2/2015/07/27/health-insurer-merger-mania-muscle-bound-competitors-and-a-new-cold-war-in-health-care/3/.

Lawrence, P., and J. Lorsch. 1967. "Differentiation and Integration in Complex Organizations." *Administrative Science Quarterly* 12 (1): 1–47.

Leask, G., and D. Parker. 2007. "Strategic Groups, Competitive Groups and Performance Within the U.K. Pharmaceutical Industry: Improving Our Understanding of the Competitive Process." *Strategic Management Journal* 28 (7): 723–45.

Lee, J. 2011. "Motivated Buyer: Highmark-West Penn Deal Illustrates the High Stakes in Integration Game." *Modern Healthcare* 41 (27): 6–7, 16.

Lee, O. F., and T. R. Davis. 2004. "International Patients: A Lucrative Market for U.S. Hospitals." *Health Marketing Quarterly* 22 (1): 41–56.

Leufkens, H., F. Haaijer-Ruskamp, A. Bakker, and G. Dukes. 1994. "Scenario Analysis of the Future of Medicines." *BMJ* 309 (6962): 1137–40.

Leventhal, R. 2015. "Report: Two More Medicare ACOs Drop Out of Pioneer Program." *Healthcare Informatics*. Published November 5. www.healthcare-informatics.com/news-item/report-two-more-medicare-acos-drop-out-pioneer-program.

Lewin, K. 1951. *Field Theory in Social Science*. New York: Harper.

Lewis, E., D. Romanaggi, and A. Chapple. 2010. "Successfully Managing Change During Uncertain Times." *Strategic HR Review* 9 (2): 12–18.

Lieberman, M., and D. Montgomery. 1998. "First-Mover (Dis)Advantages: Retrospective and Link with the Resource-Based View." *Strategic Management Journal* 19 (12): 1111–25.

LifePoint Hospitals. 2017. "Mission, Vision and Values." Accessed August 24. www.lifepointhealth.net/about-lifepoint/mission-vision-values.

Lin, D. Q. 2008. "Convenient Care Clinics: Opposition, Opportunities, and the Path to Health System Integration." *Frontiers of Health Services Management* 24 (3): 3–11.

Livingston, G., and D. Cohn. 2010. "The New Demography of American Motherhood." Pew Research Center. Published May 6. http://pewsocialtrends.org/2010/05/06/the-new-demography-of-american-motherhood/.

Livingston, S. 2016. "Ardent Health, LHP Hospital Group Enter Merger Agreement." *Modern Healthcare*. Published October 8. www.modernhealthcare.com/article/20161008/MAGAZINE/310089976/ardent-health-lhp-hospital-group-enter-merger-agreement.

Lockard, P. 2017. "5 Healthcare Marketing Trends to Watch in 2016." DMN3. Published February 14. www.dmn3.com/dmn3-blog/5-healthcare-marketing-trends-you-should-know-about.

Luke, R., S. Walston, and P. Plummer. 2004. *Healthcare Strategy: In Pursuit of Competitive Advantage*. Chicago: Health Administration Press.

MarketWatch. 2017. "HCA Healthcare Inc." Accessed June 20. www.marketwatch.com/investing/stock/hca/financials.

Martin, M. 2015. "What Is a BCG Matrix?" *Business News Daily*. Published February 3. www.businessnewsdaily.com/5693-bcg-matrix.html.

Martin, R. 2015. "Stop Distinguishing Between Execution and Strategy." *Harvard Business Review*. Published March 13. https://hbr.org/2015/03/stop-distinguishing-between-execution-and-strategy.

———. 2010. "The Execution Trap." *Harvard Business Review*. Published July/August. https://hbr.org/2010/07/the-execution-trap.

Marvasti, F., and R. Stafford. 2012. "From Sick Care to Health Care: Reengineering Prevention into the U.S. System." *New England Journal of Medicine* 367: 889–891.

Matthews, A. 2011. "The Future of U.S. Health Care: What Is a Hospital? An Insurer? Even a Doctor? All the Lines in the Industry Are Starting to Blur." *Wall Street Journal*. Published December 12. http://online.wsj.com/article/SB10001424052970204319004577084553869990554.html.

Maurer, R. 2009. "What's Happening These Days with Change?" *Journal for Quality and Participation* 32 (2): 56–66.

McDowell, T., D. Agarwal, D. Miller, T. Okamoto, and T. Page. 2016. "Organizational Design: The Rise of Teams." Deloitte University Press. Published February 29. https://dupress.deloitte.com/dup-us-en/focus/human-capital-trends/2016/organizational-models-network-of-teams.html.

McGrath, R. 2016. "The Destructive Power of Assumptions." *Fortune*. Published July 13. http://fortune.com/2016/07/13/assumptions-policy-discovery-decisions/.

McGuigan, J., R. Moyer, and F. Harris. 2017. *Managerial Economics: Applications, Strategy and Tactics*. Boston: Cengage Learning.

McKesson. 2013. "Our Company: Our Mission." Accessed August 24, 2017. www.mckesson.com/about-mckesson/who-we-are/.

McSweeney-Feld, M., S. Discenza, and G. De Feis. 2010. "Strategic Alliances and Customer Impact: A Case Study of Community Hospitals." *Journal of Business and Economics Research* 8 (9): 13–21.

Medical Group Management Association. 2005. *Physician Compensation and Production Survey*. Englewood, CO: Medical Group Management Association.

Medicare.gov. 2017. "Hospital Compare." Accessed August 10. www.medicare.gov/hospitalcompare/results.html#cmprID=140304%2C140291%2C140172&dist=25&lat=0&lng=0&state=IL& cmprDist=0.0%2C0.0%2C0.0.

Merck. 2017a. "About Us." Accessed August 1. www.merck.com/about/.

———. 2017b. "Animal Health." Accessed August 1. www.merck.com/product/animal-health/home.html.

———. 2017c. "Executive Committee." Accessed August 1. www.merck.com/about/leadership/executive-committee/home.html.

Merritt Research Services. 2017. "Hospital Medians." Accessed July 14. www.merrittresearch.com/benchmark-central/hospital.

Meyer, H. 2016. "100 Most Influential People in Healthcare: Obama's Historic Achievements Earn Him Third Time as No. 1." *Modern Healthcare*. Published August 20. www.modernhealthcare.com/article/20160820/100_MOST_INFLUENTIAL/160819926/100-most-influential-people-in-healthcare-obamas-historic.

Mihoces, G. 2015. "Bill Belichick Compares Patriots' Playoff Preparation to Dwight D. Eisenhower Quote." *USA Today*. Published January 16. http://ftw.usatoday.com/2015/01/bill-belichick-compares-patriots-playoff-preparation-to-dwight-d-eisenhower-quote.

Miles, J. 2016. "The FTC's Three Current Hospital Merger Challenges: Will the FTC Ever Lose? (Ober/Kaler)." Accessed August 1, 2017. www.bakerdonelson.com/the-ftcs-three-current-hospital-merger-challenges-will-the-ftc-ever-lose.

Miller, D. 1990. *The Icarus Paradox*. New York: HarperCollins.

Miller, J. 2008. "Old Model in New Clothes." *Pharmaceutical Technology* 32 (1). www.pharmtech.com/old-model-new-clothes-0.

Mintzberg, H. 1994. *The Rise and Fall of Strategic Planning*. New York: Free Press.

Mintzberg, H., B. Ahlstrand, and J. Lampel. 1998. *Strategy Safari: A Guided Tour Through the Wilds of Strategic Management*. New York: Free Press.

Modern Healthcare. 2016. "Hospital Systems: 2016." Published June 18. www.modernhealthcare.com/article/20160618/DATA/500036234.

Moncrieff, J. 1999. "Is Strategy Making a Difference?" *Long Range Planning* 32 (2): 273–76.

Morris, M., M. Schindehutte, J. Richardson, and J. Allen. 2006. "Is the Business Model a Useful Strategic Concept? Conceptual, Theoretical, and Empirical Insights." *Journal of Small Business Strategy* 17 (1): 27–50.

Morrison, J. 1998. "The Second Curve: Managing the Velocity of Change." *Strategy and Leadership* 26 (1): 6–11.

Murphy, T. 2006. "Hospitals Battle for Bone Biz; St. Vincent's Ortho Upgrade Ups Ante in Lucrative Niche." *Indianapolis Business Journal* 26 (51): 1.

Murray, W., M. Knox, and A. Bernstein. 1994. *The Making of Strategy: Rulers, States, and War*. New York: Cambridge University Press.

Musson, A., and E. Robinson. 1960. "The Origins of Engineering in Lancashire." *Journal of Economic History* 20 (2): 209–33.

Nam, S. 2016. "What's Disruptive and What's Not? Three Criteria for Identifying Disruptors in Healthcare." Christensen Institute. Published May 18. www.christenseninstitute.org/blog/whats-disruptive-and-whats-not-three-criteria-for-identifying-disruptors-in-healthcare/.

National Association for Proton Therapy. 2017. "Proton Therapy Centers." Accessed October 5, 2017. www.proton-therapy.org/map.htm.

National Conference of State Legislatures (NCSL). 2017. "CON-Certificate of Need State Laws." Accessed July 7. www.ncsl.org/research/health/con-certificate-of-need-state-laws.aspx.

———. 2016. "CON—Certificate of Need State Laws." Published August 25. www.ncsl.org/research/health/con-certificate-of-need-state-laws.aspx.

National Institute of Standards and Technology. 2016. "Baldrige Award Recipients' Information." Accessed August 24, 2017. http://patapsco.nist.gov/Award_Recipients/index.cfm.

Nauert, R. 2005. "Strategic Business Planning and Development for Competitive Health Care Systems." *Journal of Health Care Finance* 32 (2): 72–94.

Nelson, W., and P. Gardent. 2011. "Organizational Values Statements." *Healthcare Executive* 26 (2): 56–59.

Nexon, D., and S. J. Ubi. 2010. "Implications of Health Reform for the Medical Technology Industry." *Health Affairs* 29 (7): 1325–29.

Nike. 2017. "Our Mission." Accessed July 26. http://about.nike.com.

North, M., and C. Coors. 2010. "Avoiding Death by the Dotted Line." *Healthcare Financial Management* 65 (1): 120–21.

Novartis. 2017. "Novartis Mission and Vision." Accessed August 2. www.novartis.com/about-us/who-we-are/our-mission.

Office of Statewide Health Planning and Development. 2017a. "Hospital Annual Financial Data." Accessed August 2. www.oshpd.ca.gov/HID/Hospital-Financial.asp#Profile.

———. 2017b. "Hospital Annual Utilization Data." Updated June 9. www.oshpd.ca.gov/HID/Hospital-Utilization.html.

———. 2016. "Patient Origin and Market Share Reports." Updated July 26, 2017. www.oshpd.ca.gov/HID/POMS-Report.asp.

Ohmae, K. 1989. "The Global Logic of Strategic Alliances." *Harvard Business Review*. Published March–April. https://hbr.org/1989/03/the-global-logic-of-strategic-alliances.

O'Malley, A. S., A. M. Bond, and R. A. Berenson. 2011. "Rising Hospital Employment of Physicians: Better Quality, Higher Costs?" Center for Studying Health System Change.Published August. http://hschange.org/CONTENT/1230/.

Owens, P., E. Raddad, J. Miller, J. Stile, K. Olovich, N. Smith, R. Jones, and J. Scherer. 2015. "A Decade of Innovation in Pharmaceutical R&D: The Chorus Model." *Nature Reviews Drug Discovery* 14: 17–28.

Oxford College of Marketing. 2017. "TOWS Analysis: A Step by Step Guide." Accessed August 2. http://blog.oxfordcollegeofmarketing.com/2016/06/07/tows-analysis-guide/.

Pareras, L. 2008. "Healthcare Services Value Chain." *Healthonomics.* Published October 5. www.healthonomics.org/2008/10/healthcare-services-value-chain.html.

Park, M. 2016. "US Fertility Rate Falls to Lowest on Record." CNN. Published August 11. www.cnn.com/2016/08/11/health/us-lowest-fertility-rate/.

Parnell, J., and D. Lester. 2008. "Competitive Strategy and the Wal-Mart Threat: Positioning for Survival and Success." *SAM Advanced Management Journal* 73 (2): 14–25.

Patients Beyond Borders. 2016. "Medical Tourism Statistics and Facts." Updated August 6. www.patientsbeyondborders.com/medical-tourism-statistics-facts.

Pauly, M. V. 2011. "The Trade-Off Among Quality, Quantity, and Cost: How to Make It—If We Must." *Health Affairs* 30 (4): 574–80.

Penn Medicine News. 2016. "Penn Studies Show High Out-of-Pocket Costs Limits Access to Lifesaving Specialty Drugs." Published March 29. www.pennmedicine.org/news/news-releases/2016/march/penn-studies-show-high-outof-p.

Penner, D. 2003a. "At Wishard, Everything But Closing Is an Option." *Indianapolis Star*, July 20.

———. 2003b. "CEO Vows That Cash Woes Won't Close Wishard." *Indianapolis Star*, July 1.

Perkins, B. B. 2010. "Designing High-Cost Medicine." *American Journal of Public Health* 100 (2): 223–33.

Persico, J. 2017. "Do You Really Need a Mission Statement?" Innovation Excellence. Accessed August 2. http://innovationexcellence.com/blog/2011/05/14/do-you-really-need-a-mission-statement/.

Pesch, M. 1996. "Defining and Understanding the Focused Factory: A Delphi Survey." *Production and Inventory Management Journal* 37 (2): 32–37.

Peters, T., and R. Waterman. 1982. *In Search of Excellence: Lessons from America's Best Run Companies.* New York: Harper & Row.

Pettypiece, S. 2016. "The German Chain That's Beating Wal-Mart at Its Own Game." *Bloomberg Technology.* Published March 22. www.bloomberg.com/news/articles/2016-03-22/wal-mart-loses-everyday-low-price-edge-as-aldi-opens-across-u-s.

Pharmaceutical-technology.com. 2016. "The World's Biggest Pharmaceutical Companies." Published April 5. www.pharmaceutical-technology.com/features/featurethe-worlds-biggest-generic-pharmaceutical-companies-4853429/.

Physicians Advocacy Institute. 2016. *Physician Practice Acquisition Study: National Regional Employment Changes.* Published September. www.physiciansadvocacyinstitute.org/Portals/0/PAI-Physician-Employment-Study.pdf.

Physicians Foundation. 2016. "2016 Survey of America's Physicians: Practice Patterns and Perspectives." Published September. www.physiciansfoundation.org/uploads/default/Biennial_Physician_Survey_2016.pdf.

Pitt, M. 2001. "In Pursuit of Change: Managerial Construction of Strategic Intent." *Strategic Change* 10 (1): 5–21.

Pohl, J., A. Thomas, D. Barksdale, and K. Werner. 2016. "Primary Care Workforce: The Need to Remove Barriers for Nurse Practitioners and Physicians." *Health Affairs.* Published October 26. http://healthaffairs.org/blog/2016/10/26/primary-care-workforce-the-need-to-remove-barriers-for-nurse-practitioners-and-physicians/.

Porter, M. E. 1996. "What Is Strategy?" *Harvard Business Review* 74 (6): 54–60.

———. 1985. *Competitive Advantage: Creating and Sustaining Superior Performance.* New York: Free Press.

———. 1980. *Competitive Strategy: Techniques for Analyzing Industries and Competitors.* New York: Free Press.

Porter, M. E., and J. Heppelmann. 2015. "How Smart, Connected Products Are Transforming Companies." *Harvard Business Review.* Published October. https://hbr.org/2015/10/how-smart-connected-products-are-transforming-companies.

Porter, M. E., and R. Kaplan. 2016. "How to Pay for Health Care." *Harvard Business Review.* Published July/August. https://hbr.org/2016/07/how-to-pay-for-health-care.

Porter, M. E., and T. Lee. 2013. "The Strategy That Will Fix Health Care." *Harvard Business Review.* Published October. https://hbr.org/2013/10/the-strategy-that-will-fix-health-care.

Porter, M. E., and E. O. Teisberg. 2006. *Redefining Health Care: Creating Value-Based Competition on Results.* Boston: Harvard Business School Press.

Pourat, N. 2016. "Luxury Hospital Care Limits Care for the Less Affluent." *New York Times.* Published August 22. www.nytimes.com/roomfordebate/2016/08/22/hospitals-that-feel-like-hotels/luxury-hospital-care-limits-care-for-the-less-affluent.

Premier. 2017. "Who It Benefits." Accessed June 15. www.premierinc.com/healthcare-alliance/who-it-benefits/.

PricewaterhouseCoopers. 2016. "Joint Ventures and Strategic Alliances: Examining the Keys to Success." Accessed August 7, 2017. www.pwc.com/us/en/deals/publications/assets/pwc-deals-joint-ventures-strategic-alliances.pdf.

———. 2009. "Pharma 2020: Challenging Business Models. Which Path Will You Take?" Accessed August 7. www.pwc.com/gx/en/pharma-life-sciences/pharma2020-business-models/index.jhtml.

PR Newswire. 2006. "In Pharmaceutical Alliances, Good Partners Make All the Difference." Published September 22. www.thefreelibrary.com/In+Pharmaceutical+Alliances,+Good+Partners+Make+All+the+Difference.-a0151731274.

———. 2005. "OrthoIndy Opens Central Ind.'s First Specialty Hospital to Focus on Complete Orthopaedic Care." News release, March 1. www.prnewswire.com/news-releases/orthoindy-opens-central-inds-first-specialty-hospital-to-focus-on-complete-orthopaedic-care-53853187.html.

Qamar, S. 2014. "Direct Primary Care and Concierge Medicine: They're Not the Same." *Medpage Today*'s KevinMD.com. Published August 24. www.kevinmd.com/blog/2014/08/direct-primary-care-concierge-medicine-theyre.html.

QuoteFancy.com. 2017. "Charlie Chaplin Quotes." Accessed August 28. https://quotefancy.com/quote/1016639/Charlie-Chaplin-The-cinema-is-little-more-than-a-fad-It-s-canned-drama-What-audiences.

Radelat, A. 2017. "Anthem Not Giving Up On Cigna Merger, Is Appealing to Supreme Court." *Connecticut Mirror*. Published May 5. https://ctmirror.org/2017/05/05/anthem-cigna-gearing-for-legal-battle-over-end-of-merger-deal/.

Rajagopalan, G. 2015. "Industry Value Chain: Understand Its Importance and Application to the Mining Industry." FlevyBlog. Published November 17. https://flevy.com/blog/industry-value-chain-understand-its-importance-and-application-to-the-mining-industry/.

Ramsey, L. 2017. "A New Kind of Doctor's Office Charges a Monthly Fee and Doesn't Take Insurance—and It Could Be the Future of Medicine." *Business Insider*. Published March 19. www.businessinsider.com/direct-primary-care-a-no-insurance-healthcare-model-2017-3.

———. 2016. "The 10 Most Expensive Drugs in the US." *Business Insider*. Published September 30. www.businessinsider.com/most-expensive-drugs-in-america-2016-9/#viekira-pak-abbvie-34600-1.

RAND Corporation. 2016. "The Evolving Role of Retail Clinics." Accessed August 7, 2017. www.rand.org/content/dam/rand/pubs/research_briefs/RB9400/RB9491-2/RAND_RB9491-2.pdf.

Raps, A. 2004. "Implementing Strategy." *Strategic Finance* 85 (12): 49–53.

Reed, D. 2016. "United Airlines' Bare Bones Basic Economy Fares: Genius? Contemptible? Or Both?" *Forbes*. Published November 16. www.forbes.com/sites/danielreed/2016/11/16/united-airlines-bare-bones-basic-economy-fares-genius-contemptible-or-both/.

Regan, S. 2012. "The Impact of First Impressions on Patient Acquisition and Revenue." *Becker's Hospital Review*. Published January 18. http://go.beckershospitalreview.com/the-impact-of-first-impressions-on-patient-acquisition-and-revenue.

Rege, A. 2017. "Ardent Health Services Completes Acquisition of LHP Hospital Group." *Becker's Hospital Review*. Published March 14. www.beckershospitalreview.com/hospital-transactions-and-valuation/ardent-health-services-completes-acquisition-of-lhp-hospital-group.html.

Rein, S. 2010. "Three Keys to Improving Your Strategic Thinking." *Forbes*. Published November 9. www.forbes.com/2010/11/09/strategic-thinking-innovation-creativityleadership-managing-rein.html.

Reuters. 2009. "Merck, Schering-Plough Set to Complete Merger." Published November 3. www.reuters.com/article/us-merck-scheringplough-idUSTRE5A23YZ20091103.

Revolvy. 2017. "Indiana Orthopaedic Hospital." Accessed August 28. www.revolvy.com/main/index.php?s=Indiana Orthopaedic Hospital.

Ricketts, T. C., L. A. Savitz, W. M. Gesler, and D. N. Osborne. 1997. "Using Geographic Methods to Understand Health Issues." Agency for Health Research and Quality. Accessed August 23, 2017. http://archive.ahrq.gov/research/geomap/geomap1.htm.

Ries, A., and J. Trout. 2001. *Positioning: The Battle for Your Mind*. New York: McGraw-Hill.

Rigoni, B., and B. Nelson. 2016. "The Matrix: Teams Are Gaining Greater Power in Companies." *Gallup Business Journal*. Published May 17. www.gallup.com/businessjournal/191516/matrix-teams-gaining-greater-power-companies.aspx.

Robbins, R. 2016. "Drug Makers Now Spend $5 Billion a Year on Advertising. Here's What It Buys." STAT. Published March 9. www.statnews.com/2016/03/09/drug-industry-advertising/.

Robinson, J. C. 1999. "The Future of Managed Care Organization." *Health Affairs* 18 (2): 7–24.

Roche Diagnostics. 2011. "Roche Diagnostics, Cedars-Sinai Medical Center Enter Strategic Alliance for Center to Operate as a Roche Molecular Center of Excellence." PR Newswire. Published November 21. www.prnewswire.com/news-releases/roche-diagnostics-cedars-sinai-medical-center-enter-strategic-alliance-for-center-to-operate-as-a-roche-molecular-center-of-excellence-134240268.html.

Rodak, S. 2013. "Creating Accountability in Healthcare Strategic Plan Execution." *Becker's Hospital Review*. Published June 14. www.beckershospitalreview.com/strategic-planning/creating-accountability-in-healthcare-strategic-plan-execution.html.

Rodgers, N., and D. Dodge. 2005. *The Roman Army: Legions, Wars and Campaigns: A Military History of the World's First Superpower from the Rise of the Republic and the Might of the Empire to the Fall of the West*. Leicester, UK: Anness Publishing Ltd.

Romanelli, E., and M. Tushman. 1994. "Organization Transformation as Punctuated Equilibrium: An Empirical Test." *Academy of Management Journal* 37 (5): 1141–66.

Ronning, P. 2010. "ACOs: Preparing for Medicare's Shared Savings Program." *Healthcare Financial Management* 64 (8): 46–51.

Rose, R.V. 2015. "The Business Plan: A Must for Medical Practices." Physicians Practice. Published August 13. www.physicianspractice.com/blog/the-business-plan-must-for-medical-practices.

Rosin, T. 2016. "Hospital CEOs: 7 Core Competencies for Future Organizational Success." *Becker's Hospital Review*. Published March 24. www.beckershospitalreview.com/hospital-management-administration/hospital-ceos-7-core-competencies-for-future-organizational-success.html.

Rowe, G. 2001. "Creating Wealth in Organizations: The Role of Strategic Leadership." *Academy of Management Executive* 15 (1): 81–94.

Rowe, G., and M. H. Nejad. 2009. "Strategic Leadership: Short-Term Stability and Long-Term Viability." *Ivey Business Journal*. Published September/October.

http://iveybusinessjournal.com/publication/strategic-leadership-short-term-stability-and-long-term-viability/.

Rubenfire, A. 2016. "Logistics: The Next Target in the War on Device Costs." *Modern Healthcare*. Published May 7. www.modernhealthcare.com/article/20160507/MAGAZINE/305079980.

———. 2015. "VHA-UHC Alliance to Be Called Vizient." *Modern Healthcare*. Published November 19. www.modernhealthcare.com/article/20151119/NEWS/151119860.

Rummler, G., and A. Brache. 1995. *Improving Performance*. San Francisco: Jossey-Bass.

Sabin, G. 2017. "Cancer Treatment Centers of America: 800-Pound Marketing Gorilla." FON Consulting. Accessed August 8. https://fonconsulting.com/blog/cancer-treatment-centers-of-america-800-pound-marketing-gorilla/.

Sabria, P. 2016. "Why More Money Won't Motivate Your Employees." *Fortune*. Published March 26. http://fortune.com/2016/03/26/money-motivate-employees/.

Saebi, T., L. Lien, and N. Foss. 2016. "What Causes Managers to Change Their Business Model?" *European Business Review*. Published November 27. www.european-businessreview.com/what-causes-managers-to-change-their-business-model/.

Said, S. 2015. "A Brief History of OPEC." *Wall Street Journal*. Published June 3. http://blogs.wsj.com/briefly/2015/06/03/a-brief-history-of-opec-at-a-glance/.

Sanicola, L. 2017. "What Is Value-Based Care?" *Huffington Post*. Published February 2. www.huffingtonpost.com/entry/what-is-value-based-care_us_58939f9de4b02bbb1816b892.

Sawyer, R. D. 2007. *The Seven Military Classics of Ancient China*, reprint ed. New York: Basic Books.

Schechter, A. 2016. "The True Price of Reduced Competition in Health Care: Hospital Monopolies Drastically Drive Up Prices." *Pro-Market*. Published March 14. https://promarket.org/the-true-price-of-reduced-competition-in-health-care-hospital-monopolies-drastically-drive-up-prices/.

Scheffler, R., D. Clement, S. Sullivan, T. Hu, and H. Sung. 1994. "The Hospital Response to Medicare's Prospective Payment System: An Econometric Model of Blue Cross and Blue Shield Plans." *Medical Care* 32 (5): 471–85.

Schein, E. 2010. *Organizational Culture and Leadership*, 4th ed. San Francisco: Jossey-Bass.

Schencker, L. 2016. "DOJ Targets Hospital Contracts Barring Competitors from Top Insurance Tiers." *Modern Healthcare*. Published June 9. www.modernhealthcare.com/article/20160609/NEWS/160609904.

Schnaars, S. P. 1987. "How to Develop and Use Scenarios." *Long Range Planning* 20 (1): 105–14.

Schoenman, J. A., and N. Chockley. 2012. *The Concentration of Health Care Spending*. National Institute for Health Care Management. Published July 2012. www.nihcm.org/pdf/DataBrief3%20Final.pdf.

Schraeder, M., and D. Self. 2003. "Enhancing the Success of Mergers and Acquisitions: An Organizational Culture Perspective." *Management Decision* 41 (5/6): 511–22.

Schroeder, M. 2015. "Do Accountable Care Organizations Work?" *US News and World Report*. Published October 20. http://health.usnews.com/health-news/hospital-of-tomorrow/articles/2015/10/20/do-accountable-care-organizations-work.

Schwartz, N. 2017. "The Doctor Is In. Co-Pay? $40,000." *New York Times*. Published June 3. www.nytimes.com/2017/06/03/business/economy/high-end-medical-care.html.

Schwenker, B., and T. Wulf. 2013. *Scenario-Based Strategic Planning*. Fachmedien Wiebaden, Germany: Springer Gabler.

Schwering, R. 2003. "Focusing Leadership Through Force Field Analysis: New Variations on a Venerable Planning Tool." *Leadership and Organization Development Journal* 24 (7/8): 361–71.

Seidman, D. 2011. "Which CEOs Get 'Should'?" *Huffington Post*. Updated March 25. www.huffingtonpost.com/dov-seidman/which-ceos-get-should_b_838539.html.

Shankar, V., and G. Carpenter. 2013. "The Second-Mover Advantage." *Kellogg Insight*. Published November 4. http://insight.kellogg.northwestern.edu/article/the_second_mover_advantage.

Sharfstein, J. 2016. "Banishing 'Stakeholders.'" *Milbank Quarterly*. Published September. www.milbank.org/quarterly/articles/banishing-stakeholders/.

Shenkar, O. 2012. "Just Imitate It! A Copycat Path to Strategic Agility." *Ivey Business Journal*. Published May/June. http://iveybusinessjournal.com/publication/just-imitate-it-a-copycat-path-to-strategic-agility/.

Sherman, E. 2010. "Blockbuster's Plight Exposes a Broader Corporate Creativity Problem." CBS News. Published September 23. www.cbsnews.com/news/blockbusters-plight-exposes-a-broader-corporate-creativity-problem-update/.

Sherman, R. 2013. "Span of Control in Nurse Leader Roles." Emerging RN Leader. Published June 27. www.emergingrnleader.com/span-of-control-in-nurse-leader-roles/.

Shih, A., K. Davis, S. Schoenbaum, A. Gauthier, R. Nuzum, and D. McCarthy. 2008. "Organizing the U.S. Health Care Delivery System for High Performance." Commonwealth Fund. www.commonwealthfund.org/publications/fund-reports/2008/aug/organizing-the-u-s--health-care-delivery-system-for-high-performance.

Shortell, S. M., E. Morrison, and S. Hughes. 1989. "The Keys to Successful Diversification: Lessons from Leading Hospital Systems." *Hospital and Health Services Administration* 34 (4): 471–92.

Simpson, S. 2007. "OU to Buy Proton Cancer Treatment." *Oklahoman*. Published April 6. http://newsok.com/article/3036733.

Singer, J. 2016. "Obamacare's Catch 22." *US News and World Report*. Published August 11. www.usnews.com/opinion/articles/2016-08-11/obamacare-gave-rise-to-the-health-care-mergers-its-advocates-oppose.

Sloan, A. 1963. *My Years with General Motors*. New York: Doubleday.

Snohomish County. 2012. "Snohomish County Area Plan on Aging 2012–2015." Accessed August 28. https://snohomishcountywa.gov/DocumentCenter/View/7187.

Span, P. 2014. "Differences in Care at For-Profit Hospices." *New York Times*. Published March 3. http://newoldage.blogs.nytimes.com/2014/03/03/differences-in-care-at-for-profit-hospices/.

Spiro, J. 2011. *Leading Change Step-by-Step: Tactics, Tools, and Tales*. San Francisco: Jossey-Bass.

Squires, D., and C. Anderson. 2015. "U.S. Health Care from a Global Perspective: Spending, Use of Services, Prices, and Health in 13 Countries." Commonwealth Fund. Published October 8. www.commonwealthfund.org/publications/issue-briefs/2015/oct/us-health-care-from-a-global-perspective.

Stanford Health Care. 2016. "Stanford Health Care: Consolidated Financial Statements and Accompanying Consolidating Information." Published August 31. https://stanfordhealthcare.org/content/dam/SHC/about-us/bondholder-information/docs/consolidated-finanical-statements-august312016and2015.pdf.

Statista. 2017a. "Total Global Pharmaceutical Research and Development (R&D) Spending from 2008 to 2022 (in Billion US Dollars)." Accessed August 14. www.statista.com/statistics/309466/global-r-and-d-expenditure-for-pharmaceuticals.

———. 2017b. "Market Share of Leading Health Insurance Companies in the United States in 2016, by Direct Premiums Written." Accessed August 14. www.statista.com/statistics/216518/leading-us-health-insurance-groups-in-the-us/.

Steinhilber, S. 2008. *Strategic Alliances: Three Ways to Make Them Work*. Boston: Harvard Business School Publishing.

St. Luke's. 2013. "Find Services." Accessed August 28. www.stlukesonline.org/health-services/find-services.

St. Francis and Centura Health. 2016. *Community Health Improvement Plan*. Accessed August 11, 2017. www.centura.org/uploadedFiles/Centura/Content/Community/Community_Benefits/St-Francis-Medical-Center-CHIP-2016.pdf.

Sterling, J. 2003. "Translating Strategy into Effective Implementation." *Strategy and Leadership* 31 (3): 27–34.

Strategic Business Insights. 2017. "US Framework and VALS™ Types." Accessed August 18. www.strategicbusinessinsights.com/vals/ustypes.shtml.

Suarez, F., and G. Lanzolla. 2005. "The Half-Truth of First-Mover Advantage." *Harvard Business Review* 83 (4): 121–27.

Subcommittee on Health of the Committee on Ways and Means, US House of Representatives. 2012. Hearing on Health Care Industry Consolidation, September 9, 2011. Washington, DC: US Government Printing Office. www.gpo.gov/fdsys/pkg/CHRG-112hhrg72277/pdf/CHRG-112hhrg72277.pdf.

Sufi, T., and H. Lyons. 2003. "Mission Statements Exposed." *International Journal of Contemporary Hospitality* 15 (5): 255–62.

Sunnybrook Health Sciences Centre. 2017. "Sunnybrook's Strategic Balanced Scorecard." Published June. https://sunnybrook.ca/uploads/1/welcome/strategy/balanced_scorecard_june_2017.pdf.

Swanson, A. 2015. "Big Pharmaceutical Companies Are Spending Far More on Marketing Than Research." *Washington Post.* Published February 11. www.washingtonpost.com/news/wonk/wp/2015/02/11/big-pharmaceutical-companies-are-spending-far-more-on-marketing-than-research/.

Swiatek, J. 2003. "Hospitals Wage Battle for Market." *Indianapolis Star*, July 20.

Tarantino, D. 2005. "Positive Deviance as a Tool for Organizational Change." *Physician Executive* 31 (5): 62–63.

Taylor, B. 2016. "Catholic Health Initiatives, Dignity Health Explore Alignment." Catholic Health Association. Published November 15. www.chausa.org/publications/catholic-health-world/article/november-15-2016/catholic-health-initiatives-dignity-health-explore-alignment.

Thompson, A., M. Peteraf, J. Gamble, and J. Strickland. 2016. *Crafting and Executing Strategy: The Quest for Competitive Advantage*, 20th ed. New York: McGraw-Hill Education.

Thompson, J. D. 1967. *Organizations in Action.* New York: McGraw-Hill.

Thomson Reuters. 2011. *The Changing Role of Chemistry in Drug Discovery.* Accessed August 18. http://thomsonreuters.com/content/dam/openweb/documents/pdf/pharma-life-sciences/report/international-year-of-chemistry-report-drug-discovery.pdf.

Topolsky, J. 2016. "The End of Twitter." *New Yorker.* Published January 29. www.newyorker.com/tech/elements/the-end-of-twitter.

Tracer, Z. 2017. "UnitedHealth Agrees to Buy Surgical Care for $2.3 Billion." *Bloomberg.* Published January 9. www.bloomberg.com/news/articles/2017-01-09/unitedhealth-agrees-to-acquire-surgical-care-for-2-3-billion.

Trinh, H. Q., J. W. Begun, and R. D. Luke. 2008. "Hospital Service Duplication: Evidence on the Medical Arms Race." *Health Care Management Review* 33 (3): 192–202.

Trinity Health. 2017. "Hospitals and Facilities." Accessed August 18. www.trinity-health.org/hospitals-facilities.

Trish, E., and B. Herring. 2015. "How Do Health Insurer Market Concentration and Bargaining Power with Hospitals Affect Health Insurance Premiums?" *Journal of Health Economics* 42: 104–14.

TriStar Health. 2017. "About TriStar." Accessed August 18. http://tristarhealth.com/about/.

Tuchman, B. W. 1984. *The March of Folly: From Troy to Vietnam.* New York: Random House.

Tuttle, B. 2016. "21 Incredibly Disturbing Facts About High Prescription Drug Prices." *TIME.* Published June 22. http://time.com/money/4377304/high-prescription-drug-prices-facts/.

Tyson, B. 2015. "Why Pharma Must Change Its Model." *Forbes*. Published July 30. www.forbes.com/sites/matthewherper/2015/07/30/why-pharma-must-change-its-model/.

Ubri, P., and S. Artiga. 2016. "Disparities in Health and Health Care: Five Key Questions and Answers." Kaiser Family Foundation. Published August 12. http://kff.org/disparities-policy/issue-brief/disparities-in-health-and-health-care-five-key-questions-and-answers/.

UC Irvine Health. 2017. "Our Mission." Accessed July 26. www.meded.uci.edu/mission-statement.asp.

Ungar, L., and J. O'Donnell. 2015. "Dilemma over Deductibles: Costs Crippling Middle Class." *USA Today*. Published January 1. www.usatoday.com/story/news/nation/2015/01/01/middle-class-workers-struggle-to-pay-for-care-despite-insurance/19841235/.

UnitedHealth Group. 2016. "UnitedHealth Group Reports 2015 Results Highlighted by Continued Strong and Diversified Growth." Published January 19. www.unitedhealthgroup.com/~/media/205CB82AC7A34CBDA8361AA1C1FFA803.ashx.

United Nations. 2015. *World Population Ageing*. Accessed June 2, 2017. www.un.org/en/development/desa/population/publications/pdf/ageing/WPA2015_Report.pdf.

United Nations Population Fund. 2017. "World Population Trends." Accessed August 18. www.unfpa.org/world-population-trends.

University of Michigan Business School. 1999. "Lipitor: At the Heart of Warner-Lambert." Published December. www-personal.umich.edu/~afuah/cases/case26.pdf.

University of Utah Health. 2017. "About Us." Accessed August 18. https://healthcare.utah.edu/about/.

US Department of Justice. 1997. "Horizontal Merger Guidelines." Revised April 8. www.justice.gov/atr/public/guidelines/hmg.htm.

US Department of Labor. 2013. "General Facts on Women and Job Based Health." Published December. www.dol.gov/ebsa/newsroom/fshlth5.html.

Useem, M. 2016. "Become a More Strategic Leader by Conveying Strategic Intent." *Wharton Magazine*. Published November 2. http://whartonmagazine.com/blogs/become-a-more-strategic-leader-by-conveying-strategic-intent/.

US Navy Bureau of Medicine and Surgery. 2015. "Navy Medicine Strategic Plan FY15." Accessed August 11. www.med.navy.mil/Pages/StrategyMap/FY15%2520%2520Navy%2520Medicine%2520Strategy%2520%2520FINAL.PPTX.

Vance, A. 2010. "Microsoft Calling. Anyone There?" *New York Times*. Published July 4. www.nytimes.com/2010/07/05/technology/05soft.html.

Van Der Merwe, A. P. 2002. "Project Management and Business Development: Integrating Strategy, Structure, Processes and Projects." *International Journal of Project Management* 20 (5): 401–11.

Vizient. 2017. "A Bright Future Based on a Strong Heritage." Accessed August 28. www.vizientinc.com/about-us.

Vogt, W. B., and R. Town. 2006. *How Has Hospital Consolidation Affected the Price and Quality of Hospital Care?* Robert Wood Johnson Foundation. Published February. www.rwjf.org/content/dam/farm/reports/issue_briefs/2006/rwjf12056/subassets/rwjf12056_1.

Vollmar, H., T. Ostermann, and M. Redaelli. 2015. "Using the Scenario Method in the Context of Health and Healthcare: A Scoping Review." *BMC Medical Research Methodology* 15: 89–99.

von Clausewitz, C. 1976. *On War*, translated and edited by M. Howard and P. Paret. Princeton, NJ: Princeton University Press.

Von Lunen, J. 2011. "PMH, Kadlec Medical Center Announce 'Strategic Alliance.'" *Tri-City Herald*. Published October 11. www.tri-cityherald.com/2011/10/11/1674703/pmh-kadlec-medical-center-announce.html.

Wack, P. 1985. "Scenarios: Uncharted Waters Ahead." *Harvard Business Review* 63 (5): 72–90.

Wadhwa, V. 2014. "The Triumph of Genomic Medicine Is Just Beginning." *Washington Post*. Published March 13. www.washingtonpost.com/news/innovations/wp/2014/03/13/the-triumph-of-genomic-medicine-is-just-beginning/.

Walmart. 2017. "The Clinic at Walmart." Accessed August 18. http://i.walmart.com/i/if/hmp/fusion/Clinic_Locations.pdf.

Walsteijn, M. 2012. "6 IT Competencies That Health Insurers Must Master Post-Reform." *Insurance and Technology*. Published November 19. www.insurancetech.com/management-strategies/6-it-competencies-that-health-insurers-m/240142334.

Walston, S. 2017. *Organizational Behavior and Theory in Healthcare: Leadership Perspectives and Management Applications*. Chicago: Health Administration Press.

Walston, S. L., and A. F. Chou. 2012. "Strategic Thinking and Achieving Competitive Advantage." In *Shortell and Kaluzny's Health Care Management: Organization Design and Behavior*, 6th ed, edited by L. R. Burns, E. H. Bradley, and B. J. Weiner, 282–320. Clifton Park, NY: Delmar.

———. 2011. "CEO Perceptions of Organizational Consensus and Its Impact on Hospital Restructuring Outcomes." *Journal of Health Organization and Management* 25 (2): 176–94.

———. 2006. "Healthcare Restructuring and Hierarchical Alignment: Why Do Staff and Managers Perceive Change Outcomes Differently?" *Medical Care* 44 (9): 879–89.

Walston, S. L., and A. A. Khaliq. 2012. "Factors Affecting the Value of Professional Association Affiliation." *Health Care Management Review* 37 (2): 122–31.

Walston, S. L., J. R. Kimberly, and L. R. Burns. 1996. "Owned Vertical Integration and Health Care: Promise and Performance." *Health Care Management Review* 21 (1): 83–92.

Walston, S. L., P. Lazes, and P. G. Sullivan. 2004. "Improving Hospital Restructuring: Lessons Learned." *Health Care Management Review* 29 (4): 309–19.

Walt Disney Company. 2013. "Investor Relations." Accessed August 28. https://thewaltdisneycompany.com/investor-relations/.

Wang, D. 2017. "Successful Organizational Change Is Easier Than You Think." Tiny Pulse. Published May 20. www.tinypulse.com/blog/sk-successful-organizational-change-examples.

Warner, T. 2016. "Overcome Resistance to Change by Enlisting the Right People." *Harvard Business Review*. Published September 13. https://hbr.org/2016/09/overcome-resistance-to-change-by-enlisting-the-right-people.

Wasik, J. 2016. "How Trump's Plan to Gut Obamacare Will Take Down Medicare." *Forbes*. Published December 5. www.forbes.com/sites/johnwasik/2016/12/05/how-trump-plan-to-gut-obamacare-will-take-down-medicare/.

Watkins, S. 1997. "US Health Giant Eyes Australian Hospitals." *The Age*. Published February 27. http://newsstore.theage.com.au/apps/viewDocument.ac?page=1&sy=age&kw=health+giant&pb=age&dt=selectRange&dr=entire&so=relevance&sf=text&sf=headline&rc=10&rm=200&sp=nrm&clsPage=1&docID=news970227_0187_5722.

Weaver, J. 2013. "More People Search for Health Online." NBCNews.com. Published July 16. www.nbcnews.com/id/3077086/t/more-people-search-health-online/#.WaRuOcaQxhF.

Weil, T. 2010. "Hospital Consolidations: Do They Deliver?" *Physician Executive* 36 (5): 24–27.

Welch, D., and E. Newcomer. 2016. "GM's Alliance with Lyft Facing Rockier Road after Uber-Didi Deal." *Bloomberg Business*. Published August 3. www.bloomberg.com/news/articles/2016-08-03/gm-s-alliance-with-lyft-facing-rockier-road-after-uber-didi-deal.

Wernerfelt, B. 1984. "A Resource-Based View of the Firm." *Strategic Management Journal* 5 (2): 171–80.

Wheeler, E. L. 1988. *Stratagem and the Vocabulary of Military Trickery*. Leiden, Netherlands: Brill.

Whitler, K. 2014. "Why Strategic Alliances Fail: New CMO Council Report." *Forbes*. Published October 24. www.forbes.com/sites/kimberlywhitler/2014/10/24/why-strategic-alliances-fail-new-cmo-council-report/.

Wikipedia. 2017. "List of Mergers and Acquisitions by Microsoft." Modified August 8. https://en.wikipedia.org/wiki/List_of_mergers_and_acquisitions_by_Microsoft.

Williamson, O. 1975. *Markets and Hierarchies: Analysis and Antitrust Implications*. New York: Free Press.

Wishard Health Services. 2013. "Our Mission, Vision and Values." Accessed June 15. www.wishard.edu/about-us/our-mission-vision-values.

Wolff, M. 1999. "In the Organization of the Future, Competitive Advantage Will Be Inspired." *Research Technology Management* 42 (4): 2–4.

Yip, G., and G. Johnson. 2007. "Transforming Strategy." *Business Strategy Review* 18 (1): 11–15.

Zajac, E., T. D'Aunno, and L. Burns. 2012. "Managing Strategic Alliances." In *Shortell and Kaluzny's Health Care Management: Organization Design and Behavior*, 6th ed., edited by L. R. Burns, E. H. Bradley, and B. J. Weiner, 321–346. Clifton Park, NY: Delmar.

Zelman, W., M. McCue, N. Glick, and M. Thomas. 2014. *Financial Management of Healthcare Organizations: An Introduction to Fundamental Tools, Concepts, and Applications*, 4th ed. New York: Wiley.

Zelman, W., G. Pink, and C. Matthias. 2003. "Use of the Balanced Scorecard in Health Care." *Journal of Health Care Finance* 29 (4): 1–16.

Zetlin, M. 2013. "The 9 Worst Mission Statements of All Time." *Inc*. Published November 15. www.inc.com/minda-zetlin/9-worst-mission-statements-all-time.html.

Zuckerman, A. M. 2005. *Healthcare Strategic Planning*. 2nd ed. Chicago: Health Administration Press.

Zuckerman, H., and A. Kaluzny. 1991. "Strategic Alliances in Health Care: The Challenge of Cooperation." *Frontiers of Health Services Management* 7 (3): 3–23.

INDEX

Note: Italicized page locators refer to figures or tables in exhibits.

ABOUT THE AUTHOR

Stephen L. Walston, PhD, is a professor at the David Eccles School of Business at the University of Utah in Salt Lake City. Previously, he served as the vice president for academic affairs of the University of Utah Asia Campus at its Incheon Global Campus in Songdo, Korea, and was a professor in the Division of Public Health of the Department of Family and Preventive Medicine at the University of Utah School of Medicine. Before joining the University of Utah, Dr. Walston was a professor and associate dean for academic affairs in the Department of Health Administration and Policy at the University of Oklahoma School of Public Health. He also is a former master's of health administration program director at Indiana University and faculty member at Cornell University in Ithaca, New York. He earned his PhD from the University of Pennsylvania's Wharton School and specializes in healthcare strategy, organizational development, and leadership. In addition, he earned bachelor's and master's degrees from Brigham Young University.

Prior to his academic career, he spent 14 years as an executive in hospitals in the western United States, including 10 years as a CEO. He became a fellow in the American College of Healthcare Executives in 1993. Dr. Walston has worked in many Middle Eastern and Central American countries, helping organizations craft their strategic direction and leadership capabilities. He has published in many prestigious journals in the United States and Europe. In his free time, he enjoys woodworking, beekeeping, reading, bicycling, gardening, and helping his six children and seven grandchildren.